HYPERMOBILE AND HAPPY

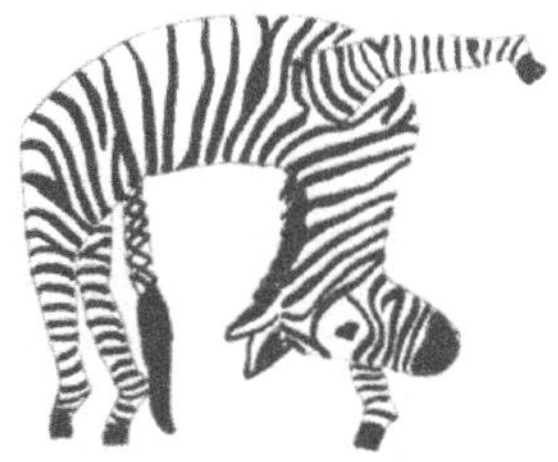

Naturally Heal Symptoms of Hypermobile Ehlers-Danlos Syndrome, Hypermobility Spectrum Disorders, and Many Secondary Conditions

SHANNON E. GALE

Hypermobile and Happy: Naturally Heal Symptoms of Hypermobile Ehlers-Danlos Syndrome, Hypermobility Spectrum Disorders, and Many Secondary Conditions

First Comes Love Publishing
Frankfort, Kentucky, USA

ISBN paperback: 978-1-965020-00-5
ISBN ebook: 978-1-965020-01-2
ISBN hardcover: 978-1-965020-02-9
ISBN large print: 978-1-965020-03-6
ISBN audiobook: 978-1-965020-04-3

All illustrations were hand drawn by Shannon E. Gale.
All figures were created by Shannon E. Gale unless otherwise attributed.
All design and formatting of the cover and book interior were accomplished by Shannon E. Gale.

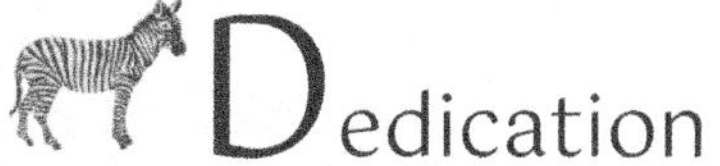

Dedication

To my husband Brandon Gale, my son Edison Gale, my mother Kathy Gale, my sisters Dr. Ashley Gale Smith and Kristin Heather Gale, my brothers-in-law Jason Smith and Joshu Goebeler, and my nephew Paxton Smith, with my love and gratitude.

In loving memory and admiration of my father Dr. Steven H. Gale.

To all of my friends from the Frankfort School of Ballet, Gale Force Dance Company, Circle Play and Learn Academy, Vibrant Life, and Helpful Editor.

And to all hypermobile people everywhere.

Table of Contents

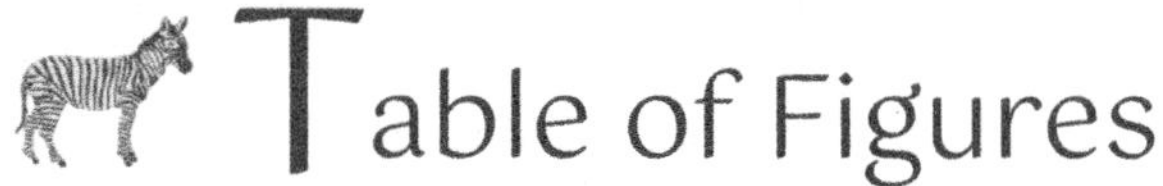

Table of Figures

Illustrations and charts are listed in bold.
All other figures are step-by-step guide boxes.

Acknowledgements

THANK YOU TO THOSE PROFESSIONALS who encouraged me to realize that my healing was possible, educated me on how to heal myself, and gave me the treatments and techniques to heal, even before we knew that my problem was hEDS. Of special note in this category are Bonnie Arndt, LMT; Dr. Tonya Cohorn, PA-C; Bear Decatur (owner of Core Pilates in Louisville, Kentucky); Dr. Emaline Fiala, L.Ac., DACM, and Dr. Joseph Fiala, L.Ac., DACM (owners of The Light Clinic in Frankfort, Kentucky); Dr. Norman A. Gale, MD; Dr. Curtis Gale-Dyer, DO (owner of Lexington Osteopathic in Lexington, Kentucky); Colleen Gehlbach; Katie Hedden, LMT, PTA; Charles Johnson; Dr. Tyler Kornblum, PT, DPT, CAPP; Jeremie Leckron; Dr. Natalie Marshall, PT, DPT; Dr. Melissa McElroy, PT, DPT, WCS; Dr. Matthew Moore, DC (owner of Westside Family Chiropractic in Frankfort, Kentucky); Candy Parrack, LMT; Shinai Angela Schindler; and Shawchyi Vorisek.

Thank you to everyone on social media who gave me useful advice and encouraged me by expressing gratitude for the ideas I shared.

Most of all, thank you to those who read earlier drafts of my book to give me invaluable feedback and later drafts of my book for editing and proofreading purposes: Brandon, Kathy, and Kristin Heather Gale. You made my book better, just as you make my life better.

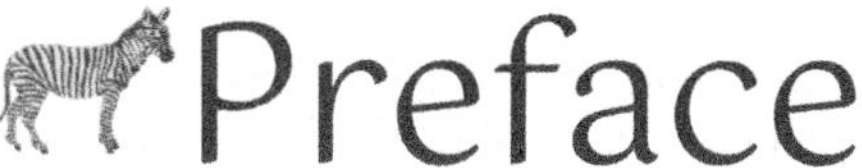

Preface

The Story of How This Book Came To Be

THIS STORY HAS A HAPPY ENDING. I want to assure you of this because at the start it is miserable, dire, and hopeless, the way many good stories are.

Invisible

My illness was invisible. Many days, I was able to struggle out of bed and brave my way into the world wearing a cute dress and a smile on my face. Most people never knew that one whiff of a neighbor's laundry vent blowing into the air, one accidental taste of a certain food, one hand washing with the wrong kind of soap, or one wrong move, and I would be laid up in bed for days, sometimes weeks.

Inexplicable, severe pain plagued me. Stomachaches, headaches, dizziness, heart palpitations, difficulty breathing, and my list went on.

I built my world around my needs. Luckily, I owned my own businesses, so I could establish my own work environment: I determined the lighting, the noise control, the cleaning products, the fragrances, the communication methods, the activities, the furniture. (So much time, money, and thought went into my careful planning!) I hired and thoroughly trained people to do the work I would not be able to do. I set my schedule – in the public location a few hours a day a few days a week at most. The rest of my work was done virtually, from home.

Even when everything was just right and I could smilingly meet with customers or friends, I felt like I was constantly suspending myself above a mire of pain. The pain never fully left, and it kept as its companions hypervigilance, confusion, and weakness. It felt as if I could never place my feet on solid ground; there was no firm foundation to walk on. My heart fluttered, my eyes watered, my stomach turned, and I just did the best I could.

But I was lucky. I had witnessed some of my clients, friends, and one of my sisters struggling to survive suffering that was worse than mine. Never will I forget when my sister, as a teenager, was hospitalized. No one knew what to do for her — we were eventually told not to expect her to wake up in the morning.

The doctors were baffled by her illness. and when she survived the night, they sent her home to live out the last of her days with her family.

When she kept waking up every morning, they were baffled by her survival, as well. For both of us, though we seemed to have two completely different conditions with unmatched symptoms, all of the medical tests that were run then and in the future came back unremarkable, normal.

My symptoms waxed and waned over the decades, and I was able to accomplish great successes and enjoy fabulous adventures throughout my life. But always there was underlying pain and a myriad of discomforts and weaknesses. And always, there were no answers.

The Miracle

One morning in August 2023, as tears rolled down my cheeks into my pillow, I had an epiphany: I had never actually asked Jesus, the most famous healer and worker of miracles, to heal me and my sister.

Many times, I had vaguely prayed to feel better or to survive a flare of symptoms, but I had never made that very simple, very specific prayer.

So, I folded my hands together, and with humility and earnestness, I said, "Jesus, please heal me and my sister." Then, I lay back down and fell into a restless daytime sleep.

By that afternoon, I was feeling a bit better. I sat up in bed, got out my phone, and typed in an online search for my symptoms. I had done this many times before, but this time, I found my answer. I was guided to click the right links, read the right articles, watch the right videos, and come to understand, finally, that all of my and my sister's varied symptoms could be explained by one condition: Ehlers-Danlos Syndrome.

And from that day on, I was guided to discover the right supplements, exercises, and treatments to heal the symptoms of this condition. Jesus worked one of his miracles on me in a very modern way. He brought me to a state of wellness, and He called me to share this information with you.

The Calling

When I first started writing this book, I wasn't writing a book at all. I was making a list of the treatments I had used and found effective so that if I needed them again in the future, I would remember them. Or, if my son or any of his future children ever develop any of these symptoms, we will know what to do.

I shared that initial list with my mother and sister, and they found it so valuable that I suddenly understood what I had. So, I sat down and prayed to Jesus again. To my surprise, I came to understand that everything I had experienced for the past twenty years had been leading to this book, qualifying me to write this book to help people all over the world.

Now, everywhere I go, I meet people who need this book. The young man working at the car repair shop who bent his fingers way back to pop his knuckles, and when I commented on his flexibility, showed me that he could bend his thumb to touch his forearm. The girl running the cash register at the toy store who exclaimed how useful ring splints like the ones I was wearing would be to prevent her fingers from hurting. The friend at the farmer's market with unbelievably soft skin who confided in me about her little girl experiencing unexplained tachycardia. The artist who posts how-to-draw videos online in which her hyperextended fingers grip her colored pencils in an unusual way. The woman at the post office who stood with her hyperextended legs crossed and became worried and dizzy as the wait in line got longer.

Whenever I ask obviously hypermobile people, "Do you have pain? Digestive problems? Headaches? Allergies?" They always affirm that they do, and usually with an exclamation of anguish mixed with a sense of reprieve. Their invisible problem has just been seen by someone who truly understands and cares.

Then, I get to inform them that I know some things that can help. It is a thrill, a blessing, and an honor so divine that it humbles me.

Visible

When I first started writing this book in January 2024, I was writing everything in present tense – describing my symptoms and treatments that I was currently doing or had only recently ended. By the time I finished the final edit of the book six months later, I had to change everything to past tense. My chronic illness was behind me.

There are still precautions I must take, nutritional supplements on my daily schedule, and exercises in my routine that are particular to my specific health concerns. But there are no more days in bed. I do not carry pain, brain fog, and weakness with me everywhere I go. Occasionally, a mild pain will pop up and want attention, but most days now, I enjoy energy, high spirits, and comfortable, nimble movement. It's strange to me after what my life was like before, but I feel good.

Today, my son and I are playing soccer together and baking cookies. My mother and I play Pickleball almost every morning. I play disc golf with my nephew. I go on adventure hikes with my husband. I cook big dinners for my family. And I do all of these things with the sensation of having my feet on solid ground; I feel strength, vitality, and peace.

I also have the clarity of mind to research, write, illustrate, and format a long, intricately detailed book about natural healing with science-backed techniques. That is no small feat.

Because my illness was invisible, I anticipated that my wellness would be invisible also. It turns out, according to my husband and my mother, my wellness is apparent.

All I want to know now is, what will your wellness look like?

Introduction

Why You Need This Book & How to Use It

I BELIEVE THAT YOU CAN HEAL. You can feel better and be happy in your life, even if you have been suffering from numerous debilitating symptoms.

If you are unusually flexible — if you consider yourself to be bendy — and you have a lot of pain and/or seemingly unrelated problems in multiple systems of the body, you might have a Hypermobility Spectrum Disorder (HSD) or Hypermobile Ehlers-Danlos Syndrome (hEDS). This book is for you.

> POSSIBLE SYMPTOMS OF HYPERMOBILE EDS OR HSD
>
> Chronic pain
> Easy bruising
> Headaches
> Stomachaches
> Dizziness
> Anxiety
> Stretch marks
> Weakness
> Diarrhea
> Numbness
> Sensitivity to chemicals
> Fatigue
> Clumsiness
> Gluten intolerance
> Sensitivity to clothing tags or jewelry
> Depression
> Slow wound healing
> Constipation
> Insomnia
> Wrinkly scars on skin
> Much, much more

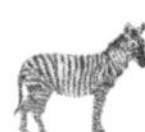

Hypermobility Conditions Are No Longer a Mystery

At this time, very few doctors know very much about hEDS/HSD, much less how to treat it effectively. Up until now, this may have made it an insurmountable challenge for you to get diagnosed and find effective help. This book will help fill in the knowledge gaps for you and your healthcare providers.

Natural Treatments Are the Answer

The few doctors who have been successful treating hEDS/HSD patients are those who recognize that pharmaceutical medications and surgeries do not usually work well for this population — and so, they prescribe some medical options as rescue treatments, but for long-term relief, they turn to natural techniques, nutritional supplements, lifestyle changes, and exercises. Still, their knowledge and experience in these realms often remain limited.

In contrast, I have spent over a decade working in the holistic healing field, and I have witnessed clients heal hypermobility-associated symptoms using a variety of natural treatments. I am hypermobile, and though mild, transitory symptoms still pop up occasionally, I have healed all of my awful and sometimes-debilitating symptoms. Although I suffered and struggled for decades, just as you may have, I am thriving and happy now, and I want you to be, as well.

What's Inside This Book

Hypermobile and Happy is a compendium of those natural techniques, nutritional supplements, lifestyle changes, and exercises that I personally have seen to be effective.

I have organized this book so that Section I gives you a solid understanding of hEDS and HSD. If you are not sure if you have hEDS or HSD, turn to Chapter 3 to see the diagnostic criteria. If you have unexplainable symptoms, turn to Chapter 4 for a list of conditions that could possibly be causing those symptoms.

Section II lets you know what it means to heal the symptoms of these conditions and gives some pointers on how to go about it.

Section III contains the most important, detailed information about how to heal the primary symptoms of hEDS/HSD so that you can live without pain and anxiety. It includes guidance on recognizing problematic hypermobile behaviors, preventing injuries and the harmful perpetual activation of the nervous system, and treating injuries.

HEDS and HSD can cause a lot of secondary conditions, and they can exist simultaneously with comorbid conditions, so in Section IV, I have listed all of those with which I have become knowledgeable. I describe the symptoms and causes of each condition, followed by a synopsis of my experience of having had the condition or treating someone else who had it, and then I provide a list of natural ways to treat it, with numbered End Notes indicating the original sources from the scientific literature that show the efficacy of each treatment.

The treatment ideas for each condition in Sections III and IV are listed in the order in which I recommend you try them. I determined this order based primarily on which treatment is the most likely to make the largest difference, but I have also prioritized easier and lower cost treatments. I want you to be able to take care of yourself without spending a lot of money.

For many of us, doctors' visits are expensive, challenging to get to because of how bad we feel, stressful because the doctors often can't help and occasionally may even harm us, and, worst of all, may lead to Migraine attacks and Allergy/MCAS/MCS reactions. Of course, if a doctor visit is easy for you, especially if you have a virtual or telehealth option or have found someone who knows how to help, you will be fortunate to rely on their guidance. Either way, the free or low-cost treatments that you can do yourself will be self-empowering, giving you that extra psychological, emotional, and spiritual strength you need to be happy with hypermobility. I have come to believe that the free and low-cost natural treatments also have a greater chance of affecting the root causes and healing the conditions altogether so that you may not have to continue taking medications for the rest of your life.

Note that Sections III and IV contain numbered lists to make it easy to see the steps to take and to refer back to them when you need to. I know as well as anyone that when you are feeling pain or experiencing brain fog, it is hard to remember what to do to feel better. It should be easy to flip through this book and find exactly the help you need at any given moment. There are numbered summary lists in boxes for each section so that you can quickly refresh your memory, and they correspond to more detailed numbered lists in the text so that you know exactly how to do what is being recommended. The summary lists can also be found in *The Hypermobile and Happy Pocket Guide*, a separate book that you can take with you wherever you go in case you get triggered or injured while you are away from home. You can purchase this at shannonegale.com

In Section V, I have thoroughly described each of the self-healing techniques that were recommended in the earlier sections. They are listed separately from the conditions because many of them can serve as treatments for multiple conditions.

Although this book is predominantly focused on what you can do for yourself, Section VI lists the professionals, both medical and alternative, whom you may want to see.

Section VII offers a simplified review of how to heal hEDS/HSD now that you understand the theory and details of the effort, as well as instruction on how to maintain your newfound health, even in the face of the occasional unexpected injuries that may occur later in your life. I also list additional health topics that you may want to investigate in case you have any remaining symptoms that do not respond to the ideas in this book, and I give my final thoughts, encouragement, and inspiration.

There are a number of different recipes that I recommend throughout the book for personal care, symptom treatment, and cleaning. I have compiled them all in Appendix A: Recipes so that you can easily find them when you are ready to make them.

There are numerous product recommendations throughout the book, and I have listed all of them, along with my notes about the products, in Appendix B: Annotated List of Recommendations. This list should make it easy for you to find the specific items in online stores. In addition to products, I have also listed experts and books so that you can easily find more information and potentially updated information in years to come. If you are reading this book on paper, you can also find this list online at shannonegale.com for ease of clicking links; I will endeavor to keep the online list updated in case the links change.

Please note that I am an Amazon affiliate and so I may receive a small commission for any purchases you make on Amazon shortly after clicking one of these links; this does not change the price for any item.

Following the appendices, I have included a Glossary of terms used in the book. This glossary will save you the trouble of searching to understand the terms. More importantly, since some terms can have different definitions depending on circumstances and who is using them, this also assures that you will know what I mean when I use a term. Additionally, familiarizing yourself with these terms may improve your ability to communicate effectively with your health professionals.

Following the Glossary are many pages of End Notes, in which I have cited scientific sources and added other details to support the information given in all of the previous chapters.

Notice that I have also included an Index so that you can easily find all subjects of interest to you. Plus, there is a short biography of me as the author, where I have included a QR code so that you can easily visit my website for more information about my offerings, including Hypermobile and Happy merchandise.

Here We Go!

I have a lot of information to share, so this is a long book. If you do not read it all of the way through because some of the conditions do not apply to you or treatment options do not interest you, please do read Sections I, II, and VII to get a good sense of the healing possibilities for someone with hEDS or HSD.

Also, I encourage you to let your loved ones read this book. It will give them a better understanding of what you have been experiencing and what kinds of treatments you are trying. They may be able to remind you lovingly to do certain treatments when you are having a flare and can't remember what to do. And, this book may give you and your loved one a starting point for a good, deep, honest, and caring conversation about your condition.

You may benefit from telling your healthcare providers about this book as well. Many of them will be happy to gain a better understanding of the hEDS/HSD experience and the natural treatments that can be effective.

I pray that this book gives you the information you need to be able to take care of your own needs, get help from loved ones, and find and communicate with the right professionals in the wellness industries. I pray that this book helps you feel better and live a more vibrant life. I pray that you thrive and feel happy being hypermobile.

Section I

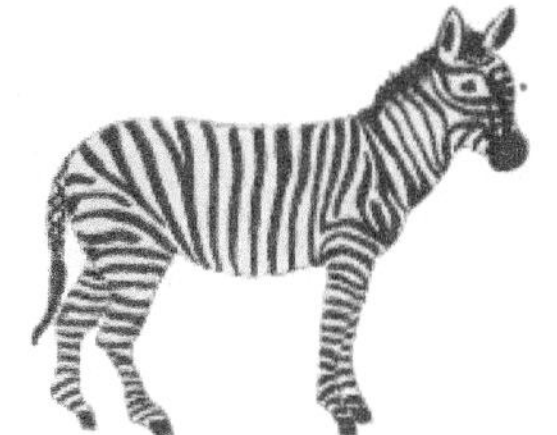

All About Hypermobility

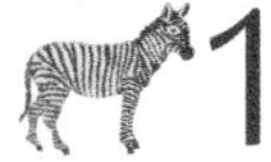

1 Are You Hypermobile?

I CAN'T COUNT HOW MANY TIMES I've heard a hypermobile person say, "I thought everybody could do that!" You may not have realized that there is something special about your flexibility. If you are hypermobile, chances are that a large percentage of your family and relatives are, too.[1] And, it is likely that you choose activities that you excel in, like dance, yoga, and gymnastics, in which case, most of the people who are participating with you are also hypermobile. [2]

Hypermobile is a fancy term for "very flexible" (hyper means excessive, and mobile means moveable). It can apply to any and every joint in the body, as well as the skin. It also applies to other tissues, but their stretchiness isn't as readily visible.

In general, flexibility is a good thing for your health and enjoyment of life, but in excess, it can present some problems.[3] There are other causes of hypermobility besides HSD and hEDS, and they may be benign or problematic. Also, the negative symptoms of HSD and hEDS may not manifest in everyone who has inherited hypermobility — and the symptoms may come and go.[4]

Being flexible does not mean that you will definitely have the symptoms of a connective tissue disorder. However, I have come to believe that awareness about both the good and bad of hypermobility is very important. When you are aware, you can take preventative measures to ensure that you enjoy as much of the good and suffer through as little of the bad as possible.

Signs of Excessive Flexibility

When determining if you are hypermobile, doctors might ask a series of questions about your current and past flexibility, such as, "When in a standing position, could you ever put your hands flat on the ground without bending your knees?"

Physical Therapists (PTs) can do a quick evaluation of the Range of Motion of any joint using a simple angle-measuring ruler called a goniometer, and they can compare that to the known average to determine if you are hypermobile in that joint. A good PT will recognize if an injury or age has reduced the native range of motion of a joint; they might look at other joints to gauge the general natural mobility that is to be expected in your body.

In practical life, your signs of flexibility may be more recognizable. You do not need to be able to say yes to all or any of the signs listed here. HEDS and HSD are diagnosed based on specific measurements of hypermobility that are different from this list. However, this list will help you figure out if hEDS or HSD is something you should consider.

Nonscientific Signs of Hypermobility

1. Rather than sitting in a chair with your back straight and feet on the floor, you sit in a variety of "childlike" positions.
2. You worry and feel anxious frequently, but you are really good in a crisis.
3. You are very aware of what is around you – smells, lights, sounds, breezes, and vibrations.
4. You are very graceful when doing a sport or art, but in regular life you're sometimes a clutz.
5. Your fingers and/or thumbs bend backwards.
6. When you are sitting and cross your legs at the knee, you wrap your crossed leg and foot all the way around your supporting leg.
7. Your fingers lock up sometimes.
8. If you pinch your skin and pull it away from your body part, it stretches pretty far and then resumes its shape.
9. You feel slightly strangled when you wear a turtleneck or shirt buttoned up to the neck.
10. People call you "bendy" or "double jointed."
11. You do tasks with your legs and feet that most people do with their hands.
12. You tend to put yourself into locked positions where one leg or arm traps the other.
13. When you're seated with your legs straight out in front of you, your knees and feet roll out to the side.
14. You can sense when the weather is about to change.
15. You can point your feet really far.
16. You can kick really high.
17. You often notice things going on inside your body like your heartbeat, muscle contractions, breathing, and intestinal movements.
18. People sometimes laugh at how strange one of your body parts looks when it is hyperextending.
19. Standing still in a line or at a museum exhibit feels like torture. You cross your legs tightly, wiggle, or crouch down.
20. You can feel and are sometimes bothered by your jewelry or the tags in your clothes.
21. You bruise and bleed easily.
22. Your veins are visible through your thin skin.
23. Things that touch your skin quickly become temporarily imprinted on your skin.
24. You feel cold all the time, but you're also intolerant of high heat.
25. You can easily do the splits and other stretches or contortions that seem impossible for some people.

There are many other possible signs that you are hypermobile. You may have never paid attention before, or perhaps you thought these little quirks about your body were part of your personality. It is likely that you had more of these quirks when you were younger and that you feel rather stiff now, although you still bend your finger or thumb backwards when you push on a button, for example.

Any of these signs could be a clue that you should consider whether you are dealing with hypermobility.

2

What Are hEDS & HSD?

HYPERMOBILITY WITH ASSOCIATED symptoms in multiple body systems was first described by Hippocrates in 400 BC when he wrote about fierce Scythian warriors, and was added to the current medical lexicon by dermatologists Edvard Ehlers of Denmark and Henri-Alexandre Danlos of France in 1908.[5] Ehlers-Danlos Syndrome is a connective tissue disorder that can affect all organs and systems of the body. Hypermobility Spectrum Disorder (HSD) is also a connective tissue disorder with the same possible symptoms, but the clinical criteria for diagnosis are less stringent; some researchers and doctors believe that they are actually a single entity.[6]

Connective tissue lends structure to tissues throughout the body — ligaments, tendons, bones, skin, muscles, fascia, organs, nerves, blood vessels, the brain — pretty much everything, and so hEDS/HSD can cause joint hypermobility, chronic pain, Digestive System Problems, allergies, dysautonomia (improper operation of the Autonomic Nervous System, which controls breathing, digestion, heart rate, temperature, vision, elimination, sweating, and more), and other symptoms. Some of the common comorbidities caused by hEDS are listed in the Table of Contents of this book, but there are many more that are not listed.[7]

Connective tissue is predominantly made of collagen, which is the most abundant protein in our bodies and is present in especially high ratios in some of our most noticeable parts: the skin and especially the ligaments.[8] When collagen is not functioning correctly in ligaments, they stretch or are lax; they do not support and stabilize the joints. For this reason, hEDS is expected to present with injuries of the shoulders, hips, ankles, wrists, etc. The neck, with its highly articulated bones, is one of the worst trouble spots for many hypermobile people, especially because improper movement of these bones can damage the nerves that serve the entire body and create a myriad of symptoms. Collagen-rich ligaments also exist in places we often don't think of as joints, such as the junctions where the ribs meet the backbone and sternum, so chest and back pain is also common.

In addition, collagen is responsible for giving the skin structure. Without this structure, the skin not only stretches and droops in unusual ways, it is prone to certain types of scars and stretch marks.[9] The commonly striped appearance of stretch marks on hypermobile people is why the mascot for hEDS is the striped zebra.

It is also said that doctors hear hoofbeats and expect a horse, when in fact the patient is a different hoofed animal — a zebra — making diagnosis elusive for many patients. Until now, hEDS has been considered a rare disease (thought to exist in 1 in 5,000 people), but recent studies have found that it is too common to reach the qualifications of a rare disease. Depending on which recent study report you read, hEDS may actually exist in 1 in 500 people[10] or maybe 1 in 100,[11] or if HSD is included, it may exist in 1 in 29[12] or even 1 in 7.[13]

Not only are visible skin abnormalities a possibility with hypermobility, skin without the proper structure normally given it by collagen is not as capable of supporting the lymph channels, which are also made with collagen.[14] These lymph vessels that run through some layers of the skin and throughout all of the body and its organs, are a very important part of the immune system, serving as microscopic tubes through which nutrients and waste molecules are transported throughout the body. Reduced lymph flow can cause a plethora of symptoms and can be implicated in serious conditions such as heart disease, neurodegenerative diseases, obesity, irritable bowel conditions, aging, obesity, lymphedema (a swelling of fluids in the soft tissues of the body[15]), and metabolic syndrome (a condition of obesity, low HDL cholesterol, and high blood sugar, blood pressure, and triglycerides that can lead to heart disease, diabetes, and stroke[16]).[17]

To make matters worse, the skin is more permeable with a connective tissue disorder. This porous nature is sometimes termed "leaky skin," and it allows potentially poisonous chemicals to be absorbed into the body that would normally be prevented from entering. This can lead to allergic-type reactions, eczema, and more.

Just as the skin can be leaky, the gut and lungs can be leaky as well, leading to numerous problems.[18, 19] Many hypermobile people have gastrointestinal distress and food allergies of some kind, as well as asthma, sensitivities to inhaled chemicals, and a number of other respiratory complaints.[20]

Collagen abnormalities in the veins can be responsible for problems with blood pressure, heart rate, temperature regulation, and more. The insufficiently supported and/or damaged nervous system can operate improperly, wreaking havoc in the gastrointestinal tract and cardiovascular system and making the body either too sensitive or insensitive.[21, 22] The bones can be prone to osteoporosis.[23] The teeth and eyes can be prone to problems of their own.[24, 25] The muscles may atrophy too easily.[26] The fascia, tendons, and other connective tissues that are responsible for holding the organs in place may not do their jobs properly.[27] And the list of potentially affected parts goes on.

For some people, the symptoms of hEDS/HSD do not appear until late in life.[28] For other people, the symptoms come and go. Doctors are not sure why this is so. A correlation with hormonal changes has been noticed — especially estrogen.[29] Women with these conditions often report that their problems started when they started menstruating, or went into perimenopause, or hit menopause, or got pregnant, or that the problems get worse every month during their period or when they ovulate. If estrogen has an impact, it seems not to be the quantity of the hormone but the fluctuation of it that matters.[30]

Fortunately, hEDS/HSD is not considered to be terminal (leading to death), nor progressive (getting worse over time). In fact, some patients with connective tissue disorders get better as they get older because flexibility naturally decreases with age. And, patients with hEDS/HSD have the same life expectancy as the general public.

Doctors have noticed a pattern of progression in hEDS/HSD, however, and it can seem to get worse over time. Most patients progress from hypermobility to pain and then to stiffness.[31] This is likely due to Joint Injuries that have not been treated or have not responded to the treatment given. My hope is that the treatments in this book will stop that progression and reverse your condition back to comfortable hypermobility, as they have for me.

> TYPICAL PROGRESSION OF CONNECTIVE TISSUE DISORDERS
>
> Hypermobility → Pain → Stiffness

HEDS is an inheritable condition, but as of yet, there is not a known genetic marker that is found in all hEDS patients. It is likely that if you have hEDS, some of your family members have it, too. However, it manifests differently in everyone. Two siblings with hEDS can have completely different lists of symptoms, even identical twins.[32] The list of all possible symptoms is extremely long, and this varying manifestation of the symptoms makes it challenging for doctors to recognize hEDS in a new, undiagnosed patient.[33]

Because hEDS is so little known and the varying manifestations of it are so difficult to recognize, many patients who have sought diagnoses have been told that their problems are psychological or psychosomatic (created by the mind).[34, 35] There is no way to think or meditate your way out of having a connective tissue disorder, and though some hEDS patients have mental health concerns and/or are helped by drugs or by behavioral changes, there is certainly an underlying biological condition.

It is still unknown what is actually happening in hEDS/HSD. Some doctors believe that these patients have faulty collagen — perhaps the molecules that make up the collagen are twisted differently than other people's collagen so that it stretches out too much.[36] Other doctors believe that numerous kinds of connective tissue, not just collagen, are either faulty or in short supply in hEDS.[37, 38, 39] Some doctors believe the collagen of hEDS is made with the wrong protein "recipe."[40] Other doctors believe that hEDS patients are deficient in certain vitamins.[41] It has also been found that other conditions (such as Lyme disease[42] or Epstein Barr virus[43]) can affect the joints, degrade collagen, and exacerbate or maybe even create hypermobility problems.

It may be that there are different forms of hEDS that have yet to be distinguished from each other. It may be that multiple factors are at play in hEDS. Sadly, doctors do not know what is going on, and there are few who have any good ideas on how to treat it. In the medical community, it is generally considered incurable and untreatable.[44] This means that the long-hoped-for blessing of a diagnosis can engender depression and anxiety.[45]

Regardless of what causes hEDS, and despite how infrequently it is diagnosed, doctors and patients have worked to determine ways to treat and cope with the condition.[46] We cannot wait for the scientific research or clinical experience to find all of the answers. We are suffering now, and we need to treat and cope with hEDS now, even if the doctors cannot help us. This book is here to help you do that.

3

The Benefits of hEDS/HSD

I KNOW, YOU MAY BE READING THIS book because hEDS is making you or someone you love feel really bad. It might even cause you to be handicapped or so sick or in pain that you might think about suicide.[47] This is serious. It is really hard to deal with. I know that you are probably living with a condition that is a 10 on the 10-point pain scale and you're trying to pretend that nothing's wrong. But we ought to look at the other side of the condition, too.

People with hypermobility conditions tend to be very attractive. First of all, flexibility is beautiful — it is sexy. Even if we reduce our hyperflexibility for the sake of our health, we will always maintain an above average range of motion that gives us grace.[48] We can move with fluidity and agility, which is enjoyable to do and pleasant to watch.

Whether we are plump or slender, we are nice to look at. We often look younger than our age.[49] We may not feel healthy, but with this "invisible illness," we usually look attractively healthy.[50, 51]

Most people with hEDS have soft skin and long limbs and fingers. We are elegant. While we may not be physically strong, we are nimble. We are beautiful dancers, gymnasts, yogis, and divers.

Not only are we physically attractive and adept, we are the kind of people everyone wants to know. People with hEDS tend to be empathetic and intelligent.[52, 53] Even when our bodies are causing us trouble, we have rich emotional and intellectual lives that are fascinating to others.

Flexibility of body leads to flexibility of mind, so we are open-minded, creative, curious, and resourceful. And, many of us have a frenetic energy that enables us, at times, to accomplish truly remarkable achievements in our careers, sports, and arts.[54]

People with hypermobility tend to be more aware of their surroundings than others, sensing subtle dynamics in light and sound, sometimes recognizing smells below normal human thresholds, and noticing even minute vibrations, breezes, and physical sensations. Our talent for observation can be an asset in understanding the world around us.

Hypermobility can also bestow upon us a more detailed understanding of our own bodies than what most people experience. We may be an enigma to some doctors, but we are attuned to and conscious of what is happening inside us and how our systems react to various inputs and stimuli. All of this self-knowledge gives us wisdom, instantaneous and instinctive responsiveness, and uncanny intuitive abilities beyond what most people can claim.

We have a tendency toward anxiety that keeps us safe but also confers upon us impressive skills of foresight, perception, and a capacity to be calm and cool-headed during a crisis — we usually respond well when others panic.[55]

Hypermobility is thought to have been around for a very long time, indicating that it is a positive evolutionary trait. Because of our unusual physical troubles, we develop an enviable ability to cope and adapt by making changes in ourselves and in our environment. It is likely that hypermobile individuals, with their specific skill set, can be credited with some of the inventions, evolutions, and leaps of progress that humankind has made that have enriched our humanity.[56]

People with hypermobility are often long-lived; the physical problems presented by the condition do not diminish life expectancy. When simple precautions are taken in response to our specific health needs, people with hypermobility can be surprisingly spry and full of vitality even when they are quite old.

I would imagine that individuals with all of these qualities of beauty, intelligence, agility, creativity, and resourcefulness (but not so much physical strength) are descended from people who were in the upper socio-economic classes, perhaps even royalty.

4

Diagnosing hEDS, HSD, & Pediatric Joint Hypermobility Spectrum Disorder

AT THIS POINT IN TIME, IT CAN TAKE A LOT of doctor's visits and many years to finally get a diagnosis of hEDS or HSD. Studies have shown that from the time a patient first seeks medical help for their hEDS symptoms to when they are finally given an official diagnosis is, on average, 14-22 years.[57, 58]

Anecdotally, it can take several decades. When my sister was a child, the doctors said that her symptoms were a result of her "wanting attention." This was the first in a list of misdiagnoses she received over four decades.

Up to 97% of people with hEDS were inaccurately diagnosed with a psychiatric condition prior to finally receiving an accurate hEDS diagnosis. Many people on social media complain of being "gaslighted" by doctors who couldn't believe they experienced the symptoms they reported. Some scientists have called the effort to be diagnosed a "diagnostic Odyssey" or "hero's journey."[59]

This challenge of achieving a diagnosis is especially problematic because these patients suffer while seeking their diagnosis, to the point that it significantly elevates their risk of suicide. Up to 31% of hEDS patients attempt suicide, and many more contemplate it, but the risk is significantly reduced when the patient receives the hEDS diagnosis, especially if that occurs before the age of 19.[60]

My hope and my prayer are that this book will help spread the word so that doctors can proffer help to the hEDS/HSD population much earlier and fully, and that people with hEDS/HSD can be empowered to take control of their health effectively.

Differentiating hEDS and HSD

Hypermobile Ehlers-Danlos Syndrome and Hypermobility Spectrum Disorder are so similar that differentiating the two is very difficult.[61] They have essentially the same symptoms and the same treatments; some doctors and scientists believe that they are the same condition and that the diagnostic criteria should be re-evaluated.[62]

However, because many doctors still adhere strictly to a list of diagnostic criteria that was developed and published in 2017,[63] and because understanding what makes up the diagnostic criteria gives you an insight to the conditions, I will explain it thoroughly.

Hypermobile Ehlers-Danlos Syndrome (hEDS)

HEDS is, as of yet, not a well understood condition. Most doctors know very little about it; it is not something they are looking for. (They usually think those hoofbeats are coming from horses, not zebras!) On average, it takes EDS patients 15 different clinicians before they finally receive an accurate diagnosis.[64] Along the way, they are likely to receive inaccurate diagnoses; the most common of these are psychological disorders, neurological disorders, Multiple Sclerosis, Fibromyalgia, Bipolar Disorder, and Ulcerative Colitis (an inflammatory bowel disease). See also Chapter 37: Other Comorbidities.

Even those doctors who are aware of it often do not know enough about it to diagnose it. Numerous professionals discounted the possibility that I could have hEDS simply because I could not touch my thumb to my forearm, when in fact I met all of the other criteria and other members of my family can do this thumb sign — I didn't know I might have hEDS until I was 48 years old because of this. I hope that other people who need this diagnosis will get it sooner because of this book.

Another obstacle to being diagnosed with hEDS is related to its inheritable nature. Everyone in my family had similarly flexible hands and bodies. The party tricks and contortions I could do did not seem unusual to me. Although I was more flexible than most of the kids in my class at school, I spent most of my physical movement activity time amongst dancers and gymnasts who also were hypermobile. I did not know how unusual my flexibility was.

Furthermore, flexibility does not seem to be related to most of the items in my long list of symptoms. Who would have guessed that the reason I felt bad was the same reason I was bendy? In my experience, being flexible had been an exceptionally good thing!

Figuring out if you have hEDS is actually a simple matter: look at the Diagnostic Criteria and determine if you meet them or not. All of the criteria are clinical, which means they are judged based on looking at you and listening to your self-reports while you are in the clinic; there are no blood tests, urine tests, or imaging tests for hEDS.

If you meet the clinical criteria, it is recommended that you get a gene panel done to rule out the possibility that you have one of the 12 other forms of EDS. An official medical diagnosis cannot be made until the gene panel has been done. Most frequently, the doctors who give official EDS diagnoses are Geneticists and Rheumatologists.[65]

Be aware that if you do not live near a really good doctor who is a specialist in hEDS, it may be better to go without an official medical diagnosis. According to what has been posted by many people in social media groups, doctors who are not familiar with hEDS are sometimes scared of it. Understandably, they do not want to lose a patient on the operating table because of something they do not understand, for example. If you have a diagnosis but no good doctor backing you up, you may have difficulty finding the medical care you need. On the other hand, a good specialist will be able to talk with any other doctors you need and give them the information that will allow them not to be afraid of taking you on as a patient while also knowing what special precautions they should take when working with you.

2017 Diagnostic Criteria

The hEDS diagnostic criteria that is used today was developed in 2017 and is organized in three parts.[66] First the Beighton Score and Hakim and Grahame Questionnaire. Then some features of the skin and organs, Marfanoid Habitus, family history, and reports of pain. And finally, all other possible diagnoses must be excluded.

The Beighton Score was developed as a research tool for a study conducted by P. Beighton, L. Solomon, and C. L. Solskone to evaluate the hypermobility of a population in Africa in 1973; their need was for a quick and easy evaluation tool, so they left many potential hypermobility signs off of it.[67] With this tool, 4, 5, or 6 or more positive signs, depending on age, indicates hypermobility. However, as it was developed as a research tool rather than a clinical diagnostic tool, time will tell if it serves the latter purpose or needs to be adjusted to be more valuable and accurate.

The Beighton Score's nine features are bending the two pinkie fingers back to or past 90 degrees, bending the two knees and two arms back to or past 10 degrees, touching the two thumbs to the wrists, and standing with the knees straight and placing both hands flat on the floor.

The Hakim and Grahame Questionnaire is a self-report of flexibility, existing or historical. Two or more out of five possible yes answers indicates hypermobility. Its five questions repeat two of the Beighton criteria but add contorting into strange shapes or doing the splits, dislocating a shoulder or kneecap, and being considered double jointed.

Some skin features that are common among hEDS patients are soft, velvety, or doughy skin; mild hyperextensibility of the skin (you can stretch it out further than most people and then it returns to its normal shape); bilateral piezogenic papules of the heel (small white bumps appear on the sides of your heels when you stand on your foot — these are tiny balls of fat that protrude through the imperfect connective tissue layers beneath the skin when pressure is applied to the area); and atrophic scars (scars that wrinkle when you press the sides of the scar together).

Some symptoms that apply to the organs that are common among hEDS patients are hernias, pelvic floor or uterine prolapse (the muscles or organs of the pelvis drop and bulge into the vagina), and rectal prolapse (the last section of the intestines bulges out of the anus).

Marfanoid Habitus, named for the typical appearance of someone with Marfan Syndrome (a different connective tissue disease) is a cluster of symptoms that indicate a connective tissue disorder. None of these features have to be present for an hEDS diagnosis if you have a family history and chronic pain. Otherwise, at least two should be noted.

The Marfanoid Habitus symptoms include stretch marks (striae distensae or rubae) that were not caused by rapid, significant weight change; high arched palate (roof of your mouth) with crowded teeth; arachnodactyly (long fingers); the Wrist Sign (wrap your thumb and pinkie finger around your other wrist; it is positive if your thumb covers the pinkie fingernail); the Thumb Sign (fold your thumb across your palm, then fold your fingers on top of it; the sign is positive if your thumb sticks out beyond your fingers); your arm span is greater than 1.05 times your height; mitral valve prolapse (the valves in the heart do not close properly); aortic root dilation (the first section of the main blood vessel of the heart is unusually large); you cannot straighten your elbows all of the way; you are remarkably tall; you are remarkably slender; you have moderate or severe Scoliosis (curvature of the spine); and you have moderate or high myopia (nearsightedness).[68, 69]

A positive family history means that you have a sibling, parent, or child who has been diagnosed with hEDS. This criterion means that the first person in the family to get diagnosed usually has severe symptoms and meets the criteria without having a positive family history. After that, it is easier for other family members to be properly diagnosed.

Reports of pain that meet the criteria for an hEDS diagnosis could be persistent musculoskeletal pain in at least two limbs for at least three months, pain throughout the body for at least three months, recurrent joint dislocations, and frank Joint Instability (excessive mobility or loss of control of a joint that is inherent to the joint and was not caused by a traumatic injury).

Differential Diagnoses

Other conditions that could look like hEDS include the 12 other types of Ehlers-Danlos Syndrome, all of which can be determined through genetic testing. These other forms of EDS are Classical, Classical-like, Cardiac-Valvular, Vascular, Arthrochalasia, Dermatosparaxis, Kyphoscoliotic, Brittle Cornea Syndrome, Spondylotysplastic, Musculocontractual, Myopathic, and Periodontal.

Additionally, other conditions that could look like hEDS are Bethlem Myopathy, Osteogenesis Imperfecta, Marfan Syndrome, Stickler Syndrome, Pseudoxanthoma Elasticum, Undifferentiated Connective Tissue Disease, Rheumatoid Arthritis, Multiple Sclerosis, Lupus, Scleroderma, Myositis, Sjogren's Syndrome, and probably others.[70, 71] See also Chapter 37: Other Comorbidities.

Some of these conditions exclude an hEDS diagnosis, while others could be determined to be comorbid (existing at the same time with it). Your doctor may want to consider and test for all of these possibilities before confirming a diagnosis.

Drawbacks to the 2017 Diagnostic Criteria

Although the diagnostic criteria makes it easy to determine if you have hEDS, there are some drawbacks to the criteria. It works well for young adults, but not so well for children and older adults. Fortunately, to combat this discrepancy, many doctors are not asking older patients if they can do the things on the Beighton Score but if they have ever been able to do them, and a separate set of criteria has been determined for children.

In my opinion, the Beighton Score is not a sufficient measure of whether a person is hypermobile — flexibility varies from joint to joint in all people, and some may be extremely hypermobile in joints that are not on the Beighton Score while they are not hypermobile in the hands, elbows, hips, or knees. Also, hypermobility is not invariable; it can change within any given joint due to a number of different factors. Nevertheless, if someone meets many but not all of the clinical criteria, they can be diagnosed with Hypermobility Spectrum Disorder (HSD), which has essentially the same symptoms and treatments as hEDS.

In fact, some people with HSD seem to have even more symptoms and more severe symptoms than some people with hEDS. I expect that in the future the diagnostic criteria will be revisited, and that the distinction between HSD and hEDS will be dissolved.

I would love for doctors to understand that if their patient has a greater-than-average range of motion in some of their joints, it is an indication that they should watch out for the common symptoms and comorbidities of hEDS/HSD so that the patient can take steps to prevent problems and can be treated as soon as any problems begin.

Do You Have hEDS According to the 2017 Diagnostic Criteria?

On the next page is the form your doctor might fill out when deciding on your diagnosis.

There are numerous YouTube videos that explain the diagnostic criteria thoroughly so that you can determine for yourself if you meet the criteria. I especially like this one: "Hypermobile EDS Diagnostic Criteria on 5 People w/ Ehlers-Danlos" by Izzy K DNA https://www.YouTube.com/watch?v=HkEHAXgEjaA .

Hypermobility Spectrum Disorders (HSDs)

HSD is usually diagnosed when someone almost meets the criteria of hEDS but not quite. A spectrum disorder is a condition in which the symptoms and severity of symptoms can vary widely from person to person.[72]

There are four different types of HSD: Generalized, Peripheral, Localized, and Historic. These distinctions indicate the type of hypermobility that can be observed by the doctor in the clinic. Generalized means hypermobility in joints throughout the body, though not necessarily passing the Beighton Criteria. Peripheral hypermobility is mainly focused in the hands and feet. Localized hypermobility would be in one or two joints or joints in one area of the body. Historic hypermobility is based on the patient's report of having been more flexible in the past.

Just like hEDS, all four types of HSD may include symptoms like chronic pain, mild skin hyperextensibility (skin can stretch when pinched and pulled), recurrent joint dislocations, cardiovascular autonomic dysfunction (problems with heart rate), Marfanoid Habitus (see previous part), stretch marks, and atrophic scarring. The difference with hEDS is that it would also potentially include mild cardiovascular findings and a family history.[73]

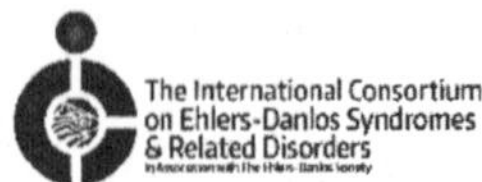

Diagnostic Criteria for Hypermobile Ehlers-Danlos Syndrome (hEDS)

This diagnostic checklist is for doctors across all disciplines to be able to diagnose EDS

Distributed by

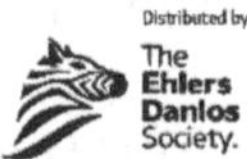

Patient name: ______ DOB: ______ DOV: ______ Evaluator: ______

The clinical diagnosis of hypermobile EDS needs the simultaneous presence of all criteria, 1 ***and*** 2 ***and*** 3.

CRITERION 1 – Generalized Joint Hypermobility

One of the following selected:

- ☐ ≥6 pre-pubertal children and adolescents
- ☐ ≥5 pubertal men and woman to age 50
- ☐ ≥4 men and women over the age of 50

Beighton Score: ____/9

If Beighton Score is one point below age- and sex-specific cut off, two or more of the following must also be selected to meet criterion:

- ☐ Can you now (or could you ever) place your hands flat on the floor without bending your knees?
- ☐ Can you now (or could you ever) bend your thumb to touch your forearm?
- ☐ As a child, did you amuse your friends by contorting your body into strange shapes or could you do the splits?
- ☐ As a child or teenager, did your shoulder or kneecap dislocate on more than one occasion?
- ☐ Do you consider yourself "double jointed"?

CRITERION 2 – Two or more of the following features (A, B, or C) must be present

Feature A (five must be present)

- ☐ Unusually soft or velvety skin
- ☐ Mild skin hyperextensibility
- ☐ Unexplained striae distensae or rubae at the back, groins, thighs, breasts and/or abdomen in adolescents, men or pre-pubertal women without a history of significant gain or loss of body fat or weight
- ☐ Bilateral piezogenic papules of the heel
- ☐ Recurrent or multiple abdominal hernia(s)
- ☐ Atrophic scarring involving at least two sites and without the formation of truly papyraceous and/or hemosideric scars as seen in classical EDS
- ☐ Pelvic floor, rectal, and/or uterine prolapse in children, men or nulliparous women without a history of morbid obesity or other known predisposing medical condition
- ☐ Dental crowding and high or narrow palate
- ☐ Arachnodactyly, as defined in one or more of the following:
  (i) positive wrist sign (Walker sign) on both sides, (ii) positive thumb sign (Steinberg sign) on both sides
- ☐ Arm span-to-height ratio ≥1.05
- ☐ Mitral valve prolapse (MVP) mild or greater based on strict echocardiographic criteria
- ☐ Aortic root dilatation with Z-score >+2

Feature A total: ____/12

Feature B

- ☐ Positive family history; one or more first-degree relatives independently meeting the current criteria for hEDS

Feature C (must have at least one)

- ☐ Musculoskeletal pain in two or more limbs, recurring daily for at least 3 months
- ☐ Chronic, widespread pain for ≥3 months
- ☐ Recurrent joint dislocations or frank joint instability, in the absence of trauma

CRITERION 3 – All of the following prerequisites MUST be met

1. Absence of unusual skin fragility, which should prompt consideration of other types of EDS
2. Exclusion of other heritable and acquired connective tissue disorders, including autoimmune rheumatologic conditions. In patients with an acquired CTD (*e.g.* Lupus, Rheumatoid Arthritis, etc.), additional diagnosis of hEDS requires meeting both Features A and B of Criterion 2. Feature C of Criterion 2 (chronic pain and/or instability) cannot be counted toward a diagnosis of hEDS in this situation.
3. Exclusion of alternative diagnoses that may also include joint hypermobility by means of hypotonia and/or connective tissue laxity. Alternative diagnoses and diagnostic categories include, but are not limited to, neuromuscular disorders (*e.g.* Bethlem myopathy), other hereditary disorders of the connective tissue (*e.g.* other types of EDS, Loeys-Dietz syndrome, Marfan syndrome), and skeletal dysplasias (*e.g.* osteogenesis imperfecta). Exclusion of these considerations may be based upon history, physical examination, and/or molecular genetic testing, as indicated.

Diagnosis: ______

v9

Figure 3: Diagnostic Criteria for Hypermobile Ehlers-Danlos Syndorme. Reprinted with permission of The Ehlers-Danlos Society.[74]

Pediatric Joint Hypermobility Spectrum Disorder

In 2023, scientists determined a separate Diagnostic Criteria to be used for children.[75] If they meet these criteria, their diagnosis is not actually hEDS but Pediatric Generalized Hypermobility Spectrum Disorder, and there are eight different subtypes:

1. Pediatric generalized joint hypermobility;
2. Pediatric generalized joint hypermobility with skin involvement;
3. Pediatric generalized joint hypermobility with core comorbidities;
4. Pediatric generalized joint hypermobility with core comorbidities and with skin involvement;
5. Pediatric generalized hypermobility spectrum disorder, musculoskeletal subtype;
6. Pediatric generalized hypermobility spectrum disorder, musculoskeletal subtype with skin involvement;
7. Pediatric generalized hypermobility spectrum disorder, systemic subtype; and
8. Pediatric generalized hypermobility spectrum disorder, systemic subtype with skin involvement.

This diagnostic criteria for children has very strict standards, necessary because children in general are more hypermobile than adults. It also has strict standards regarding pain experience, which I anticipate will be tricky because children's pain is so often dismissed by adults.[76] Not only that, but children do not always understand their pain nor recognize that it is abnormal if it has always been their experience (this is true for adults, too, but usually the adults who are seeking a diagnosis have finally come to recognize that their pain is not ordinary). Additionally, children heal quickly — their pain may not become chronic even if it is frequent. I expect that adults may also neglect and misunderstand children's experiences of fatigue and anxiety.

I pray that any families who are seeking a diagnosis for their children will be blessed with a good doctor who understands these concerns. The following two pages are the worksheets for the Pediatric Joint Hypermobility Spectrum Disorder diagnosis.

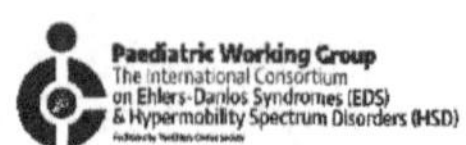

Diagnostic Criteria for
Paediatric Joint Hypermobility

This diagnostic checklist is to support doctors to diagnose paediatric joint hypermobility and hypermobility spectrum disorder

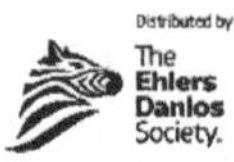

Patient name: ____________________ DOB: ____________ DOV: ____________ Evaluator: ______________

Joint Hypermobility in Children from 5 Years

L☐R☐ L☐R☐ L☐R☐ L☐R☐ ☐

Beighton Score: _____/9
Must be a minimum of 6

Skin and Tissue Abnormalities

- ☐ Unusually soft skin – unusually soft and/or velvety skin
- ☐ Mild skin extensibility
- ☐ Unexplained striae distensae or rubae at the back, groin, thighs, breasts and/or abdomen without a history of significant gain or loss of body fat or weight
- ☐ Atrophic scarring involving at least 1 site and without the formation of truly papyraceous and/or haemosideric scars as seen in classical EDS
- ☐ Bilateral piezogenic papules in the heel
- ☐ Recurrent hernia in more than one site (excludes congenital umbilical hernia)

Score: _____/6
Must be a minimum of 3

Musculoskeletal Complications

- ☐ Episodic activity related pain not meeting the chronic pain frequency and duration criteria
- ☐ Recurrent joint dislocations, or recurrent subluxations in the absence of trauma, and/or frank joint subluxation on physical exam in more than one joint (excludes radial head <2yrs)
- ☐ Soft tissue injuries – one major (needing surgical repair) and/or current multiple minor tendon, and/or ligament tears

Score: _____/3
Must be a minimum of 2

Co-Morbidities

- ☐ Chronic primary pain
- ☐ Chronic fatigue
- ☐ Functional GI disorders
- ☐ Functional bladder disorders
- ☐ Primary dysautonomia
- ☐ Anxiety

Any number causing distressor disability?
Y / N

Prerequisites:

1. This framework can only be used after exclusion of other Ehlers-Danlos syndrome subtypes, heritable disorders of connective tissue, syndromic conditions, chromosomal microdeletions, skeletal dysplasia's, or neuromuscular disorders. From biological maturity or the 18th birthday, whichever is earlier, the 2017 Adult criteria should be used.

2. If a child has a biological parent with a current hEDS diagnosis and a confirmed disease-causing genetic mutation and they also have the same mutation with GJH (although large genetic discovery projects are underway these genes are currently yet to be identified) that diagnosis should be used.

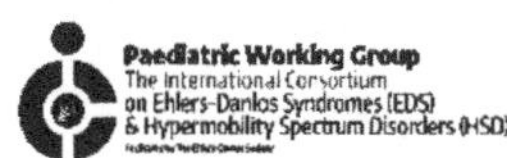

Diagnostic Criteria for Paediatric Joint Hypermobility

This diagnostic checklist is to support doctors to diagnose paediatric joint hypermobility and hypermobility spectrum disorder

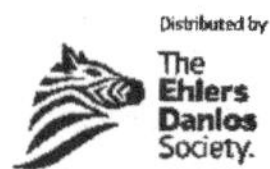

	Generalized Joint Hypermobility	Skin and tissue abnormalities	Musculoskeletal complications	Core comorbidities
Asymptomatic conditions				
Paediatric Generalized Joint Hypermobility	Present	Absent	Absent	Absent
Paediatric Generalized Joint Hypermobility with skin involvement	Present	Present	Absent	Absent
Symptomatic conditions				
Paediatric Generalised Joint Hypermobility with core comorbidities	Present	Absent	Absent	Present
Paediatric Generalised Joint Hypermobility with core comorbidities with skin involvement	Present	Present	Absent	Present
Paediatric Hypermobility Spectrum Disorder, Musculoskeletal subtype	Present	Absent	Present	Absent
Paediatric Hypermobility Spectrum Disorder, Musculoskeletal subtype with skin involvement	Present	Present	Present	Absent
Paediatric Hypermobility Spectrum Disorder: Systemic subtype	Present	Absent	Present	Present
Paediatric Hypermobility Spectrum disorder: Systemic subtype with skin involvement	Present	Present	Present	Present

Diagnosis: ______________________________

Figure 4: Diagnostic Criteria for Paediatric Joint Hypermobility. Reprinted with permission of The Ehlers-Danlos Society.[77]

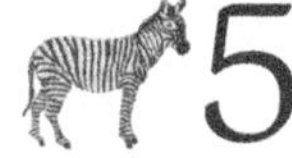

5

Common Symptoms & Their Causes Among hEDS/HSD & Their Secondary Conditions

THIS LIST REFERS ONLY TO THOSE conditions covered in this book. Other conditions could be responsible for any of these symptoms. An important part of the diagnostic process is ruling out other possible causes, but it is beyond the scope of this book. If you suspect that you might have any of these conditions, it is recommended that you talk about it with your doctor, who should be qualified to do the appropriate tests to rule out other possibilities and confirm the correct diagnosis.

Anxiety, Depression, Irritability, Mood Swings — Allergy/MCAS/MCS, Digestive System Problems, Joint Injury (see also pain), Lymph Congestion, Migraine, MTHFR, Peripheral Neuropathy, POTS, Sinus Congestion

Arm Pain or Numbness — CCI, Joint Injury (in the wrist, elbow, or shoulder or referred from the neck or back), Myofascial adhesions, Peripheral Neuropathy, Thoracic Outlet Syndrome

Back Pain — CCI, Digestive System Problems, Joint Injury (in the back, hip, shoulder, or neck), Lymph Congestion, Myofascial adhesions, Pelvis Complaints, Rib Subluxation, Thoracic Outlet Syndrome

Bleeding During Pregnancy — Subchorionic Hematoma

Brain Fog, Difficulty Concentrating, Aphasia (inability to remember words), Forgetfulness — Allergy/MCAS/MCS, Digestive System Problems, Joint Injury (especially in neck, back, or shoulders), Lymph Congestion, Migraine, Motion Sickness, MTHFR, Peripheral Neuropathy, POTS, Thoracic Outlet Syndrome, TMJ

Breast Pain — Lymph Congestion

Burning Sensation on Skin — CCI, Peripheral Neuropathy, Sensitive Skin, Thoracic Outlet Syndrome

Cellulite — Lymph Congestion, Collagen Deficiency

Clumsiness — CCI, Cerebellar Ataxia, Dystonia, Essential Tremor, Joint Injury, POTS

Cold Hands and/or Feet — Lymph Congestion, Migraine, Peripheral Neuropathy, Thoracic Outlet Syndrome

Desire to Sit Down with Feet Up, Desire to Lie Down — Digestive System Problems, Joint Injury, Migraine, POTS (see also Fatigue)

Difficulty Breathing — Allergy/MCAS/MCS, Digestive System Problems, Forward Head Posture, Joint Injury, Rib Subluxation, Sinus Congestion

Dizziness — CCI, POTS

Euphoria — Migraine, POTS (especially with fainting), Vasovagal Syncope (especially following fainting)

Eye Pain, Poor Vision, and Light Sensitivity — Allergy/MCAS/MCS, Eye Strain, Migraine, Occipital Neuralgia

Fatigue, Lethargy, Drowsiness — Allergy/MCAS/MCS, Digestive System Problems, Dystonia, Joint Injury, Lymph Congestion, Migraine, Motion Sickness, Peripheral Neuropathy, POTS

Finger Pain or Numbness — Allergy/MCAS/MCS, CCI, Dupuytren's Contracture, Joint Injury (in the hand or referred from the elbow, shoulder, neck, or back), Peripheral Neuropathy, Thoracic Outlet Syndrome

Food Cravings — Allergy/MCAS/MCS, Digestive System Problems, Migraine, POTS

Foot Pain or Numbness — Bunion, CCI, Joint Injury (in the foot or referred from the ankle, knee, hips, or back), Lymph Congestion, Peripheral Neuropathy, Plantar Fasciitis, Tailor's Bunion

Frequent Viral Illnesses — Digestive System Problems, Healing Crisis, Lymph Congestion, MTHFR

Headache — Allergy/MCAS/MCS, CCI, Joint Injury (in the neck or referred from shoulders or back), Lymph Congestion, Migraine, Motion Sickness, MTHFR, Peripheral Neuropathy, POTS, Scoliosis, Thoracic Outlet Syndrome

Insomnia, Difficulty Sleeping — Allergy/MCAS/MCS, Growing Pains, Joint Injury, Migraine, MTHFR, Peripheral Neuropathy, Thoracic Outlet Syndrome, TMJ, Threatened Joints (if a joint is slipping or at risk of hyperextending, you may wake up with a jerk)

Joint Pain — Bunion, CCI, Joint Injury, Lymph Congestion, Muscle Injury, Myofascial Adhesion, Pelvis Complaints, Peripheral Neuropathy, Rib Cage Pain, Scoliosis, Tailor's Bunion, TMJ, Thoracic Outlet Syndrome

Knee Pain — Joint Injury (in the knee, ankle, or hip), Lymph Congestion, Myofascial Adhesion, Peripheral Neuropathy

Leg Pain or Numbness — CCI, Joint Injury (in the ankle, knee, hip, or referred from the foot or back), Peripheral Neuropathy

Light Sensitivity — Allergy/MCAS/MCS, Eye Strain, Migraine, Peripheral Neuropathy

Muscle Pain — Allergy/MCAS/MCS, Dystonia, Joint Injury, Lymph Congestion, Migraine

Nausea, Indigestion, Bloating, Vomiting, Diarrhea, Constipation — Allergy/MCAS/MCS, CCI, Digestive System Problems, Food Allergy or Sensitivity, Gluten Intolerance, Hyperemesis Gravidarum, Lymph Congestion, Migraine, Motion Sickness, MTHFR, Pelvis Complaints, POTS

Neck Pain — Allergy/MCAS/MCS, CCI, Dystonia, Joint Injury, Lymph Congestion, Migraine, Peripheral Neuropathy, Rib Subluxation, Scoliosis, Sinus Congestion, Thoracic Outlet Syndrome, TMJ

Numbness — CCI, Joint Injury, Migraine, Peripheral Neuropathy, Thoracic Outlet Syndrome

Pain in the Arms or Legs of Children — Growing Pains, Joint Injury, Thoracic Outlet Syndrome

Shaking — Allergy/MCAS/MCS, Cerebellar Ataxia, Dystonia, Essential Tremor, Joint Injury, Migraine, Peripheral Neuropathy, POTS, Thoracic Outlet Syndrome

Shoulder Pain — CCI, Joint Injury, Peripheral Neuropathy, Rib Subluxation, Thoracic Outlet Syndrome

Sinus Congestion — Allergy/MCAS/MCS, CCI, Digestive System Problems, Eye Strain, Lymph Congestion, Migraine, MTHFR, TMJ

Skin Problems, Rashes, Sores, Dandruff, etc. — Allergy/MCAS/MCS, Digestive System Problems, Lymph Congestion, MTHFR, Sensitive Skin

Sound Sensitivity — Allergy/MCAS/MCS, Eye Strain, Joint Injury, Lymph Congestion, Migraine, Motion Sickness, Peripheral Neuropathy, POTS, TMJ

Stiffness — Allergy/MCAS/MCS, Bunion, CCI, Dupuytren's Contracture, Joint Injury, Lymph Congestion, Migraine, Myofascial Adhesions, Pelvis Complaints, Rib Subluxation, Thoracic Outlet Syndrome, Tailor's Bunion

Sweating, Hot Flashes — Allergy/MCAS/MCS, Migraine, Motion Sickness, MTHFR

Swelling — Allergy/MCAS/MCS, Digestive System Problems, Joint Injury, Lymph Congestion, Thoracic Outlet Syndrome

Tingling — CCI, Joint Injury, Migraine, Pelvis Complaints, Peripheral Neuropathy, Rib Subluxation, Thoracic Outlet Syndrome

Tinnitus (Ringing in the Ears) — Allergy/MCAS/MCS, CCI, Lymph Congestion, Migraine, Sinus Congestion, TMJ

Twitches, Spasms, and Cramps — Allergy/MCAS/MCS, CCI, Digestive System Problems, Dystonia, Female Reproductive Concerns, Joint Injury, Lymph Congestion, Migraine, Pelvis Complaints, Peripheral Neuropathy, Thoracic Outlet Syndrome, TMJ

Urinary Frequency and Urgency, Incontinence — Allergy/MCAS/MCS, Digestive System Problems, Female Reproductive Concerns, Lymph Congestion, Migraine, Motion Sickness, Pelvis Complaints

Weakness — Allergy/MCAS/MCS, CCI, Cerebellar Ataxia, Digestive System Problems, Dystonia, Essential Tremor, Female Reproductive Concerns, Growing Pains, Joint Pain, Migraine, Pelvis Complaints, Peripheral Neuropathy, Scoliosis, Thoracic Outlet Syndrome

Weight Gain or Loss —Allergy/MCAS/MCS, Digestive System Problems, Lymph Congestion, TMJ

Yawning — MCAS, MCS, Migraine, POTS

Section II

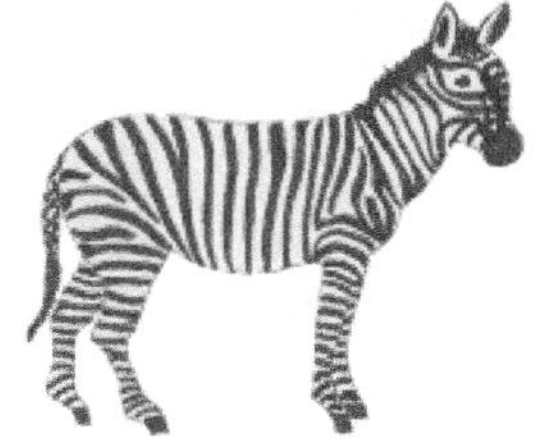

Learn About Healing hEDS/HSD

6

What it Means to Heal Symptoms of hEDS/HSD

FOR MOST OF US WITH A HYPERMOBILITY syndrome, our connective tissue is problematic due to our inherited genetic profile. We will always have these genes. Still, there are ways to reduce and prevent the symptoms caused by the connective tissue disorder.

Even more encouraging is the fact that genes can express themselves in different ways. This ability is called epigenetics, and it explains why identical twins with identical genes can have different behaviors and health profiles.[78] What we experience, what we do, the foods we eat, the toxins and viruses we are exposed to — all of these factors and many more could potentially turn genes on or off or change the way they are expressed.

No matter what mechanism is responsible for changes in our bodies, I truly believe that at least some of us can make the changes that equate to recovering from the symptoms of hEDS/HSD. In order to do this, we need to turn our focus from treating symptoms, even though that will still be important. We need to take responsibility for ourselves and focus on teaching our bodies to work in a different way.

Most of the medications available to us treat only symptoms and bring along a host of undesirable side effects; sometimes they even make the diseases they treat progress more quickly, though possibly less miserably. While I was writing this book, I learned about a young woman with hEDS who died of liver failure, leaving behind a grieving husband and young son. The woman's heartbroken mother said that the liver failure was brought about by all of the medications the woman was taking due to her hEDS. I pray that from now on, we can be successful in treating our hypermobility condition with natural techniques so that no family has to experience that sadness again.

Natural treatments are generally safer, though subtler, than most medications and over time can make real changes in our bodies. Be cautious, though, as even natural treatments can have adverse effects and might be dangerous. You must take responsibility for learning the risks and evaluating them.

Fortunately, we are designed for this. Although people with hEDS often have diminished proprioception (sense of the body's position and movement) that can make us clumsy, we tend to have heightened interoception (sense of the condition inside the body) that can make us wise about our own bodies. Doctors sometimes inappropriately blame our strong interoception for our extreme though accurate reports of pain, but in fact, having heightened interoception can be a useful tool in determining if the treatments we use are working or not. We can recognize our pain, and we can also pay attention to our heart beat, breath, hunger, muscle contractions, and everything that is going on inside us.

In a nutshell, if we:

1. get the nutrients our bodies need to make sufficient amounts of connective tissues, even though it may still be faulty,
2. prevent injuries, whether severe or microscopic, to our joints, blood vessels, and nervous system,
3. avoid exposures to substances and experiences that are harmful to us in our vulnerable condition, and
4. heal and soothe our bodies into a condition of safety and happiness,

we can potentially train our bodies to be healthy. Our nervous systems will start operating normally so that we won't experience dysautonomia, anxiety, gastrointestinal distress, and heightened immune system activation. Our muscles will be strong and well trained so that we will move comfortably without harming ourselves. It may even be possible for us to affect how the genes express themselves.

I have been naturally treating myself for hEDS/HSD for only months, and already, it feels so weird to feel healthy. Most of all, it feels good.

Natural Healing Treatments are Accessible for Everyone

The treatments in this book are mostly inexpensive, easy to find, and easy to use. None of them are likely to be a magic bullet for you, though. Natural treatments are subtler than medical ones, so you have to give them time to work.

You also have to anticipate that things will change in unexpected ways over time. Things that work for you this week may not be what you need next week. You might get bumped by a kid who is running down the sidewalk, and you'll be set back to the pain you were feeling last month. The time of perimenopause might arise and your hormone fluctuations will be unpredictable, making your body feel unfamiliar.

My Physical Therapist told me that our bodies don't stop changing as soon as we grow up. We keep growing in different ways throughout our lives. You'll never be the same for long, and you're not meant to be.

Fortunately, there are a plethora of natural treatments for every different circumstance.

Go with the Flow, Roll with the Punches, and Ride the Tide

Getting better with natural treatments will likely not be a straight-line trajectory. Just as you have gotten used to having flares and remissions (better days and worse days) during your chronic illness, you will probably try some treatments that help a lot, some that cause problems, and everything in between.

In fact, even getting better sometimes has minor or temporary drawbacks. For example, whenever I finally got a long-misbehaving joint realigned, with the muscles strong enough to hold it, my lifestyle temporarily built around protecting it, and the supplements tightening the ligaments, I felt a sudden and elating relief from pain. The next day, though, inevitably I experienced a day of fatigue. It was always a surprise that the pain was gone but the fatigue was weightier. My guess is that when the joint was in a state of malposition with pain, my body reacted by releasing adrenaline or cortisol. Once the condition was resolved, there was a sudden drop in stimulating hormones, and my body got busy repairing whatever damage had occurred. My body needed a day of rest in order to recover, and so I experienced fatigue.

Fortunately, I usually rebounded within a day, but then I had to be cautious because my new freedom of movement could lead me to re-injure the joint. Fortunately, in time, I got stronger and was able to forget about that old injury. That kind of forgetfulness is what we are here for.

Similarly, it is possibly to experience what seem to be backward steps when starting new supplements. A famous example of this is called a Herxheimer Reaction; it occurs when you successfully kill off spirochete bacteria (like the cause of Lyme Disease), and then get flu-like symptoms even though you are, technically, suddenly well. Similarly, accomplishments like ridding the body suddenly of candida yeast overgrowth, returning blood flow to a frozen body part, or replenishing the body with a previously deficient nutrient can cause new symptoms and/or an exacerbation of existing symptoms; this is considered a Healing Crisis.

Going slowly in your healing process can reduce these Healing Crises. You can do this by starting with small doses of supplements and increasing the dose slowly over time. Do the same slow build with exercise and lifestyle changes. Most importantly, know that you are on the right path; have patience as you go through the Crises if they occur. They won't last for long, and you will feel better soon.

Another up-and-down of healing is that once you have healed whatever is your worst condition — the one that has been causing you so much trouble that it almost seems like the only problem you have — you will feel better for a little while, but before long, you will notice another condition. This will be a condition that is not as severe as the first one was but that has been lingering silently in the background. Now that the worse condition is out of the way, this one will start acting like the squeaky wheel.

You will probably have to go through the healing process on subsequent conditions many times. Don't let this get you frustrated. Remind yourself that you are raising your baseline of comfort and ability with every step. Every time you heal another condition, you are learning more about yourself so that you can feel more fulfilled and confident in life, and you will be better equipped to handle whatever needs your body develops in the future.

Keep going, and you will feel better and better and be able to do more and more over time.

My Investigation and Discovery of Natural Treatments for hEDS/HSD

This book is a summary of my experiences, knowledge gained, and effective treatments of symptoms related to hEDS since I learned that I have this condition and in the decades preceding this, as I was searching for answers to my health issues as well as those of my family, friends, and clients at Vibrant Life, the holistic healing center I opened in 2012 after working independently as a professional healer for 4 years.

Over the years of my training and professional career in holistic healing, the method I have utilized to develop my extensive base of techniques and treatments is first to learn of potential techniques and treatments from books, teachers, doctors, professionals, scientific articles, and occasionally from my own intuition or spiritual guidance. If the evidence was compelling, I then tried the treatment on myself, and if the treatment was successful and safe, I communicated it to my clients, family, and friends who were in need of it. I then followed up with them to make sure that it was also successful and safe for them, especially considering the different circumstances in which they used it.

At the time that I was gathering these treatments, I did not know that I was going to write a book — I did not keep track of all of the original sources of information. So, during the process of writing this book, when I have been missing a source to back up information or a treatment listed, I have gone seeking confirmation in the scientific articles available online. In almost every case, the confirmation was readily available and convincing. I have put all of those source citations into the End Notes. In a very few cases, the treatment seems not to have been studied scientifically, so it could neither be confirmed nor denied. Most of these cases regarded the use of an Ayurvedic, Traditional Chinese Medicine, or other alternative or complementary method of treatment that has been used successfully for centuries or more, and so I linked articles from specialists in those areas in the End Notes. On occasion, I have also made a comment in the End Notes regarding my personal experience if it fills in holes in the scientific literature.

Specifically regarding hEDS, my research was largely limited to online searches due to the dearth of doctors who specialize in it in my area of the country. This research included hospitals' and doctors' websites; YouTube channels of self-proclaimed specialists of hEDS in the medical, Physical Therapy, and personal training fields; and social media groups of people with hypermobility and connective tissue disorders. This unconventional approach to treating hEDS has enabled me to assemble a very well-rounded knowledge base. Individual doctors with different patients and different educational foci have addressed their uniquely informed perspectives, mostly in isolation from the other viewpoints around the world; I have been able to consider all of them. My approach has also been informed by thousands and thousands of self-reports from people with hEDS across the world, and therefore it is able to preempt clinical practices that are based solely on published findings from a limited number of research studies.

I expect that some of the treatments that have been successful for me will be supplanted in the future by other more effective treatments, as hEDS becomes more recognized and researched by the medical and scientific communities. It is important to me to record my findings thus far, at this time when I have made an initial remarkable progress, so that my experience can inform my son, relatives, and friends in the event they have similar symptoms in the future. My condition has improved to the point that already I have put aside many of these treatments and habits in favor of living a more normal, comfortable, free lifestyle, yet I do not want to forget the things that helped me get to this point.

I began writing this summary of my effective self-treatments in January of 2024, less than 5 months after I figured out that I have hEDS. I made distinctive progress in a short amount of time, thanks in great part to the support of my husband, who gave me the opportunity to be a homemaker so that I could focus on my health and who was always willing to give me massages, recommend exercises for my various ailments, and provide whatever help with chores I needed. I am also indebted to my mother, who has been my constant supporter, was always willing to discuss the hEDS condition, has always encouraged me every day, and continues to bring joy to our family at every turn, and to my sister Heather, who perpetually shared hEDS-related information with me and let me talk out ideas and discoveries as if it were a full-time job.

My Experience of hEDS/HSD Diagnosis, Treatment, and Healing

I have had various signs and symptoms of hEDS my entire life. I have always been very flexible and excelled at gymnastics and dance. In fact, I was a dance and acrobatics teacher and professional performer from the age of 16 to 47. I have also had a few "party tricks" of finger and body flexibility that I would alternately proudly show my friends or feel embarrassed about because my hands or body looked so strange.

When I was 15, I became a cheerleader and the hyperextension in my elbows caused my arm positions to look bad, so I spent many, many hours hitting straight arm positions while looking in the mirror. I actually trained my muscles so well that I lost the hyperextension in my arms. Since I have started protecting my fingers from hyperextending and have started taking some of the supplements on the Cusack Protocol (see Chapter 42: Cusack Protocol), my finger joints, though still hypermobile, cannot hyperextend as far as they used to.

Although I have had a variety of hEDS symptoms throughout my life, it was not until shortly after my baby was born in 2013 that I became periodically debilitated by my symptoms. I struggled through being a single mother of a baby for two years with health support only from a Chiropractor and a Reiki healer, before a new friend recommended I go to a Physical Therapist. This was the beginning of 8 years of intense effort to heal my body.

The PTs at this center were specialists in pelvic PT, and in my work with them over the next three years, they immensely improved the state of my hips and back. They, as well as several other PTs at other clinics, recognized that I was hypermobile, flexible, and had a larger range of motion than most people.

Because medical professionals are not typically given very much training about EDS, oftentimes the sole diagnostic criteria they use for hEDS is the ability to touch the thumb to the forearm. Numerous times, I was asked by a PT if I could touch my thumb to my forearm, but as soon as they saw that I could not, they discounted the possibility that I might have EDS. At the time, I did not know that one of my sisters can easily touch her thumbs to her forearms on both sides, and my mother could when she was younger; I have often wondered if I was able to do this prior to breaking both of my wrists as a child, especially considering that I always had wrist pain prior to them breaking and healing. Regardless of the PTs' mistaken understanding of the hEDS diagnostic criteria, the ability to touch the thumb to the forearm is not a required criteria — I clearly qualified for a diagnosis even without that specific flexibility.

Simultaneously with doing a lot of PT during those 8 years, I was addressing the needs that were created by a genetic variation I have of the MTHFR gene, which caused terrible Multiple Chemical Sensitivity (MCS) symptoms. I owned a holistic healing center that I had opened in 2012 after having practiced as a professional spiritual and energy healer since 2008, and where I hired dozens of practitioners of various alternative therapies. In addition, I owned a dance studio (which I opened in 1997) and a forest school (which I opened in 2018) and an editing service (which I began with my father's support when I was 8 years old), and I implemented a wholesome, healthy lifestyle.

During this time, I researched numerous possible causes and conditions that could explain the symptoms I was having. I tried many different supplements, treatments, doctors, and alternative modalities. Most of what I tried helped a little bit, though some made everything worse, and nothing could explain it all until I learned about hEDS.

As soon as I recognized that I had hEDS, or at least HSD, I began researching and focusing my self-healing and making better progress than ever before. As you will see from my list of symptoms, I was in a great deal of pain and misery, but after just 5 months of treating hypermobility, most of my pain was gone. It seems like a miracle, and in fact, my discovery that I have hEDS came immediately after I prayed to Jesus, the most famous healer and worker of miracles of all time, to heal me.

hEDS-related Symptoms I Personally Have Experienced

- Allergy/MCAS/MCS (awful reactions in all systems of the body, immediate and delayed and prolonged, to foods and chemicals in the air or on the skin)
- Auditory Processing Disorder (difficulty understanding and tolerating sounds that come through electrical amplification such as Public Address system speakers and telephones)
- Brain Fog (forgetfulness, lack of clarity, difficulty making decisions, etc.)
- Bruising easily
- Bunion and Tailor's Bunion (painful misshaping of the bones of the feet and toes)
- CCI (neck instability causing nerve damage and pain)
- Cerebellar Ataxia (loss of coordination of movement, causing extreme clumsiness)
- Dandruff and skin conditions, including Tinea Versicolor (skin discoloration)
- Digestive System Problems including bloating, indigestion, nausea, constipation, diarrhea, severe stomach pains, and stomach protrusion
- Earaches frequently, along with inflamed tonsils (leading to tonsillectomy) likely caused by poor drainage of the Eustachian tubes
- Edema, bloating, swelling, water retention, and swollen lymph nodes caused by poor drainage of the lymph system
- Essential Tremor (in tongue and, during flares, in fingers and hands) and Dystonia (cramps, spasms, twitches, and tremors in various body parts)
- Excessive ear wax
- Eye strain (causing pain and blurry vision)
- Fatigue
- Finger and thumb joint pain and swelling caused by accidental hyperextensions
- Ganglion Cysts (bumps inside wrist during childhood, sometimes painful)
- Headache (plus face and neck pain, tingling, and itching) due to Occipital and Trigeminal Neuralgias and Migraine (with all prodromal, aura, and postdromal phases including severe headache, nausea, indigestion, sinus congestion, constipation, diarrhea, mouth sores, skin rashes, brain fog, joint and muscle aches, muscle spasms and twitches, etc.)
- Hip Upslip and Pelvic Torsion (painful misalignments of the pelvic bones), Coccydynia (pain in pelvis, back, and legs caused by hypermobile tailbone), and Pubic Symphysis misalignment
- Hyperemesis Gravidarum (extreme nausea and vomiting during pregnancy)
- Hypertonicity (tension) in muscles in numerous parts of the body
- Insomnia (inability to sleep through the night)
- Lhermitte's Sign (a sudden, intensely painful sensation of electric shock originating in the neck and radiating into the head, face, spine, and arms)
- Malocclusion (teeth that were crowded, crooked, and moved, painfully, frequently), and high, narrow palate
- Motion Sickness (extreme at times — could not sit in a rocking chair without nausea)
- Mouth sores (caused by fragile oral mucosa — the inside of the cheeks and the gums and frenula) and swollen salivary glands (very painful)
- Pain throughout body, persistent and chronic (mostly referred from joint hyperextensions and inflammation but sometimes of undetermined source)
- Pelvic dysfunction, hemorrhoid, pelvic organ prolapses, urinary incontinence (inability to control urination), urinary frequency (need to urinate very frequently, sometimes as often as every 15 minutes), and urinary urgency (urge to urinate that comes on suddenly and must be relieved immediately)
- Peripheral Neuropathy (frequent unrelenting itchiness and occasional pain in left big toe and inside of left ankle, right big toe, and burning on the skin of the thighs)
- Plantar Fasciitis (tightness and pain in the heel and sole of the foot) and turf toe (broken sesamoid bone of the foot)
- POTS, Vasovagal Syncope, Postprandial Syncope, Exercise-Induced Syncope, and Postural Syncope (or near syncope), usually resulting in presyncope (causing painfully racing and pounding heart, headache, dizziness, weakness, nausea, and

trembling, and preventing me from standing for lengths of time, bending over, exercising, or climbing stairs or hills, and requiring me to lie down during episodes)
- Rib Subluxations (partial dislocations)
- Shoulder pain (inability to lift arms above shoulders)
- Skin sagging, thinning, and crepey texture prematurely
- Sprains of various joints
- Subchorionic Hematoma in pregnancy (bleeding under the placenta)
- Swallowing difficulty and pain (high dysphagia if head is not perfectly positioned when drinking or eating; low dysphagia when taking pills)
- Tennis elbow (pain in the forearm)
- Thoracic Outlet Syndrome (pain, numbness, and tingling in the arms and hands and swelling in the chest and neck)
- TMJ (jaw pain and loss of movement)
- Transient Ischemic Attack (mini-stroke that caused almost complete loss of vision for a matter of hours)
- Upper Crossed Syndrome (painful stooped posture with forward head) and Military Neck (stiff and painful condition in which the cervical curve is lost and the neck vertebrae are lined up inappropriately straight)
- Vocal Cord Dysfunction (inability to speak or breathe due to vocal cords tightening and closing the airway)
- Wrist pain during childhood due to frequent accidental hyperextending

Due to the plethora of symptoms I have experienced since I was a young child, I have always been interested in medical and wellness matters. Due to my dance career, I have had a focus on the body. I also have had a robust spiritual life as a follower of Jesus Christ, a seeker and mystic, a Waldorf/Steiner-style teacher, and an honorary member of the Native American Hopi Community — these spiritual experiences led me to discover a number of alternative and complementary healing methods.

I began professional healing work after becoming a Certified Reiki Master and Teacher in 2005, and over the years, I added a variety of healing modalities to my professional offerings. Through that work, I gained much clinical experience with clients with a huge variety of ailments, and I expanded my professional network to a large number of professionals in different fields of alternative medicine. As the director of a healing center, I contracted with dozens of these professionals, and I always learned as much as I possibly could about each modality and each professional's way of working before and after hiring them.

I love learning new things about health, and more than anything, I love seeing people I care about recover from their ailments and gain a sense of self-empowerment for having accomplished this. I am very hopeful that this book can help others who have been suffering to find a more comfortable way to live and thrive.

7

You Do You

THIS BOOK IS FULL OF TECHNIQUES that have worked for me or someone I know. Some of them I learned from an expert, some from other hEDS patients, some from combining my years of experience and knowledge in the dance and alternative wellness industries, and some I figured out on my own through trial and error.

When you try out these recommendations, you also will be experimenting on yourself as I did. Always ask your doctor first (but know that whatever you try will still be an experiment considering how differently hEDS/HSD individuals' bodies react). Be careful not to do anything dangerous. Some of the ideas in this book might be contraindicated for you due to other health conditions you have, medications you are taking, allergies you have, pregnancy or breastfeeding, etc. Be thoughtful about what your own body needs — it is different from every other body in the world.

Not only is your body unique, your living situation is unique, and each day, everything you experience and eat and smell and do is a little bit different. This will affect your healing needs. For example, many times throughout this book, I recommend taking electrolytes, specifically a brand that I get great results from, but the electrolytes you need will be based on what you have eaten, what your body's propensity is for absorbing and using specific minerals, what minerals are in the water and food you ingest, and what specific stresses your body has experienced recently.

Keep in mind that one of the greatest challenges in figuring out what works is separating the effects of one healing technique from everything else that is going on in your life. It is impossible to do a true control study of a specific treatment on your own body due to the number of variables in your environment and experience. Over the course of even a day, you will experience both stresses and joys, which affect how your body works. Your hormones will fluctuate. The foods you buy this week might come from different farmers or a different part of the same farmer's field than what you bought last week. The weather changes, and the pollution and other chemicals in the air change. The new supplement you are taking might interact with a different supplement you are taking in a way that varies from how it would be if you weren't taking the other supplement. The multitude of variables make the task before you a tricky one, but I figured out a lot of helpful treatments for my body and you can too.

I pray that this book helps you. At the very least, I pray that it helps you to think of things in new ways, even if you end up needing to do everything differently than I did.

You know your own body better than anyone else does. I believe you can find the right answers for you.

Do your own thing!

Important Disclaimer

The entirety of this book is intended for educational purposes only; it does not constitute medical advice. Readers are strongly encouraged to discuss the ideas in this book with their trusted medical professional and follow only the medical professional's advice. Any actions undertaken based on information in this book, whether with or without the supervision of a doctor, are at the reader's own risk. The author has neither liability nor responsibility to any person or entity in regards to any adverse effects caused or alleged to be caused as a direct or indirect result of this book and the information herein.

Furthermore, any links provided in this book are for convenience but do not indicate an endorsement of the website owner for this book. The author and publisher of this book do not have any control over the content of the linked websites, which may have changed since they were mentioned in this book. The author and publisher bear no responsibility for any aspect of the linked websites.

Section III

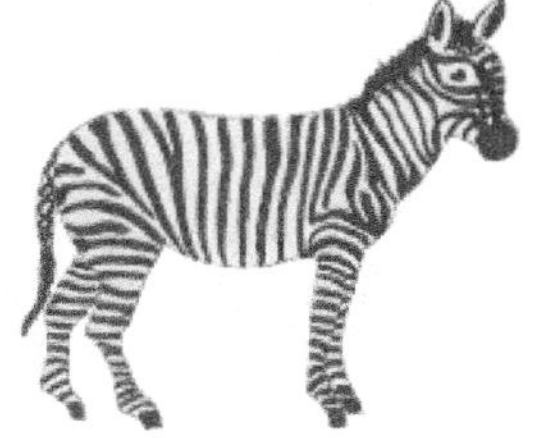

Heal Symptoms of hEDS/HSD

8

You Can Heal

HYPERMOBILE EHLERS-DANLOS SYNDROME and Hypermobile Spectrum Disorder, as explained above, are conditions in which the connective tissue is somehow disordered. Although faulty connective tissue may be present throughout all tissues of the body, Joint Instability and the resulting pain are actually the only required symptom of the conditions. All other symptoms fall under secondary diagnoses that are either caused by the connective tissue disorder or comorbid (co-existing) with it.

It is very important to address Joint Instability in hypermobile people even if it is not causing a problem right now. It is very likely to lead to pain, if not now, then in the future, when injured joints may deteriorate into arthritic conditions.[79]

Joint Instability may also damage muscles, tendons, ligaments, nerves, and blood vessels. The effect of Joint Instability on the nervous system is especially concerning, as it can lead to symptoms throughout all of the other bodily systems. Joint Injuries even make long-lasting changes in the brain, making it harder for the brain to judge the position of the joint and thus affecting proprioception (the sense of self-movement and body position).[80]

It is important to treat your symptoms as soon as they arise because if they go untreated, they may give way to more serious, seemingly unrelated symptoms. If you have not had a satisfactory diagnosis to explain these specific symptoms, the delay and resulting increase in symptoms can obfuscate the real problem and prevent an accurate diagnosis.

Fortunately, there are means of reducing Joint Instability and Pain. Even better, the most effective treatments are natural, which means that there are few, if any, adverse side effects. Some of the treatments are simple and easy to implement. Other treatments will take some effort and dedication on your part, but it is worth it. Focus and work hard through the initial stages of stabilizing your joints, and then the maintenance of joint stability will be easier, plus you will be rewarded with freedom of movement and comfort.

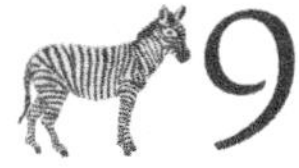

9

Joint Instability & Pain

THE DEFINING FACTOR OF A HYPERMOBILITY disorder is joint pain, but the instabilities in the joints create many more problems than just pain in the affected joints. Frequently, the pain of Joint Instability is felt in other tissues and body parts; sometimes pain is not even felt in the joint.

The body reacts to instabilities by creating stability elsewhere — to protect a threatened joint, the body will cause muscles and/or fascia to tense up around the joint, even if that causes pain.

Furthermore, joint dislocations (separations of the bones from their correct position where they meet), subluxations (partial dislocations), and strains (stretches of the ligaments), can pinch or tear nerves, causing Peripheral Neuropathy (pain and other sensations caused by nerve damage).

This damage to peripheral nerves can decrease a person's proprioception in that joint (ability to recognize its location and movement in space). Additionally, significant Joint Injury can make changes in the brain that further reduce proprioception.[81] With limited proprioception, a person is likely to become somewhat clumsy. They are more likely to injure themselves in the future.

Also and perhaps most importantly, when a joint is stretched beyond its natural range of motion, the nervous system reacts whether it hurts or not. Nociceptors are nerves whose job it is to recognize when the body is in danger, even before damage occurs or pain is felt.[82] When recognizing danger, such as a joint at risk of being moved beyond its safe range of motion, the nociceptive nerves immediately send messages to various parts of the brain to involve the fight/flight response, the emotional response, the pain response, and more.

The threat of a joint being moved beyond its range of motion is a serious threat to the body, and if it happens repeatedly, it can cause the nervous system to get stuck in the fight/flight mode. In actuality, there are a number of different ways for the Sympathetic Nervous System to meet a threat, some of which escalate activity and some of which diminish it, and so this mode is also known as the

Fight/Flight/Freeze/Feed/Friend/Fornicate Mode.[83]

This nervous system state can be responsible for a variety of symptoms, such as slowed digestion or diarrhea, heightened or reduced sensitivity to pain, sensory processing disorders, heightened sensitivity to environmental and/or food molecules, Insomnia or fatigue, and much more.

Many of these symptoms of an activated Sympathetic Nervous System are on the list of common complaints among people with hEDS/HSD. Some of them may be caused by faulty connective tissue, but some of them may be caused by the nervous system. Certainly, both causes may occur at the same time and exacerbate each other.

Obviously, it is extremely important that we stop harming the joints through our own activity.

My Experience with Joint Instability and Pain

For many years, I experienced constant pain throughout my entire body, and I was surprised to find that it diminished as I did Physical Therapy work for misalignments in my skeleton. As my hypertonic (excessively tense) muscles relaxed and my skeleton came into proper alignment, the pain decreased in area, shrinking in a radius around the responsible joints.

For example, pain in my arms was radiating from a perpetually subluxed (partially dislocated) rib in the middle of my back; pain in my legs and feet was radiating from a hip upslip; head and torso pain was radiating from my unstable cervical spine (neck). When the condition was corrected, the pain disappeared.

In another example, my hands used to swell and feel painful whenever I was in a flare, but once I started wearing ring splints, that swelling and pain stopped. In fact, I had not realized that my fingers hurt all of the time — it was a milder pain than what I was feeling elsewhere, after all — until the use of ring splints made my hands stop hurting and the difference was noticeable.

The Joint Injuries also caused other symptoms: Migraine attacks, burning sensations on the skin of my thighs, swelling and pain in my hands, and intense itching on my ankles and toes. These injuries also had some responsibility in causing my MCAS, Digestive System Problems, and Insomnia.

One of the most interesting aspects of healing Joint Injuries has been discovering that I frequently did not feel pain at the location of the injury but instead in the muscles and fascia that surrounded it. Sometimes, I did not even feel pain in the surrounding tissues but in the ones that were adjacent to them. As I healed, areas that had been pain free would frequently be found to be frozen, with taught fascia and/or hypertonic muscles. As the fascia and muscles were released from their stiffness, these tissues would begin to hurt. Sometimes healing was agonizing, but I could always tell that it was necessary. Soon, treatment would relieve that pain, and I would be amazed at the return of mobility and comfort to the entire area.

Recognize Joint Instability

In my experience, any one of these conditions will indicate that a joint has been pushed too far and should be returned to a normal position. You do not have to experience all of them; just one is enough to serve as a warning.

Recognize When a Joint Is Threatened or Hyperextended

1. **The joint hurts.** Pain is the body's most obvious warning sign not to do that![84]

2. **Body parts near the joint hurt — sharp stabbing, dull ache, throbbing.** If you have hypermobility, you may not know this, but it is not normal for a joint or the muscles around it to hurt.
3. **Muscle cramps or spasms near the joint.** The muscles are trying exceptionally hard to keep the joint safe and are fatiguing.
4. **The joint locks up.** If you must use outside force (from another body part or stationary object) to move the joint, then it is probably in a hyperextended position.
5. **Tingling or numbness in the joint or another body part.** The hyperextension may be compressing blood vessels or nerves in body parts adjacent to the joint or downstream from it.
6. **Weakness or trembling.** When your joint is within its appropriate range of motion, it will be strong, so a loss of strength or stability is an indication to stop what you are doing.
7. **Breathlessness or fatigue.** Suddenly feeling worn out might mean that your body is using all of its reserves of strength or energy to protect a threatened joint.
8. **Your body looks funny (to you or someone else).** An overly extended joint sometimes looks strange or wrong — because it is.

Repetitive hyperextending of joints causes microscopic tears that will cause arthritis and other kinds of pain in the future.[85, 86, 87] If you can learn to recognize when a joint is being threatened and stop yourself before you get to that point, you may be able to continue unscathed even with activities that take advantage of your flexibility. You will first need to spend some time going slowly and training yourself to stay within your limits

RECOGNIZE WHEN A JOINT IS THREATENED OR HYPEREXTENDED

1. The joint hurts.
2. Body parts near the joint hurt —sharp stabbing, dull ache, throbbing.
3. Muscle cramps or spasms near the joint.
4. The joint locks up.
5. Tingling or numbness in the joint or another body part.
6. Weakness or trembling.
7. Breathlessness or fatigue.
8. Your body looks funny (to you or someone else).

Ask your doctor before trying anything new.

Prevent Joint Injury

In people with hypermobility, the ligaments are weak and cannot stabilize the joints as they should. The body compensates by involving the muscles.[88] This works for a short time, but this is not the work the muscles were designed for, and they fatigue quickly. Once the muscles have fatigued, they may begin to hurt. They will likely allow the joint to slip out of place, causing damage to the components of the joint and any blood vessels and nerves that thread through it, and creating a trauma state in the nervous system. Most likely, the muscles and/or fascia will freeze up in their effort to protect the joint, possibly resulting in pain, trigger points (painful knots in the muscle that refer pain to other locations as well), hypertonicity (muscle tension), and a reduction in mobility. (The fascia is a connective tissue that gives structure to the body; it both separates and holds in place the bones, muscles, organs, blood vessels, lymph channels, and nerves.) Thus, we must give special attention to the muscles and fascia as well as the joints, to keep them strong, healthy, and able to give support to the joints.

Sometimes, hyperextending, especially when done in a controlled way like stretching, can feel good and release feel-good brain chemicals in response to the trauma,[89] but it is still trauma that should be prevented unless done in specific ways (See Chapter 57: Range of Motion Exercises and Dynamic Stretching). This is a great challenge for many hypermobile people because Joint Injury or instability has led to excessive muscle tension, and when our muscles are tense, we want to stretch them out. Stretching is something we've always been good at, so it is emotionally pleasing, too. It is a vicious cycle that takes dedication to change.

It is worth it to make the change, though. By not stretching or otherwise overextending the joints, we can give the ligaments an opportunity to heal and to tighten up as much as they can, making the joint more stable and reducing the workload on the muscles. Because stretching does a lot of good for the muscles — releasing tension and knots, allowing built-up waste to be flushed out, stimulating and maintaining the tissues to do what they were designed to do, and more — we must find other ways of doing these good things for the muscles.

I have listed here some ideas with which to accomplish these good things, garnered from my time working with professionals, reading doctors' and patients' accounts online, and experimenting on my own. I was surprised and pleased to discover how quickly after I began taking these steps that my joints stabilized and my nervous system became regulated.

Avoid Joint Injury

1. **Stop purposefully or accidentally stretching/hyperextending**. Pay attention to what your joints look and feel like. Do not bend them past straight. Do not put them in a position that is painful. When exercising, to start with, do slow movements through the natural range of motion. Do not hold stretches nor try to increase flexibility. Some of the flexibility in the joint will reduce and the ligaments will tighten up somewhat if you stop challenging that joint. It will be easier for the joints to maintain their proper position the longer you keep them in their proper position. *Also, even if you are used to the hyperextension, due to nociception (the recognition of a threat), your nervous system will go on alert every single time you hyperextend, which will make you more susceptible to pain, allergies, MCAS, dysautonomia, digestive problems, etc.*
2. **Change position every 2 minutes**. The change can be subtle, but after 10 minutes and 5 position changes, even subtle changes will make a difference. If you feel a pulling sensation, slipping sensation, or pain in a joint, go ahead and change position even if fewer than 2 minutes have passed. Because the ligaments of hypermobile people are weak, the muscles compensate to hold your joints in place, but muscles fatigue quickly and may become overfatigued since they are doing work they weren't really designed to do. *By changing position before the muscle begins to fatigue, you will not risk the joint moving out of place and you will not get an overall sense of fatigue.*
3. **Analyze all of your movement patterns throughout the day and work to improve them**. Do not push drawers in with your hips or feet. Do not turn your head while drinking or eating. Square up your body before pulling or pushing a door open or closed (especially car doors and commercial building doors). Do not lean on one leg (e.g. when shaving legs in the shower, keep your balance on the supporting leg and do not lean into the shelf or shower wall where the lifted leg is placed). Do not lean on the handrail when going down stairs. Do not lean against the counter while working in the kitchen. Do not carry a bag on one shoulder. Sit

squarely on the toilet seat (a Squatty Potty toilet stool may be helpful), and do not hyperextend your fingers when you flush. Do not hold the leash in one hand when walking a dog who pulls. Hold the vegetables with rounded fingers, not hyperextended, when chopping them. Sweep with a Vietnamese Grass Fan Broom so that you won't twist your body while sweeping. Watch out especially for the little joints tending to hyperextend and give them extra support. Trim your fingernails, especially thumbnails short so that they can hold a rounded position instead of bending backwards when you use them. *Keep the skeleton squared up and straight so that you have the strength of both sides of the body keeping your joints aligned instead of pushing against one side of the body.*

> **AVOID JOINT INJURY**
>
> 1. Stop purposefully or accidentally stretching/hyperextending.
> 2. Change position every 2 minutes.
> 3. Analyze all of your movement patterns throughout the day and work to improve them.
> 4. Improve posture from head to foot.
> 5. Use braces, ring splints, SI belts (for the sacroiliac joints of the hips), etc. as needed for weak joints.
> 6. Use tools that make the job easier.
> 7. Opt for clothing with zippers rather than snaps and buttons.
> 8. Do Strength Training very carefully.
> 9. Cross train.
> 10. Sleep toes and nose to the ceiling.
> 11. In the car and other places where you must sit still, use small pillows or other tools to support the body.
> 12. Follow the Cusack Protocol of supplements.
> 13. Eliminate infections.
> 14. Be more cautious when other symptoms flare up due to triggers.
> 15. Be more cautious at times of changing hormone levels.
> 16. Follow a "Life Hacks" social media group.
> 17. Stand up for yourself.
>
> Ask your doctor before trying anything new.

4. **Improve posture from head to foot.** The most important area to focus on is the neck, aiming to avoid "military neck" and "forward head posture." However, your foot posture will affect your neck posture, as will your pelvis, back, and shoulders. Use exercises and conscious positioning to fix any posture habits that are causing the skeleton not to be square and tall and are inhibiting the proper operation of the nervous, circulatory, digestive, and respiratory systems. When you are anxious or stressed, you may have a tendency to clench the abdominal muscles and let the upper body fall in — endeavor not to do that. See Chapter 56: Posture. Weak joints allow posture to deteriorate, and this inhibits the health of all parts of the body. *HEDS makes it easier for our posture to slip out of alignment, so we need to be more conscientious and work a little harder than the general population to keep our posture strong.*
5. **Use braces, ring splints, SI belts (for the sacroiliac joints of the hips), etc. as needed for weak joints.** You can purchase these on your own or, even better, through a Physical Therapist. When a joint is weak, wear the support item all day long and continue movement as normal. Ideally, get help from a Physical Therapist to strengthen the joint and release any hypertonic muscles related to the weakness. (Note that improper use of braces can weaken the body and cause unhelpful movement patterns to develop. It is wise to have the help of a PT when implementing braces.) *The joint will strengthen and tighten itself while the support*

item is being worn, and the reduced pain will keep the nervous system calm; eventually, you may be able to stop wearing the support item.

6. **Use tools that make the job easier**, such as jar openers, rolling chairs for working in the kitchen, specialty pencil grips or pens for easier writing, book supports or openers, and periscopic glasses for reading without tilting your head. I have seen a lot of people with hEDS use brilliant ingenuity to cope with their condition — like the woman who used salad tongs to reach the clothes at the bottom of her washing machine or the woman who used her two children's swim goggles on either side of her thighs in the driver seat of her car to prevent her thighs from opening too far. *Be creative and do what works for you.*
7. **Opt for clothing with zippers rather than snaps and buttons.** These are generally easier for hypermobile hands to manage. *Choose ways to make your movement life easier so that you can exert energy on activities that you enjoy.*
8. **Do Strength Training very carefully**. Whealth, Jeannie di Bon, and other online videos made by EDS specialists can be very helpful, but always listen to your own body and do not endanger your joints. Go slowly while building strength, never working through pain. See Chapter 62: Strength Training. *Strength Training is important for giving your muscles the ability to support the joints without fatiguing.*
9. **Cross train**. If there is a certain kind of activity that you do much more than others, take time to do activities or movements that are opposite of what you usually do. If you are an athlete or dancer, especially if you are professional, you really need to cross train. For example, one of the most important cross training activities for ballet dancers is to do various movements with the legs in parallel or turned in since ballet is done with the legs turned out, which is not a natural position and weakens the ligaments and muscles that normally support the hips when in a neutral position. *Use cross training that balances the body so that the muscles will support the joints' integrity even when forces work against them from one direction.*
10. **Sleep toes and nose to the ceiling.**[90] Sleep on your back with your legs straight, feet neutral, arms at your sides, and head straight. Use a pillow or rolled-up towel to support your neck, and pillows and blankets to prevent your head from turning and your legs from falling outward. To keep your feet and toes from being pressed into a pointed or hyper-flexed position put pillows under the blankets at the soles of your feet. It may be acceptable to sleep in other positions well supported by pillows, and it may take some time to get used to sleeping on your back, but try it for short periods during the night and gradually increase the time spent sleeping in this position. While asleep, it is very easy to lapse into a position that challenges and injures joints. *The straight position is easiest for the body to maintain, but it must be supported by bedding.*
11. **In the car and other places where you must sit still, use small pillows or other tools to support the body.** (Do not put your feet on the dashboard or tie yourself; these positions would be dangerous in the case of an accident.) *Moving vehicles challenge the joints constantly with every bump and turn, so you must find ways for your body to be held in place while staying safe.*
12. **Follow the Cusack Protocol of supplements.**[91] See Chapter 42: Cusack Protocol. These supplements do not help everyone, but it is worth trying to find out if they will help you. *Certain nutritional supplements can reduce all types of symptoms of EDS.*
13. **Eliminate infections**. Olive leaf extract is a powerful herb for immune health, as well as many other aspects of health and can eliminate infections whether they are active or silent.[92, 93, 94] It should not be taken for more than three months at a time,

and for most people, 10 days is sufficient. *Many people with hEDS have found that their joints were much more likely to pop out of place when they were sick or had an infection.*

14. **Be more cautious when other symptoms flare up due to triggers.** In my experience, smelling fragrance (one of my Allergy/MCAS/MCS/Migraine triggers) can cause my joints to be a lot "slipperier" and sublux more easily. Probably, these other conditions increase inflammation in the tissues throughout the body; as my Physical Therapist told me, the inflammation will cause the muscles and other tissues to behave in suboptimal ways. *Whenever symptoms flare in any system of the body, it can increase Joint Instability, so be more cautious in your daily movements and exercise.*
15. **Be more cautious at times of changing hormone levels.** All hypermobility symptoms seem to flare up at certain times of a menstrual cycle, when starting puberty, getting pregnant, going into perimenopause, etc. This is especially true for women of childbearing age, whose bodies make and elevate specific chemicals to increase flexibility for reproductive purposes. Make plans around any expected or noticed hormonal events — for example, do not plan to go ice skating for the first time in your life on the day of your menstrual cycle that is always worst for you (or, if you really don't want to miss out, stay in touch with the walls of the ice rink and take frequent breaks). *We cannot always anticipate when our joints might get injured, but if we know they might be more susceptible to injury at certain times, it is our responsibility to protect them as much as possible.*
16. **Follow a "life hacks" social media group.** Watching a group like this will help you learn ways to manage the physiologically challenging tasks in your life — read other people's ideas in their posts and ask the community for ideas to solve your problems. *Hacks that improve your movement habits and allow you to manage tasks will allow you to thrive in your life.*
17. **Stand up for yourself.** Ask for help when you need it. Refuse to do things that you know will hurt you. *Everyone has different needs; your strength comes in knowing what your needs are and how to get them met.*

Treatments and Coping Strategies for Joint Injury

Once I started avoiding Joint Injuries, I got angry at myself (or whomever I thought was to blame) anytime I injured a joint despite my best efforts. These things happen, though. You have to accept it and move on to treating the injury so that you can heal quickly.

Recover From Joint Injury

1. **Use ice to prevent and reduce inflammation.** When a tissue is injured, the body sends lots of fluids to help protect and repair it. Although the fluids are helpful, too many fluids are harmful and painful. However, too much icing will slow healing and could potentially cause damage to the skin and nerves. *Cold therapy will reduce the swelling, as well as numb the area temporarily.*[95, 96]
2. **Apply comfrey to the skin at the site of the injury.** Comfrey is an herb that has been used for centuries under the folk name "bone knit," and it helps rebuild collagen structures. I have seen it heal numerous of my friends, relatives, and clients much more quickly than what the doctors had told them their healing would be, and I rely on it for both pain relief and quick healing. There are many creams, ointments, cold-pressed oils, and teas available for purchase; the oil is especially

convenient and effective. Comfrey is easy to grow in my region, on a sunny hillside, and the leaf can be used fresh as a poultice. *Comfrey can speed healing of all kinds of body tissues, as well as reducing pain.*[97]

3. **Apply heat to relax muscles**. Heat can be especially soothing for hypertonic muscles after a Joint Injury, and it can also quicken the healing of the injured parts.[98] Wait until after the swelling has stopped since heat can increase swelling. When you are ready to relax the muscles, use a heating pad multiple times throughout the day. Moist heat is especially helpful, so take a bath — use magnesium bath flakes for extra healing.[99, 100] However, be cautious not to use heat too much, as extremely excessive use can cause damage to the skin cells, resulting in discoloration and eventually potentially cancer.[101, 102] Keep in mind that after a hyperextension, sprain, or dislocation, the tissues will be slightly damaged, and it will take some time for them to heal. *Treat the tissues gently and use heat to quicken the healing.*
4. **Massage.**[103] Numerous types of massage, including deep tissue, gentle, trigger point, Myofascial Release, and more are good for your muscles, especially after Joint Injury and in exchange for stretching. Our muscles all want to stretch because stretching is good for them — it lets them experience the extent of their range of motion, it releases tension, adhesions, trigger points, and build-up of chemicals and waste, and it activates the nerves. However, if a joint has been overstretched, the muscle needs to shrink, so no stretching should be done until the muscle has shrunk; also, if a blood vessel or nerve has been compressed, you may harm it more if you press on it. It is wise to withhold from massaging the joint itself until it has had some time to heal, but you can probably safely massage the tissues around the joint as soon as the injury has occurred. Once the tissues of the joint have nearly healed, massage can be implemented to increase blood flow to the area to ensure total healing as well as decrease any overactive pain messages from the Sympathetic Nervous System.[104] See Chapter 52: Myofascial Release Massage. *Massage can give the benefits that stretching would during this recovery time.*
5. **Keep moving, but do not move in ways that hurt**. After an injury, a joint will be prone to freezing up — it is the body's protective measure; however, allowing it to freeze completely can lead to more harm than good. After an initial, short rest, start moving again.[105] You may find that other joints and muscles get injured if the tightness around the injured joint pulls on them, reduces their range of motion, and/or requires them to do work they are not well suited for. Limit your movements and weight bearing to those that do not hurt so that the tissues have an opportunity to heal. *Give your tissues an opportunity to heal by not asking too much of them, but gently and slowly, day after day, increase the amount of movement and weight bearing you do with the affected joint.*
6. **Use KT Tape, a brace, splint, or a sling to stabilize the affected joint**. You can purchase these on your own or through a Physical Therapist. *In addition to stabilizing a joint, KT Tape, braces, and slings will help you limit your movements to a safe range.*[106]
7. **Use Near-Infrared and Red Light Therapy to heal injuries and tighten skin.**[107, 108, 109] Place the glass of the light box against the skin for best results, and keep it there until the body beneath the glass begins to feel uncomfortably warm. See Chapter 53: Near Infrared and Red Light Therapy. (Far-infrared light therapy is potentially more effective, but the devices are more expensive.) *NIR can reduce fatigue, heal injuries, and make your skin look younger and feel softer.*
8. **Follow the Pilates videos by Jeannie di Bon or another hypermobility movement specialist**. YouTube is a treasure-trove of help. Be very careful — use your own brain to determine how intelligent the advice given is, and go very slowly

and thoughtfully when trying any exercise recommended on YouTube. *Fortunately, a lot of the exercises recommended by Jeannie di Bon are so mild that it might look like you're sleeping while you are doing them, but they will be just what you need to relax your muscles.*

9. **Use Earthing Therapy Patches applied to the affected area**. Although electrodes are the most effective, other earthing/grounding devices will work, and being in contact with the earth itself with your skin will work and is free, too. See Chapter 45: Earthing. *Earthing will reduce inflammation and promote healing.*[110]
10. **Apply magnesium oil to the skin where muscles are tight**. Coping with stress uses up magnesium, and a lack of magnesium can increase muscle tension and twitching. Magnesium oil is actually just magnesium in water — it feels oily, and thus the name. You can purchase it in spray bottles or make your own using some of the Ancient Minerals magnesium flakes and a tiny bit of water. If you are severely deficient in magnesium, topical application will make your skin sting and it will take a while for the stinging to go away. Another way to use magnesium topically is to put a magnesite stone inside your sock or your underwear or bra — anywhere that it will be touching the skin; the closer to the injured joint, the better. Your body will absorb what it needs. *Magnesium is important for the health of your muscles and can help heal joint and nerve injuries more quickly.*[111]
11. **Meditate.** There are many different ways to meditate, and virtually all of them calm the mind, which then calms the nervous system, which then calms the muscles. This can be very helpful in allowing tense or frozen muscles around an injured joint to relax. Simply closing the eyes and clearing the mind can sometimes help — if a thought comes up, set it aside to consider at another time. Don't be alarmed, though, if clearing your mind gives you anxiety. In this case, focus on a mantra — a short sentence or word, perhaps "I am safe" or "Peace" or "I can relax" or "I have already healed." Some studies have shown that it is even more effective to use spiritual phrases, such as "God is good," "God is love," "God is peace," or "God is joy."[112] Sometimes it is possible to use meditation to relax the muscles that are hypertonic — just encourage them in your thoughts to relax. One of Louise Hay's Affirmations can help. See Chapter 40: Affirmations and Chapter 64: Medical Professionals & Complementary & Alternative Medicine Professionals Who Treat Symptoms of hEDS/HSD. *Our minds are very powerful and sometimes can enact*

RECOVER FROM JOINT INJURY

1. Use ice to prevent and reduce inflammation.
2. Apply comfrey to the skin at the site of the injury.
3. Apply heat to relax muscles.
4. Massage.
5. Keep moving, but do not move in ways that hurt.
6. Use KT Tape, a brace, splint, or a sling to stabilize the affected joint.
7. Use Near-Infrared and Red Light Therapy to heal injuries and tighten skin.
8. Follow the Pilates videos by Jeannie di Bon or another hypermobility movement specialist.
9. Use Earthing Therapy Patches applied to the affected area.
10. Apply magnesium oil to the skin where muscles are tight.
11. Meditate.
12. Find good, reliable professionals who are familiar with hEDS and HSD.

Ask your doctor before trying anything new.

tremendous healing; even if this is not one of those times, your mind can calm and relax you, which will reduce the amount of pain and tension in your body.

12. **Find good, reliable professionals who are familiar with hEDS and HSD**. In my experience, the most essential professional to have on hand in case of any need is an Osteopath. A Massage Therapist is pretty important, too. Physical Therapists are the most important when injuries occur, but you may need a different one for different injuries. Find a good health insurance plan that will cover the things you need, and find a good Primary Care Physician who will give you the referrals that will help you. See Chapter 64: Medical Professionals & Complementary & Alternative Medicine Professionals Who Treat Symptoms of hEDS/HSD. *Professional help can serve you well when you need more than you can do for yourself.*

LINKS FOR PRODUCTS MENTIONED IN THIS CHAPTER

Squatty Potty https://amzn.to/4aRQjvg
Jar Opener https://amzn.to/3Sz2S8I
Rolling Chair https://amzn.to/3HJiS1p
Book Support https://amzn.to/4bqRUt6
Book Opener https://amzn.to/3Umrl2j
Lie Down Glasses https://amzn.to/3vUcdyP
Olive Leaf Extract https://amzn.to/3OxpILh
Comfrey Oil https://amzn.to/3TDV4D9
Magnesium Bath Flakes https://amzn.to/3HrNIvn
KT Tape https://amzn.to/47YF0zy
NIR Light Therapy Box https://amzn.to/3S8vLXG

Section IV

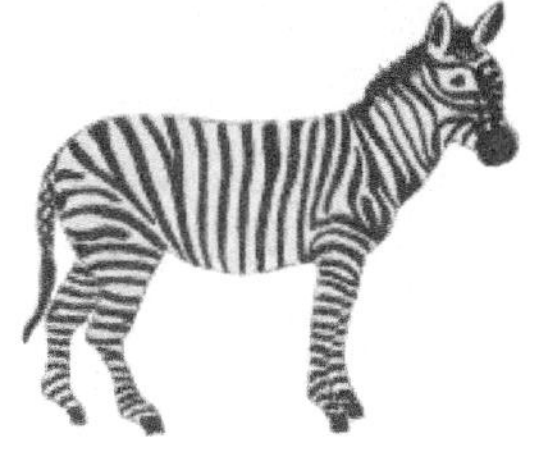

Heal Symptoms of Secondary Conditions of hEDS/HSD

10

You Can Heal Symptoms of Secondary Conditions & Comorbidities of hEDS/HSD

IN ADDITION TO JOINT INSTABILITY, connective tissue disorders can manifest in a number of different ways. Connective tissues are ubiquitous throughout the entire body, providing structure to the skin, blood vessels, nerves, lymph channels, bones, and organs. Understanding this, it is not surprising that every system of the body can exhibit symptoms of hypermobility. Patients with EDS have an average of 6.32 additional diagnoses.[113]

Although virtually every person with hypermobility will experience Joint Injuries, the other symptoms they might experience are less predictable. It is unknown why some people will have particular trouble with their gastrointestinal system while others are plagued with nervous system disorders or environmental allergies. Even within a family, even among twins, the specific symptoms of hEDS/HSD will be different.[114]

Fortunately, the systemic symptoms of hEDS/HSD tend to present as conditions that have names and, often, treatments. Doctors call these "secondary conditions" because they are caused by hEDS/HSD, or "comorbidities" because they exist at the same time as hEDS/HSD. Being able to label these symptoms makes it easy to discuss ways of healing them.

Do not forget that these conditions are likely caused by faulty collagen — the same underlying cause of hypermobility, Joint Instability, and pain — or by Parasympathetic Nervous System activation caused by unstable joints. The most important thing to do is treat Joint Instability. (See Chapter 9: Joint Instability & Pain.) Sometimes, this alone can reduce the symptoms of the secondary conditions and comorbidities even without a need to address the specific conditions.

It can also be the case that treating some of the secondary conditions and comorbidities will give the joints opportunities to heal and become stronger. Many of our conditions are exacerbated by other conditions that we have comorbid. They form feedback loops for each other, making each other worse. We need to treat all of the conditions and the entire body, mind, and soul so that we can interrupt the feedback loops wherever we can.

I pray for total healing for you.

11

Allergy, MCAS, & MCS

IT IS VERY COMMON FOR PEOPLE with hypermobility to have Allergies, MCAS (Mast Cell Activation Syndrome), and/or MCS (Multiple Chemical Sensitivity). This may in part be because people with connective tissue disorders can be expected to have leaky guts, leaky skin, and leaky lungs.[115, 116] This allows molecules to enter the body that normally would be kept out, and it leads to both IgE- and non-IgE-mediated allergic reactions.[117] IgE stands for Immunoglobin E, which is an antibody that incites the immune system to respond to threats; in the case of allergies, IgE activates in response to non-threatening chemicals (or overreacts to small amounts of dangerous chemicals).

Another component of the immune system that also responds to threats and is responsible for allergic and allergic-like reactions is mast cells. Mast cells can be found in the connective tissues of the skin, gastrointestinal tract, lungs, bone marrow, and most other body tissues. They are the sentinels on guard, watching for substances in the body that do not belong there — viruses, bacteria, parasites, and toxins. When they notice one of these invaders, they "degranulate," which means that they release chemicals from granules inside the cells, most famously histamine, that incite an inflammatory response so that the body can be on alert for more of the invaders and remove them from the body. Mast cells actually can release thousands of mediators, any of which can create allergic-type symptoms.

Mast cells also respond to non-substance dangers, including tissue injury (such as joint dislocations or skin wounds) and stress (such as strenuous exercise or getting bad news). And, mast cells respond not only to present harm but also to threats of harm. This ability in the body is called nociception, and nociceptor nerve cells can recognize when a danger is approaching or about to occur. They will react, for example, when a joint has begun to hyperextend, even before any damage has been done, and they will get the mast cells involved.

The fact that some hypermobile people experience mild hyperextensions and severe Joint Injuries on a daily basis may explain part of why mast cells over-proliferate, get over-excited, and/or react too strongly and too frequently, sometimes creating chronic (long-lasting) inflammation in numerous symptoms in the body. Also, considering that mast cells reside in connective tissue, their operation may be affected by the faults inherent to the connective tissues of people with hEDS/HSD.

There are some scientists who have alternatively hypothesized that there is a genetic variant that causes mast cells to overreact, and the subsequent action of the inflammatory chemicals creates hypermobility and laxity in the connective tissues. It has further been hypothesized that MCAS could be the underlying cause of depression, diabetes, fibromyalgia, POTS, sleep apnea, Insomnia, chronic kidney disease, miscarriage, headache, dental problems, irritable bowel syndrome, and more.[118]

It is thought by some doctors that Allergy, MCAS, MCS, and mastocytosis, are all forms of Mast Cell Activation Disease (MCAD). Some doctors think there may be even more forms of MCAD. Much more research needs to be done, but there are many overlapping natural treatments that can be helpful for all of these conditions.

All of these allergic and allergic-like conditions are unpleasant and dangerous because they can induce anaphylaxis. Anaphylaxis is not as simple as you may have thought, if you have heard of it when someone couldn't breathe after eating an allergen. It is a transient illness that develops in reaction to a food or environmental chemical and that includes two or more body systems. Symptoms of Level I Anaphylaxis include hives, swelling of the face, nausea, runny nose, sore throat, tingling, etc. Level II includes vomiting, diarrhea, dizziness, coughing, difficulty breathing, etc. Level III includes tongue swelling, difficulty swallowing, sleepiness, fainting, noisy breathing, confusion, etc. Level IV, which is considered Severe Anaphylaxis, can be fatal because it constricts airways and leads to collapse and cardiac failure.[119]

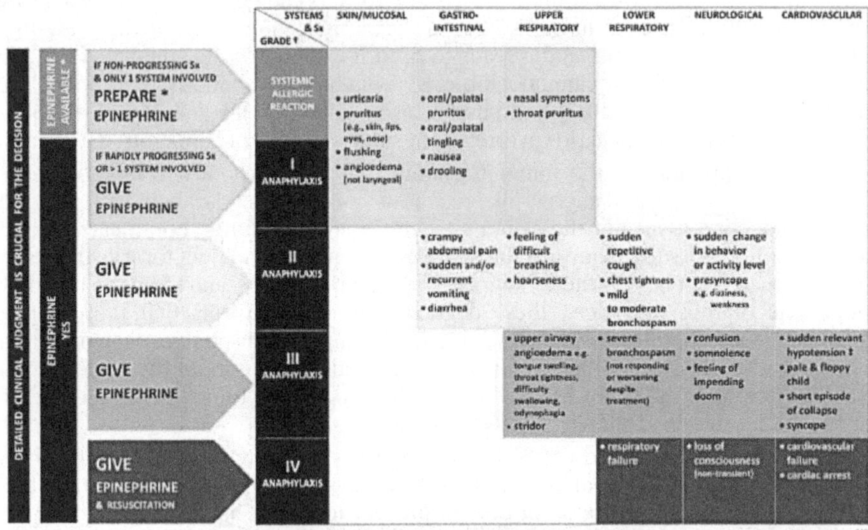

Figure 8: Anaphylaxis Severity Grading System. Reprinted with permission of Błażowski, Łukasz & Majak, Pawel & Kurzawa, Ryszard & Kuna, Piotr & Jerzyńska, Joanna. (2021).[120]

Over the longer term, anaphylactic reactions of any level can lead to more problems in the body. For example, they create inflammation that leads to joint pain and arthritis, Lymph Congestion, Migraine, and more. They disrupt the gastrointestinal system in ways that can cause malnutrition, impair elimination, and disrupt the microbiome in the gut. They can cause tightening and cramping of muscles all over the body, which is painful and most notably problematic in the intercostal muscles around the ribcage, which can lead to poor posture, Thoracic Outlet Syndrome, Rib Subluxations, Costochondritis, and breathing problems. The inflammation can even cause increased laxity in the connective tissues, which exacerbates the hEDS/HSD condition.

It is important to try to eliminate or minimize these kinds of reactions and develop a healthy but not overactive immune system.

Allergies

IgE reactions are the traditionally recognized allergies that occur within minutes after exposure and induce hives, swelling, vomiting, and potentially severe anaphylaxis. This type of allergy has been well studied and is well understood by most allergy doctors.

Currently, there are well-proven tests to determine IgE-mediated allergies in a person, and allergy specialist doctors have many treatments available to help patients manage the condition. In some cases, they are even able to use immunotherapy to cure the allergies.[121, 122] Immunotherapy is a method of giving a patient food or shots containing miniscule amounts of an allergen to desensitize them to the substance. This method is not always successful and is sometimes very unpleasant or dangerous, but it works often enough that it remains the medical method of choice for medically curing allergies.

There are also alternative means of treating and curing allergies, as practiced in Traditional Chinese Medicine, Ayurveda, and herbalism.

Mast Cell Activation Syndrome

Two Mast Cell Activation Diseases (MCADs), Mastocytosis and Mast Cell Activation Syndrome (MCAS), are common among people with hEDS/HSD.[123, 124] It is thought that up to 20% of the general population and 89% of people with hEDS/HSD have MCAD.[125, 126, 127] Mastocytosis is a condition in which a person has too many mast cells. MCAS is a condition in which the mast cells are normal in number but are overactive.[128]

A FEW OF THE POSSIBLE MCAS SYMPTOMS		
Nervous System	**Circulatory System**	**Face**
Headache	Chest pain	Watery eyes
Brain fog	Racing heart	Congested nose
Numbness, tingling	Dizziness	Mouth sores
Nerve pain	**Reproductive System**	Red ear(s)
Anxiety	Genital pain	**Body**
Anger	Genital swelling	Joint pain
Digestive System	**Respiratory System**	Muscle pain
Bloating	Difficulty breathing	Fatigue
Stomach pain	Hoarseness	**Skin**
Diarrhea	Inflamed throat	Hives
Constipation	Coughing	Flushing
Incontinence	Wheezing	Itching

It is very important to take MCADs seriously because not only can they be miserable and debilitating, they can cause or contribute to many of the other conditions that are common among people with hEDS: Peripheral Neuropathy, Sinus Congestion, Rheumatoid Arthritis, POTS, Migraine, Gastrointestinal Disorders, Celiac Disease (intolerance of gluten), Infertility, Dysmenorrhea (lack of menstruation), Menorrhagia (excessive menstrual bleeding), Dystonia (muscle spasms), and more.[129] There is also evidence that MCAS may be an underlying cause of Alzheimer's Disease.[130]

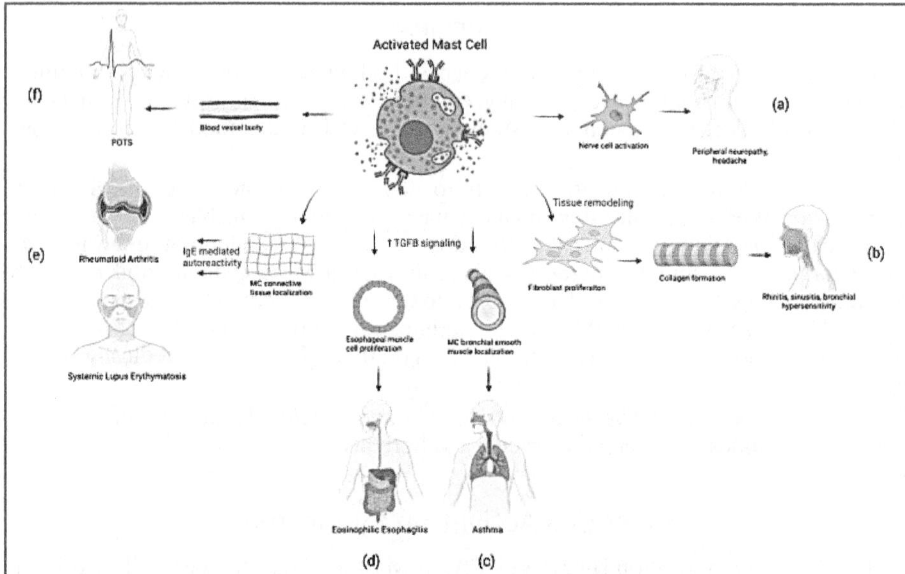

Figure 10: Association of Mast Cell Related Conditions with Hypermobile Syndromes. Reprinted according to the PMC Open Access Subset from the article by Monaco, A., Choi, D., Uzun, S., Maitland, A., & Riley, B. (2022).[131] Aberrant mast cell (MC) activation can produce inflammatory changes at the connective tissue level leading to dysfunction in multiple organ systems. In peripheral nerves, MC can localize to epineurium, perineurium, and endoneurium and release mediators which may activate nociceptors producing symptoms such as peripheral neuropathy and headache (a). MC-mediated upregulation of cytokines can lead to dysfunctional fibroblast proliferation in nasal and bronchial tissue leading to rhinitis and sinusitis (b). MC-induced TGFB upregulation and localization within bronchial smooth muscle cells can cause modification of matrix proteins of bronchial parenchyma contributing to tissue damage and Asthma (c). MC-induced TGFB upregulation in esophageal tissue can cause proliferation and smooth muscle contraction contributing to eosinophilic esophagitis symptoms (d). When MCs are localized to connective tissues, they can cause microenvironmental changes to the extracellular matrix, inducing IgE medicated autoreactivity and contributing to rheumatologic conditions such as rheumatoid arthritis and systemic lupus erythematosus (e). MC-induced changes may contribute to laxity within blood vessels, causing pooling of the blood in extremities, contributing to postural tachycardia syndrome (POTS) in which patients experience increase of heart rate with standing, a finding commonly associated with hEDS (f).

MCAS is a form of non-IgE-mediated allergy; it can occur immediately or hours or even several days after exposure to a trigger. It tends to incite symptoms in the digestive system, the nervous system, the skin, or other bodily systems, and can occasionally result in severe anaphylaxis.

There has been a lot of research about MCAS in recent years, but this condition continues to be not very well understood by medical research scientists or doctors. For this reason and also because of the drastically varying range of possible symptoms in a syndrome such as MCAS, diagnosis and treatment can be elusive for many people with the condition.

In fact, there are more than half a dozen markers in the blood that can be tested for to diagnose MCAS, but unfortunately, many of the blood markers are chemicals that are released from mast cells following triggers on varying schedules. To top it off, many of these chemicals remain in the blood for a very short time, so catching the markers on a test is very challenging. A bone marrow test is more reliable for diagnosing MCAS, but many patients decline such an intrusive and painful procedure. Also, some people with MCAS have none of the known markers, so negative test results do not negate a diagnosis; rather, the diagnosis is based on clinical signs and symptoms.

To make diagnosis and treatment even more challenging, not only can MCAS manifest with very different symptoms in different people, the triggers can be very different for different people as well. In fact, whereas allergy triggers are consistent, MCAS triggers — and resulting symptoms — can vary within a person from day to day.

In one study, each MCAS patient had anywhere from 2 to 85 symptoms, though the average was 20 symptoms in each person. Even so, most of the patients appeared normal for their age and much healthier than would be expected considering that they were chronically ill.[132] Their relatively healthy appearance also proved to delay diagnosis for many patients.

Some of the most common symptoms of MCAS are fatigue, Fibromyalgia, fainting, dizziness, headache, hives, itching, tingling, numbness, nausea, chills, swelling, eye irritation, indigestion, reflux, brain fog, Dystonia, rashes, abdominal pain, throat irritation, heart palpitations, sweating, fever, easy bruising, constipation, diarrhea, difficulty swallowing, flushing, mouth sores, swollen lymph glands, interstitial cystitis (bladder pain, urinary frequency and/or urgency), incontinence, nasal inflammation, weight gain, dental problems, weight loss, cough, anxiety, depression, lax joints, joint dislocations, seizures, and tremor. Dermatographia, in which the skin becomes inflamed and red following a minor scraping, as with a fingernail, is thought to be the most common symptom; however, it is not present in all people with MCAS. Some also have frequent bouts of severe, life-threatening anaphylaxis.

Among the many triggers of MCAS are mold, viruses, toxins, airborne synthetic fragrances, stress, joint and other injuries, exercise, natural odors, insect bites and stings, vibrations, cold, heat, hormone fluctuations, exhaustion, sunlight, hunger, and foods.[133, 134, 135] Many people with MCAS react to almost all foods and are able to eat only a very small number of foods; they often experience frightening weight loss and nutritional deficiencies.[136] Numerous people in social media groups have reported that they even react to their own bodily fluids when they are released or get on their skin: tears, blood, and sweat can cause burning, itching, redness, and swelling.

Triggers can vary for people with MCAS, and reactions seem to be "dose dependent," meaning that exposure to a trigger may not create a reaction if it is minor and there have been very few exposures recently. However, if the exposures add up, the person may react to something that they normally are not sensitive to. Anecdotally, many people with MCAS talk about their "histamine bucket" filling up more and more with each trigger exposure, and once it's full, they begin to experience a flare. Often, exposure to a trigger is unexpected and unplanned for, so people with MCAS usually do best when they avoid their environmental and food triggers as much as it is in within their control to do so. Unfortunately, when a person's "histamine bucket" is full, it can instigate sensitivity to new triggers that will cause reactions in the future as well.

Most people with MCAS react to both noxious chemicals (especially fragrance) and to high-histamine containing foods. For this reason, and to keep the number of triggers low, many people choose to follow a low-histamine diet. This can be risky, as it can limit the number of nutritious foods available, but some doctors recommend avoiding at least the highest-histamine-containing foods: cured or smoked meats or fish and spinach.[137] Another complication in the low-histamine diet is the fact that food ripening, storage, and cooking can affect histamine content.

Only 5% of the histamine in the body comes from foods or intestinal bacteria; so the avoidance of histamine-containing foods will probably make very little difference for most people with MCAS most of the time.[138] It is a good thing to keep in mind when already in a flare, though. More important is to avoid any specific food allergens or foods that you are intolerant to due to a lack of the specific enzyme for digesting it.

Medications also can cause problems for people with MCAS. Sometimes, the fillers and other ingredients in medications are also problematic. A list of medications to avoid can be found on the Histamined website:

https://www.histamined.com/post/medications-to-avoid-with-mcas .

Fortunately, some doctors, like Paul Anderson, who shares information about MCAS on his YouTube channel, have been having clinical successes. However, Dr. Anderson explains that the treatments must be individualized for each patient.

People with MCAS can often find relief by being treated with antihistamines or mast cell stabilizers. Although antihistamines give immediate relief to some people, it can be challenging for a patient to find the right antihistamine; many people try numerous ones and never find one that they can tolerate and that works for them. Also, although antihistamines are generally well tolerated, they do have potential adverse effects, especially with long-term use; MCAS and hEDS/HSD patients tend to react badly to medications more often than the general public.[139, 140, 141, 142]

It is important to use antihistamine medications and/or nutritional supplements or natural antihistamine herbs to reduce the severity of reactions in an effort not only to bring comfort but also to calm down the system overall. Among helpful nutritional supplements are B vitamins, which can help break down histamine and other hormones so that they can be removed from the body. Diamine Oxidase (DAO) is an enzyme that breaks down histamine that you can take as needed; for many people with MCAS, it helps to take DAO 5-15 minutes before each meal. Anecdotally, and in my experience, it can also be helpful to take DAO immediately after a trigger exposure, right before going to sleep, and during the night any time you wake up.

However, histamine is not the only chemical at play; mast cells also release cytokines, interleukins, prostaglandins, and chemokines, all of which can create symptoms similar to those attributed to histamine; antihistamines are not sufficient for everyone with MCAS.

In fact, 25% of the chemicals released by mast cells are neurotoxic (they harm the nerves and brain).[143] Not only that, but mast cell activation increases the permeability of the Blood Brain Barrier, which then puts the brain at increased risk for damage from toxins made by the body or exposed from outside of the body. Additionally, some of the chemicals (like Substance P and Tumor Necrosis Factor), promote and create sensations of pain.[144] So, it is even more important to stabilize the mast cells not only during flares but also prophylactically (in advance) on a daily basis so that they will be less likely to react to triggers.

Some pharmaceutical medications have mast cell stabilizing effects. This may even be why so many hEDS/HSD patients respond well to benzodiazepine medications like Diazepam or Valium, which are prescribed for anxiety, depression, and muscle spasms. Unfortunately, these medications can have serious adverse effects, especially when used over the long term.[145]

Fortunately, there are also a number of non-pharmaceutical mast cell stabilizers that are readily available, inexpensive, and generally have fewer adverse effects: Quercetin, Berberine, Chinese Skullcap, Milk Thistle, Aspirin (in small doses), baking soda, B Vitamins, Vitamin C, oregano, feverfew, nettle, parsley, thyme, and many others.[146, 147, 148, 149] Note that although culinary herbs are included in this list, many people with MCAS do not do well with jarred spices, perhaps because of the potential for mold, a very common MCAS trigger; fresh herbs for cooking are best for these people.

Some weeds are mast cell stabilizers and anti-inflammatory too — like broad-leaf plantain and purple dead nettle. [150] In many parts of the world, they are easy to find fresh, but do not harvest them from roadsides where they could be contaminated with exhaust fumes and oil spills, nor from yards that could have been sprayed with any kinds of chemicals. Plantain is also beneficial for healing and reducing the pain of minor wounds and insect stings; chew it up so that your saliva activates it, and put the resulting paste on the affected skin. The taste of purple deadnettle really grows on you if you eat it daily; Europeans brought it here when they came to settle because they valued it as a food.

Another angle for treating MCAS that is even more effective for me is to prevent mast cell degranulation even earlier in the cascade of events following a trigger. Often, the body's signal for mast cells to activate initially comes from prostaglandins. Every cell in the body is capable of releasing prostaglandins, which the cells make using COX molecules.[151] Furthermore, mast cells also produce prostaglandins, and these prostaglandins incite inflammation as well. Whereas histamine is responsible for the symptoms felt immediately upon being triggered, prostaglandins are responsible for the delayed symptoms.[152] Fortunately, there are some easily available COX inhibitors: aspirin or willow bark and grape or tart cherry juice.[153, 154] Willow bark is the inspiration for aspirin and can be taken as a tea; aspirin is easily carried and taken as needed, but aspirin is a mast cell activator when taken at high doses.

MTHFR can also exacerbate MCAS because it weakens the body's ability to break down histamine and other chemicals and get them out of the system, so methylated B vitamins may be of benefit during MCAS episodes for some people.[155] See Chapter 24: MTHFR.

On the next page, you will find a chart showing my theory of why people with hypermobility are prone to MCAS and how we can respond.

MCAS Solutions *My current theory is that MCAS in people with hypermobility is caused mainly by these 7 problems, which create feedback loops with each other so that the condition amplifies itself.*		
	PROBLEMS	SOLUTIONS
1	Mast cells mostly live in connective tissue, so the connective tissue faults inherent in hEDS/HSD may activate mast cells.	Intake foods (especially those high in protein) and nutritional supplements (such as those recommended in the Cusack Protocol) to generate the healthiest connective tissues we can despite our condition.
2	Leaky skin, gut, and lungs common in hEDS/HSD allow our bodies to be bombarded with dangerous substances that the mast cells have to be on constant alert for.	Avoid toxins by doing things like eating organic, whole foods; using non-toxic, supportive soaps and moisturizers on our skin; breathing clean air; and choosing all-natural toiletries and cleaning products.
3	Mast cells respond to injuries so that the body will send the repair team in - people with hEDS/HSD frequently get Joint Injuries, vein injuries (bruises), and nerve injuries — we might need repairs on a constant basis, so the mast cells work overtime.	Keep the muscles strong and make efforts to avoid injuring yourself; also work to heal any injuries as quickly as possible.
4	Even when the joints aren't injured, threats to them get the nociceptor cells activated, and they in turn get the mast cells involved.	Do not hyperextend even when it doesn't hurt.
5	Joint Injuries, neurotoxic chemicals released by mast cells, invasion of noxious substances, and the stress of living with hEDS/HSD engage the sympathetic nervous system, which tells the mast cells to be on alert.	Avoid stress, find joy, and stimulate the Vagus Nerve to activate the Parasympathetic Nervous System.
6	The faulty connective tissues cause problems in the detox pathways, so toxins in the body are more upsetting and last longer and so get the attention of mast cells more.	Use supplementation to keep the detox pathways working, and avoid toxins and stress so that they don't have too much work to do.
7	Inefficient detox pathways prevent us from eliminating histamine and the other mediators from our body once they are no longer needed, and so they linger and continue to cause symptoms as well as activate more mast cells.	Use supplementation to move hormones through the detox pathways more quickly.

Multiple Chemical Sensitivities

Similar in its presentation but less well understood than MCAS is Multiple Chemical Sensitivity (MCS). MCS is the name most frequently used to describe a non-IgE allergy that is not recognized in the usual Allergy or MCAS tests. Previously, MCS was called Environmental Illness (EI) or Chemical Intolerance (CI). Some doctors, scientists, and holistic practitioners think — and I agree — that a more appropriate name for this condition would be Toxicant Induced Loss of Tolerance (TILT).[156] Another suggested name is Symptoms Associated with Environmental Factors (SAEF),[157] but the name MCS has been used for about 25 years and is well recognized.

Nearly 60% of people with MCAS may have MCS; some scientists have hypothesized that MCS actually is MCAS, most likely initiated by an episode of exposure to high levels of a toxicant, rather than being endogenous (originating due to factors within the body).[158] Examples of responsible toxicants include pesticides, building and renovating materials, mold, medical treatments, combustion products, and fragranced personal care and household items. The exposure to one or more toxicants may have been short-lived or transpiring over a long period of time; the toxicants can enter the body via the breath, skin or genital contact, food or drink, or medical procedures.

As any of the condition's names indicate, MCS constitutes non-IgE-allergic reactions to a variety of chemicals, even in miniscule doses. Generally but not always, the chemicals that people with this condition react to are noxious (poisonous or harmful to the human body), but these chemicals usually do not bother healthy people in the doses typically found in daily life. In fact, many doctors believe that the rise of chemical sensitivities is caused by the increasing number and quantities of poisonous chemicals that humans are being exposed to today.[159]

Most people with MCS believe that they are like the canaries in the coal mines of American history. It used to be that miners took caged canaries with them into coal mines because they had no scientific testing equipment for detecting potentially fatal fumes that could be released underground during the mining process. The canaries sang in their cages throughout the day, but if the singing stopped, it was usually because the canary had dropped dead due to exposure to dangerous fumes. When the silence of the canaries warned them, the miners would evacuate immediately before they came to harm. People with MCS posit that the ubiquitous chemicals in our modern environment are potentially fatal and that those who are already getting sick from them should be considered the early warning sign.

In both the case of MCAS and MCS, the chemical to which people most commonly react is "fragrance," which is indeed noxious and responsible for a great deal of health problems. It is a good idea to avoid fragrances even if they are not currently triggering you, as they are neurotoxic (damage the brain and nerves), mutagenic (permanently change the genes), endocrine disrupting (upset the hormonal balance), and more.[160] Unfortunately, fragrance is present in most mainstream cleaning products, toiletries, and scented products. See Chapter 44: Detox for more information about fragrance.

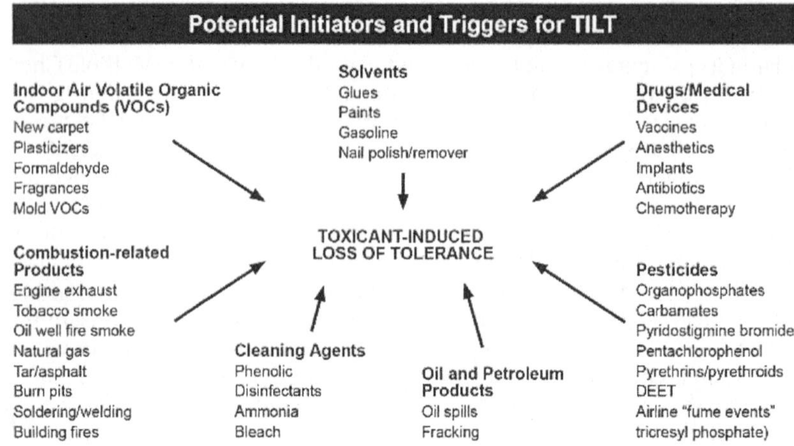

Figure 12. Reprinted under Creative Commons License, by Palmer, R. F., Dempsey, T. T., & Afrin, L. B. (2023).[161]

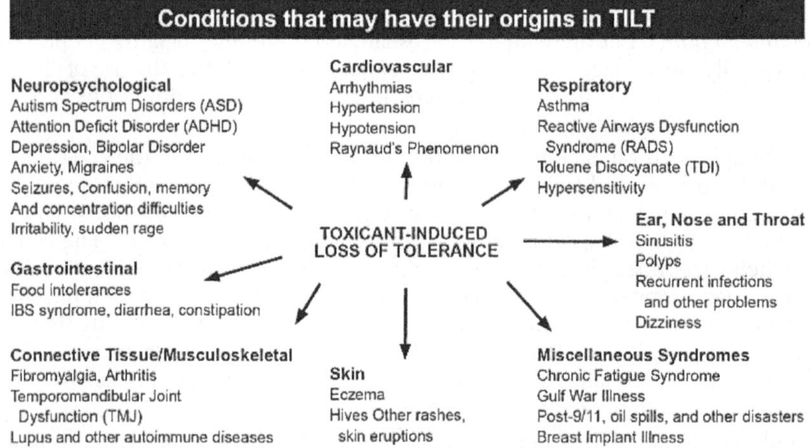

Figure 13. Reprinted under Creative Commons License, by Palmer, R. F., Dempsey, T. T., & Afrin, L. B. (2023).[162]

Often, people with chemical sensitivities also exhibit symptoms due to exposure to electromagnetic frequencies (EMFs).[163] Electromagnetic Hypersensitivity (EHS) can also exist without chemical sensitivity. EMFs have been shown to increase the number and size of mast cells in the skin. EMFs are also recognized to be responsible for increases in ADHD, cancerous tumors, Infertility, and neurodegenerative diseases such as Alzheimer's Disease.[164] A number of countries in the world have restricted the use of devices that emit certain forms of EMFs, such as WiFi in nurseries, or have required disclosure of the EMF risks, such as with the sale of mobile phones. For those of us living in countries with no such restrictions, we must take responsibility ourselves for our protection from excessive exposure to dangerous forms of EMFs.

Other than avoidance and general health considerations, no standard treatments (or tests) for MCS or EHS have been developed. Because the cause of these sensitivities and symptoms are as of yet unknown, patients are often dismissed or considered to have a psychological disorder rather than a somatic (biological) condition. However, scientists have found that there are legitimate differences in the way sensitive people's bodies react to chemicals and EMFs — differences in the activation of neurons in certain parts of the brain, lack of blood flow in certain parts of the brain, changes in the mucous membranes of the nasal passages, unusual activation of mast cells, reduced detoxification ability, glutathione deficiency, lower odor-detection thresholds, genetic mutations, pre-existing pain disorders, Insomnia, and inflammation.[165, 166, 167, 168, 169, 170, 171, 172]

My Experience with Allergies/MCAS/MCS

When I and my staff treated clients in my holistic center, we found so overwhelmingly that fragrances were problematic for so many people that we decided to require all staff, clients, and guests to be fragrance-free when they came into the building. In fact, 90% of those who came in with physical or emotional complaints significantly resolved their problems simply by removing fragrance from their lives. A large part of our work was guiding them in how to stop using and exposing themselves to fragrances.

My Allergy/MCAS/MCS symptoms have ranged from mildly annoying when I was a child to severe when I was in my late 30s and early 40s. Before I learned to avoid my triggers and discovered some of the treatments for these conditions, I felt so bad that I could hardly get out of bed for months at a time.

During a period of time when I felt bad but was able to go about my life, there were a couple of weeks one winter when I stayed home to care for my son who had the flu. For the first time, I experienced two weeks without an exposure to any of my triggers. I then caught the flu, and even with all of the flu symptoms (fever, vomiting, diarrhea, congestion, body aches, etc.), I felt so much better than I had with my allergic reactions that I was energetically catching up on laundry, house cleaning, dishes, and playing with my son.

Fortunately, I have made a great deal of progress, and when I most recently had the flu, I felt much worse than I do during the relatively mild and infrequent Allergy/MCAS/MCS reactions I have experienced most recently.

Especially relevant to the hEDS/HSD condition is my experience of Joint Injuries causing MCAS flares. This sometimes occurred immediately in response to a dislocation or hyperextension, but it was sometimes delayed. Whenever I had an injury that did not improve over a few days time, even if it was not severe enough to create an MCAS flare at the time of the injury, I would begin to get MCAS symptoms, regardless of my avoidance of all other triggers. Fortunately, if my injury improved steadily over the following days, it did not induce MCAS even if there was still pain and inflammation at the site of the injury.

It was also interesting to understand that sometimes, upon exposure to an environmental or food Allergy/MCAS/MCS trigger or allergen, some of my joints would instantly "go out". Any of my joints could be affected, most notably my hips and my neck, and it frequently led to Trigeminal or Occipital Neuralgia or a Migraine attack. Sometimes, the joints would go out because of Dystonia muscle spasms; Dystonia in my neck was usually my very first symptom after being triggered. This risk and consequence may be important for people with hEDS/HSD to be aware of so that you can take measures to protect your joints after being triggered.

Below is a list of symptoms I have experienced due to exposures to my triggers/allergens:

Allergy/MCAS/MCS Symptoms

- Acne on face and body
- All over body achiness
- Brain fog, difficulty concentrating, decreased intuitive abilities, forgetfulness, aphasia
- Chapped lips
- Chest congestion
- Clumsiness and proneness to injury (my hands became covered with scratches, bruises, and burns, but all body parts could be affected)
- Daytime chills and nighttime sweats
- Diarrhea and cramping alternating with constipation, bloating, indigestion, nausea, stomach pains, gassiness
- Dystonia
- Ear pain (both from congestion and extreme muscle tightness and inflammation with redness)
- Excessive ear wax and eye discharge, itchy ears, burning eyes
- Exhaustion and fatigue, sudden inability to stay awake
- Eye pain and blurred vision
- Flare ups of Hip Upslip, Rib Subluxation, TMJ, Plantar Fasciitis, Tennis Elbows, and other prior injuries
- Flushing, redness and puffiness of face, sallow/pale/green skin, dark circles under/around eyes (Allergic Shiners), droopy eyelids, deepened creases on face
- Fluttery, shaky, buzzy feeling
- Grimacing (involuntary frowning)
- Gum abscesses and mouth sores
- Hair shedding
- Headache and Migraine
- Heightened sensitivity to smells, motion, allergens, chemicals, light, sound (increased Auditory Processing Disorder), touch (light touch was painful)
- Increased laxity in joints
- Insatiable appetite
- Insomnia
- Joint swelling, stiffness, and pain (especially in fingers)
- Loss of will power: intense cravings for foods and activities that were not the most health bringing
- Menstrual cramps when menstruating, back pains when ovulating
- Mucous membrane irritation and sore throat
- Muscle tightness, trigger points, and weakness
- Neck pain (sometimes leading to face pain)
- Sense of dullness, slowness, heaviness
- Sinus congestion and pressure and runny nose
- Skin rash (tinea versicolor on torso and itchy, flaky rash on scalp)
- Sneezing, coughing, hoarse voice
- Swollen painful salivary glands and excessive salivation
- Swollen tongue (and sores on tongue from biting it because it didn't fit in my mouth)
- Tinnitus
- Tooth movement leading to greater crowding and misalignment
- Tremor, spasms, twitches, cramps
- Unpleasant body odor under arms
- Unstable emotions: worry, hopelessness, overwhelm, anger, anxiety, depression
- Urinary Frequency, Urgency, Pain, and Incontinence

Since I was never able to find a doctor who knew how to diagnose and treat my MCAS condition, I treated myself for MCAS for a long time. I achieved consistent improvement for years, and then when I started taking DAO, I experienced a big jump in improvement. It was the first time in my life that I experienced being relaxed. I do not know if it would have created the same boost if I had added it early on.

I prefer to reduce my histamine load with DAO rather than antihistamines because it feels better to my body. Perhaps this is because DAO is derived from foods (usually pork kidney or legumes), whereas antihistamines are synthesized from petroleum (or chemicals that were synthesized from petroleum), which is known to be poisonous to humans.

Also, antihistamines do not decrease the amount of histamine in the body; they attach to receptors on cells so that histamine cannot. Sometimes the body reacts to this by creating even more histamine — after all, histamine plays a part in many non-allergy functions of the body, including sleep cycles, brain activity, hunger, thirst, the menstrual cycle, and more. For this reason, patients often find that antihistamines become less effective over time, and frequently, people who take antihistamines get a rebound effect when the antihistamines wear off, in which their symptoms come back worse than they started.

DAO, on the other hand, is an enzyme that our bodies make to decrease the amount of histamine in the body. Since histamine can act as a signal to other cells to make more histamine, it is optimal to reduce the amount of histamine in the body; otherwise, if the histamine remains in the body, you can get trapped in a feedback loop. Plus, histamine is a signal for cells to make not only more histamine but also other chemicals that mast cells degranulate, many of which are harmful to the body (remember, some of the chemicals that mast cells release are neurotoxic).

Some people have a genetic profile that causes them not to make enough DAO, and whether we are among them or not, we are probably among those who make so much histamine that our bodies can't make enough DAO to take care of it all. The histamine is going to have to get processed out eventually, so the DAO will have to be on board at some point to get that done.

Some antihistamines have severe adverse effects if taken over the long term, especially dementia, and also blurred vision, constipation, dependence/withdrawal, anxiety, and increased risk of falls. Some of the newer antihistamines are safer, but all of them have some adverse effects. I have not been able to find any adverse effects listed for DAO. That might mean that DAO has not been studied thoroughly enough, or it might mean that it is a chemical that is native and necessary to the body, and any excess is simply excreted in urine.

Everything we do for our health is a risk/benefit decision, and it probably makes sense to take antihistamines sometimes. It might make even more sense to take DAO at the same time as antihistamines, when the problem is too bad for the DAO to take care of it. I have never yet heard of anyone taking so much DAO that it was a problem, and so I just take more DAO when what I've taken isn't enough. However, I'm at a point that my MCAS isn't nearly as bad as it used to be, so I am not the best experimental case study.

Over the years since I began treating myself with natural remedies for Allergy/MCAS/MCS and especially over the months after I learned about hEDS, I have become much less sensitive. As I write this, I am still cautious about not over-exposing myself to my triggers; this is a problem that prevents me from participating in some aspects of life that I would like to enjoy. However, after previously having been completely debilitated by chemicals, I now live a fairly normal lifestyle. My prayer is that you will be able to soon, too.

Preventions, Treatments, and Coping Strategies for Allergies, MCAS, and MCS

Healing symptoms of MCAS will be done through four main tactics. First of all, calm your system down as much as possible so that the immune system is less likely to react to benign triggers. Second, make sure that your detox pathways are open, supported, and not overtaxed so that they can quickly process out the chemicals that the mast cells degranulate. Third, use herbs, foods, and supplements that are COX inhibitors and mast cell stabilizers to further prevent the immune system from overreacting. And fourth, give your body time to re-establish nutrient levels that may have become deficient, rebuild structural weaknesses that might have developed, and get used to a new way of life.

To make it simpler for practical use, I have organized the details for doing those four things into calming the body every day, preparing for risky situations, and responding to having been triggered. Some of these things you will only have to do until you got better, while some of them will become simple habits that you will continue indefinitely, and others you will do only when you experience an extreme trigger.

Note that it has been my experience as well as that of some of my clients that the sensitivity symptoms are significantly reduced by treating for MTHFR. The genes associated with MTHFR can decrease methylation, which is a process in the body that is important for processing chemicals like histamine to remove them from the body. If you have these genes, you may require supplementation of folate, B12, P5P, and/or riboflavin. This is of special importance because a recent clinical study about hEDS found that folate supplementation helped significantly, sometimes completely alleviating patients' symptoms of the connective tissue disorder.[173] I self-treated myself for MTHFR about six years ago and noticed a great deal of improvement but continued to have numerous symptoms of hEDS; other people on the hEDS social media groups have given similar testimonials. Clearly, the two conditions can be comorbid and can exacerbate each other's symptoms, but there is a lot more to hEDS than folate deficiency. (See Chapter 24: MTHFR.)

Reduce the Unpleasant Effects of Allergies/MCAS/MCS

1. **Figure out what environmental components, household chemicals, and foods you are sensitive to.** Use diaries and elimination diets. The most challenging aspect of this is that it can take time for a reaction to build, and the amount of time can vary. It can take only minutes or seconds, but it also may take 24 hours or even 3 days for the symptoms to become noticeable. Also, allergens may be hidden, such as coconut in water filters and rosemary as a preservative in foods and supplements. Most people with sensitivities react to synthetic fragrances. Other common sensitivities for those with hEDS are gluten, essential oils, artificial sweeteners, artificial food dyes, preservatives, and poisonous household chemicals. People with MCAS may benefit from a low-histamine diet. I have designed a *Hypermobile and Happy Health Diary* to help you on this step; you can purchase it at shannonegale.com . *Knowing what your triggers are is the most important first step in reducing symptoms.*
2. **Avoid anything you are allergic or sensitive to.**[174, 175] You may be strong enough to be able to experience an exposure for a certain amount of time before you have recognizable symptoms, but exposures are usually dose-dependent and cumulative. You may not reach your threshold during an exposure, but then an unplanned and unexpected exposure to the same trigger or a different one later may put you over your threshold. Also, you may be having subtle symptoms that you don't relate to the exposure but that are harming your body. Stand up for yourself and protect your body from anything that may harm it. You need all of the strength you can get. *You may not have to avoid your triggers forever, but avoiding them now is the best way to reduce symptoms.*
3. **Choose organic, all-natural, fragrance-free toiletries and cleaning products.** Most importantly, avoid fragrances. *Nurture yourself with health-giving, not health-compromising household and personal products.*
4. **Eat only organic, all-natural foods**. Some people in the MCAS social media groups report that they react to foods in the USA that are grown with chemical

fertilizers and pesticides but not to foods in the UK that are grown with safer methods. Avoid artificial flavors, dyes, and preservatives, as well as hydrogenated or partially-hydrogenated oils and other ingredients commonly found in processed foods but not in whole foods. *A whole-foods, made-from-scratch diet of fresh meats, vegetables, fruits, legumes, and grains that were grown on biodynamic farms is usually best.*

5. **Avoid toxic chemicals, even if they are not harmful in small doses to most people.** Toxic chemicals include or are found in gasoline, bleach, ammonia, hair dye, tattoos, fingernail polish, powerful cleaning agents, paints, glues, new furniture, building supplies, and more. *Keep the load of toxins you are exposed to as low as possible so that your body can process them without becoming overwhelmed.*
6. **Avoid having anything implanted into your body**, like earrings, birth control devices, breast augmenters, lip fillers, and dental implants. *Sometimes an implant will be medically necessary, but if it is not, play it safe and don't get it.*
7. **Avoid Electromagnetic Frequency Radiation (EMFs).**[176, 177] Some people are so sensitive to EMFs that they can sense them; many get headaches or malaise from exposure to them. However, scientists have found that in some cases, EMFs have harmed even those people (and animals) who did not sense them. Turn off the Wi-Fi while you sleep, and do not sit close to your router. Do not carry your phone in your pocket. If possible, turn off all of the electricity in your bedroom while you sleep. Do not stand close to a microwave. Do not hold your laptop on your lap. It is possible to use special paints and other materials to turn your bedroom or your entire home into a Faraday Cage through which no radiation can enter, but if you do it wrong, it will act as an antenna instead, so do your research before making changes. The kinds and quantities of EMFs that we are exposed to are increasing all of the time. No one on Earth has been exposed to these levels of EMFs in all of history, so we really do not know what effect they might have on us. Our entire nervous system is electric, and all of our cells have ion channels, so it is reasonable to assume that there is some kind of effect, even if it has not been measured yet. *Consider that those of us who are sensitive and made physically uncomfortable by EMFs may be like canaries in the coal mines, warning others of dangers they haven't yet sensed.*
8. **Keep the air in your home clean.** Do not bring noxious chemicals or anything you might react to into your house. If you live in an area with clean outdoor air, open your windows frequently to allow the house to air out. If you do not, invest in

REDUCE THE UNPLEASANT EFFECTS OF ALLERGY/MCAS/MCS

1. Figure out what environmental components, household chemicals, and foods you are sensitive to.
2. Avoid anything you are allergic or sensitive to.
3. Choose organic, all-natural, fragrance-free toiletries and cleaning products.
4. Eat only organic, all-natural foods.
5. Avoid toxic chemicals, even if they are not harmful in small doses to most people.
6. Avoid having anything implanted into your body.
7. Avoid Electromagnetic Frequency Radiation (EMFs).
8. Keep the air in your home clean.
9. Keep your vehicle scent-free.
10. Request accommodations at your workplace, school, and church.

Ask your doctor before trying anything new.

a high-quality air filtration system. Get any ductwork in your house professionally cleaned yearly, but insist that the contractor you hire does not use any chemicals and does only mechanical cleaning; also request that they use new filters and bags on their machines. Use an allergy-grade filter on your furnace if you have a forced-air heating-and-cooling system, and change the filter monthly even though the package probably says to change it every three months. If smells come into your house from outside, turn off any bathroom or stove vents that are blowing air out because this draws air in through any tiny cracks in the house; if this is a persistent problem, get a small air intake machine with a good filter that can draw air in from outside and create pressure in the house that will prevent air coming in through cracks.[178] Be alert to the dangers of mold in the house, and if you discover any mold, have it professionally mediated. When you buy new furniture or household items, they may need to off gas outside or be washed with vinegar before bringing them into the house. Always put new clothes and linens directly into the washing machine as soon as you bring them home. In cases when smells get into the house, use an ozone generator to purify the air, but do so cautiously, following all of the guidelines in the instructions that come with the machine; ozone is very good at breaking down VOCs and ozone itself breaks down into oxygen quickly, but ozone is harmful to people, animals, and plants. *Let your home be your sanctuary.*

9. **Keep your vehicle scent-free.** Keep your vehicle interior clean, using only products that are safe for you. If you go to a carwash, request that they do not put air fresheners into your car; take your own cleaner for them to use on surfaces. Change your cabin air filter when you get your oil changed. Switch your AC system to recirculating the cabin air whenever you are in an area with pollution, but when you are in an area with fresh air, use outside air or open the windows. In the summer when it is hot, the heat may cause the plastics in the vehicle to off gas, so open the windows for a few minutes before you get in. When you pump gas, step 10 feet away from the tank so that you do not breathe the gasoline fumes, and in case the previous person who used the pump left fragranced lotion on the handle, protect your hand with a paper towel, which you can throw away in the gas station trash can. Alert repairmen to your sensitivities so that they do not spray anything in your car; most repair shops have plastic steering wheel covers and paper seat covers that can protect your vehicle from contamination. *Let your vehicle always be safe for you.*
10. **Request accommodations at your workplace, school, and church.** Any place where you spend a lot of time should be safe for you, so follow the guidance for keeping your home scent-free, and make these requests elsewhere. You may also need to make requests regarding the lighting and EMFs. *If the people you make the request of will not comply, try to find another place with people who will comply.*

Calm Your System Every Day to Reduce Sensitivity to Food, Chemicals, Stress, and Sensory Inputs

Some of these recommendations are inspired by Ayurvedic, Anthroposophical, Hopi, and Christian principles.

1. **Prevent your joints from hyperextending**. (See Chapter 9: Joint Instability & Pain.) The hyperextension or dislocation of a joint is a serious trauma to the body, even if it has happened frequently to you. *Prevent these threats and injuries, and you will give your nervous system a chance to calm down and allow your body to function in the rest-and-digest state.*

2. **Follow a daily rhythm that works for you.** Go to bed and wake up at about the same time every day. Eat your meals, go outside, do your work, play, and relax at about the same time every day. You do not need a strict time schedule; in fact, it is best to keep flexibility in your rhythm, but do things in the same order each day. Try to arrange your rhythm so that it breathes in and out with low-energy activities alternating with high energy activities and introspective activities alternating with social activities. Daily rhythms help keep your circadian rhythm and many other bodily processes regulated. They also reduce the number of decisions you have to make in a day, which is beneficial for your mental health. *Make sure to plan joy and gratitude into your rhythm.*
3. **Follow a weekly rhythm.** Do the same thing or same kind of thing each Monday, and so on. Rudolf Steiner developed a theory and practice regarding which kinds of activities, meditations, attitudes, and food grains are best on which days of the week — it might inspire you.[179] Or, you might start with the things you can't control like the day you go to church, the day your baseball team plays, the day your child has piano lessons. Then figure out when you want to do which household tasks, when you want to go someplace fun, when you want to watch movies with the family. *A weekly rhythm ensures that you divide your time appropriately between social, home, work, play, nature, music, or whatever activities you want to include; it helps keep you comfortable and lets your subconscious self know what to expect.*

CALM YOUR SYSTEM EVERY DAY TO REDUCE SENSITIVITY TO FOOD, CHEMICALS, STRESS, AND SENSORY INPUTS

1. Prevent your joints from hyperextending.
2. Follow a daily rhythm that works for you.
3. Follow a weekly rhythm.
4. Follow a yearly rhythm that is inspired by the seasons.
5. Avoid any foods and environmental substances that trigger you.
6. Eat warm, soft foods, and drink warm beverages.
7. Limit foods like peppers, onions, and garlic that are known to excite the immune system.
8. Do not eat leftovers or overripe foods.
9. Take DAO right before eating and sleeping.
10. Get massages or give them to yourself.
11. Tap the thymus.
12. Take warm baths.
13. Feel gratitude.
14. Spend time in nature.
15. Snuggle and cuddle with someone you care about or a pet.
16. Keep warm.
17. Avoid electronics.
18. Play.
19. Sing.
20. Listen to music, and if you feel like it, dance like no one is watching.
21. Don't rush.
22. Eliminate infections.
23. Take quercetin or berberine to stabilize mast cells.
24. Eat culinary and wild-grown herbs.
25. Drink AllergEase Tea daily.
26. Detox your body and your lifestyle.
27. Take trace minerals.
28. Get auricular acupuncture.

Ask your doctor before trying anything new.

4. **Follow a yearly rhythm that is inspired by the seasons**. To an extent, everyone in our society does this, especially in places where the seasons change noticeably — shorts in summertime and sweaters in winter, pumpkin spice in the fall, peppermint at Christmas time. Still, it might be helpful to conscientiously take this further. Eat food that is in season at your local farmer's market. Plan celebrations that honor the holy days and seasons. *A yearly rhythm keeps you healthy by being in tune with nature, and it opens up a lot of opportunities for us to appreciate this miraculous world we live in.*
5. **Avoid any foods and environmental substances that trigger you**.[180] Keep a diary of foods, activities, and exposures so that you can see if there are any patterns and figure out what you are reacting to. You can use the *Hypermobile and Happy Health Diary* to make this easy yet comprehensive; find it at shannonegale.com . Some common triggers for people with MCAS are gluten, histamine-containing foods, oxalates, salicylates, mold, lectins, cooking smells, and fragrance, but your specific triggers could be anything. *Whether it makes sense or not for your body to react to a certain substance, eaten or inhaled, you will probably not be able to get your system to calm down until you have avoided it for some time.*
6. **Eat warm, soft foods, and drink warm beverages.**[181, 182, 183] The digestive system requires heat to work, so it is easier on it if you add the heat in. It is also easier to digest soft foods rather than crunchy ones. *You do not need to restrict yourself to warm and soft foods and drinks all of the time, but it will be helpful when you are not feeling your best.*
7. **Limit foods like peppers, onions, and garlic that are known to excite the immune system.**[184] Allergy/MCAS/MCS conditions generally indicate an overactive immune system. *If your immune system is overactive, do not try the things that most people are seeking to strengthen their immune systems.*
8. **Do not eat leftovers or overripe foods.** *As food ages, its histamine and mold contents increase, both of which are common MCAS triggers.*[185]
9. **Take DAO before eating and sleeping.** *DAO helps the body process out excess histamine, so it can make you less sensitive to foods and more likely to sleep through the night.*[186, 187, 188, 189]
10. **Get massages or give them to yourself.**[190] *Human touch is a miraculous healing tool.*
11. **Tap the thymus.**[191] The thymus is a thyme leaf-shaped gland in your upper chest, above your heart, and it is responsible for immune system regulation. You can do this like Tarzan, beating your chest with your fists and yelling, or you can do it more gently with your fingertips. *Tapping the thymus will activate it so that it will do its job of regulating the immune system, which is responsible for Allergy/MCAS/MCS reactions.*
12. **Take warm baths**. Add Ancient Minerals and you will also be absorbing magnesium and other minerals that get depleted during physically and/or emotionally stressful times.[192] *Warm water relaxes the muscles and nervous system.*
13. **Feel gratitude**. Pay attention to what feels good, what is wondrous, what gives your life meaning, what makes your day easier, what comes as a pleasant surprise, what you can always rely on. *Gratitude and a positive outlook are both good for your health and wellbeing, so pay attention to all of the good you can possibly find.*[193, 194, 195, 196]
14. **Spend time in nature**. There are countless scientific studies proving that nature is healing.[197, 198, 199, 200] Just looking at a photo of a tree makes a measurable improvement. Make opportunities for yourself to get out into the wild spaces near where you live or around the world. When you have a busy day in the city, see if

you can find the hidden bits of nature in the cityscape — I think you'll be surprised (and if you can't find them, ask a child — they are very good at this). See Chapter 48: Forest Bathing. *Nature is healing and calming.*

15. **Snuggle and cuddle with someone you care about or a pet.** [201, 202, 203] As I've said before, physical touch is a miraculous healing tool, but it doesn't have to be purposefully healing. It can even be lazy! *When you cuddle a loved one or friend, not only will you get a big dose of increased health, your loved one will, too!*
16. **Keep warm**. It takes quite a bit of effort for the body to keep its temperature regulated. Although some people will sometimes be too hot, the more common and stressful condition is being too cold. Wear a scarf around your neck — this is really important during the change of seasons. Drink warm drinks. Dress for the weather. Soak up some sunlight.[204] *Warmth is life giving.*
17. **Avoid electronics**. Electromagnetic Frequencies (EMFs) have been shown to harm our bodies, so spend as little time close to electronics as possible.[205] Turn off your cell phone, the WiFi, and power strips at night. Keep your cell phone at a distance from your body when it is turned on. Step away from the microwave and other high-powered electronic devices when they are running. *Spend time in nature away from EMFs; living in the real world, in natural ways, brings a calmness to your body.*
18. **Play**.[206] Play board games, play on a jungle gym, play childhood games, play act. Do stuff that is fun and reminds you what it was like to be a kid. *When we are not feeling fulfilled and inspired by life, play can bring back the meaning.*
19. **Sing**. No matter where or whom you sing with, because the Vagus Nerve touches the larynx, it activates the Vagus Nerve, bringing balance to your nervous system.[207] Sing in the shower, sing while you're cleaning the house, sing along to the radio while you drive your car, sing in the church choir, sing with a child. Make sure that the kind of singing you do makes you feel good, not nervous (like performing a solo in front of a crowd if you aren't confident about your singing voice).[208] *Sound healing is a powerful thing to experience at a concert or a personal session; it can be even more healing to create the sounds yourself.*
20. **Listen to music, and if you feel like it, dance like no one is watching.** Calming music that you enjoy can improve mood, blood pressure, and heart rate. The music's wellbeing effect is amplified if you dance to it.[209] *Listen to music that is cheerful but not too fast, and your body will respond.*
21. **Don't rush**. Move slowly and stop to breathe deeply if you're feeling the need to rush. Pray for things to happen in perfect timing and then let them unfold as they will. Appreciate the little moments of rest throughout the day, like the minute it takes for your glass of water to fill up, or the two minutes you sit at a traffic light, or the five minutes you wait for your child to get their shoes on. Rushing is possibly the leading cause of disease for our culture[210], and when you rush, you miss out on so much. *Take control of your wellbeing by adopting a slow lifestyle, easy like a Sunday morning.*
22. **Eliminate infections**. If you have or suspect an infection that is mild or that the doctor has not been able to eliminate, try taking olive leaf extract.[211, 212] This supplement is also shown to fight off flus and colds, regulate blood pressure and blood sugar levels, kill excessive yeast, bacteria, and fungi (without harming the beneficial gut flora), prevent cancer, and reduce inflammation. *Olive leaf extract is a powerful herb and should not be taken for a very long time, but its benefits will often last after you stop taking it.*
23. **Take quercetin or berberine to stabilize mast cells**, which are the producers of histamine and other hormones that create the reaction when you have been

exposed to an allergen or trigger. Quercetin also supports the immune system and the cardiovascular system and is neuroprotective, among many other health benefits.[213, 214, 215, 216] However, I don't notice any differences in how I feel when I take Quercetin, but I find that Berberine makes me feel energized and relaxed at the same time. Also be aware that quercetin can affect your body's iron levels.[217] Many doctors recommend that MCAS patients take antihistamines, but it can be a challenge to find the right antihistamine, and it might have unpleasant side effects. Quercetin is found in foods like apples and grapes; berberine comes from certain berries. They are relatively safe and stop the body from producing histamine in excessive quantities in the first place. *These natural plant substances are good for overall health.*

24. **Eat culinary and wild-grown herbs** that are mast cell stabilizers. Many culinary herbs, like oregano, basil, turmeric, and parsley are delicious used fresh in your cooking.[218] Backyard weeds like broadleaf plantain, purple dead nettle, and chickweed are anti-inflammatory or stabilize mast cells, and they are free;[219] if you leave an empty pot on your back patio, the herbs you most need may volunteer themselves there. *Let healthy, fresh, organic food be your first medicine.*
25. **Drink AllergEase Tea daily**. I have cured many clients and relatives of seasonal pollen allergies by prescribing them to drink a cup of this tea each day with a spoonful of local honey, preferably produced at the same time of year as when their allergies strike. This herb tea has also significantly cut down on my reactions to fragrance, especially in eliminating the stomach bloating I used to get. AllergEase Tea by Health King includes scute, astragalus, polygonatum, angelica daburica, polygala, eleuthro, green tea, and jasmine. *Herbs can help calm the system and reduce allergic sensitivity.*
26. **Detox your body and your lifestyle**. (See Chapter 44: Detox.) *Pure, clean living will keep your system calm.*
27. **Take trace minerals**. I have used ION* Intelligence of Nature Gut Support Liquid (just a few drops, not a whole dosage), as well as some varieties of fulvic and humic acids, which taste delicious mixed in hot tea and can give me energy and improve my skin, fingernails, and hair. *Trace minerals reduce inflammation, reduce allergic-type immune responses, maintain gut health, and more.*[220, 221, 222]
28. **Get auricular acupuncture**. I have not tried this myself, but there are many reports on social media that a specific kind of acupuncture, called SAAT, is particularly effective at putting an end to MCAS for some patients. SAAT is Soliman's Auricular Allergy Treatment, a protocol developed by Dr. Nader Soliman using a tiny needle, inserted into the outer ear and left in place for 3 weeks, to treat allergy. Some practitioners use Ear Seeds, which are tiny seeds, beads, or stickers, instead of needles. *Auricular acupuncture, when practiced by a licensed acupuncturist, is a low-risk treatment that has been shown to be effective for the majority of allergy patients.*[223, 224]

Take Preventative Measures for Risky Situations When You Anticipate Being Exposed to Environmental Allergens

Keep in mind that although the worst reactions develop from either touching contaminants or inhaling environmental allergens, airborne chemicals can also cause reactions when absorbed through the skin. Often, people with MCS develop hypersensitive smelling abilities, but even then, being distracted can prevent you from noticing scents. In addition, the congestion and inflammation of reactions can reduce smelling abilities.

1. **Take supplements.** These are known to be helpful for allergic and mast cell reactions:
   a. One baby aspirin every 12 hours. Aspirin in low doses is a COX inhibitor, so it prevents the production of prostaglandins (which in turn degranulate mast cells); however, aspirin in high doses is a mast cell activator.[225, 226, 227, 228, 229, 230]
   b. Grape juice has high concentrations of resveratrol, which is also a COX inhibitor, as well as being anti-inflammatory and neuroprotective, among many other benefits.[231] Tart cherry juice also contains polyphenols, quercetin, and other beneficial nutrients which allow it to be anti-inflammatory and mast cell stabilizing.[232, 233]
   c. Vitamin C with bioflavonoids or ascorbic acid has an antihistamine effect and supports the immune system.[234, 235, 236]
   d. Magnesium is deficient in many people with Allergy/MCAS/MCS.[237]
   e. Homeopathic *Ignatia amara* is also beneficial for reducing anxiety.[238]
   f. Astragalus supports the immune system without activating it.[239, 240]
   g. Milk thistle supports the liver so that it can detoxify the body of toxins and hormones like histamine.[241]
   h. Methylfolate[242] and Methylcolbalmin[243] at the same time are imperative for the removal of excess histamine from the body.
   i. Bioplasma cell salts help balance the body's mineral and electrolyte content.[244]
   j. DAO helps the body digest excess histamine.[245, 246, 247, 248]
2. **Rebound or do Lymph Drainage Massage.** Rebound is a fancy way of saying jump on a trampoline to get lymph flowing. (See Chapter 51: Lymph Drainage Massage.) *This will process toxins out of your body more quickly.*
3. **Wear a personal ionizer** (worn under a scarf tied loosely around the face when in highly fragrant places). *Ions break down VOCs (Volatile Organic Compounds), which are the molecules that you can smell and that you would react to.*[249, 250]

TAKE PREVENTATIVE MEASURES FOR RISKY SITUATIONS WHEN YOU ANTICIPATE BEING EXPOSED TO ENVIRONMENTAL ALLERGENS

1. Take supplements.
   a. One baby aspirin.
   b. Grape Juice or tart cherry juice.
   c. Vitamin C with bioflavonoids or ascorbic acid.
   d. Magnesium.
   e. Homeopathic *Ignatia amara.*
   f. Astragalus.
   g. Milk thistle.
   h. Methylfolate and Methylcolbalmin.
   i. Bioplasma cell salts.
   j. DAO.
2. Rebound or do Lymph Drainage Massage.
3. Wear a personal ionizer.
4. Wear a mask when you do not have a personal ionizer.
5. Wrap hair or wear a hood or hat so that your hair won't absorb scent, and bring a change of clothes.
6. Apply refined shea butter on any exposed skin to protect against getting allergens on the skin.
7. Wear sunglasses to filter out too-bright or flickering lights.
8. Wear specialty ear plugs to filter out background noise.

Ask your doctor before trying anything new.

4. **Wear a mask when you do not** have **a personal ionizer**. The benefit of the mask or other cloth over your face is that it will filter out larger particles, like pollen, that you may react to, but it is not very effective against fragrances and other chemicals.[251, 252] *Avoid inhaling anything that you might react to.*
5. **Wrap hair or wear a hood or hat so that your hair won't absorb scent, and bring a change of clothes**. *Reactions are often dose dependent, so being able to get away from the smell instantly is helpful, which you can't do if the scent is attached to your clothing or hair.*
6. **Apply refined shea butter on any exposed skin to protect against getting allergens on the skin.**[253] Shea butter, and sunflower seed, jojoba, and coconut oils are known to support the skin's barrier against absorbing noxious chemicals. Shea butter is nice and thick for a good protective coating. *The shea butter can be scrubbed off after exposure and take the chemicals away with it instead of letting them absorb into your body.*
7. **Wear sunglasses to filter out too-bright or flickering lights**. Although sunglasses are not recommended for all of the time when you are outside in natural light,[254, 255] they may be helpful when you are photosensitive or sensitive to flicker.[256]
8. **Wear specialty ear plugs to filter out background noise.**[257, 258] If you reduce the noise that your brain has to cope with, you will have more capacity to deal with other threats like chemicals.

Prevent and Reduce Symptoms of Allergy/MCAS/MCS After Exposures

1. **Wipe skin down with a wet cloth immediately after exposure**. As soon as possible bathe and wash your hair. *Do not carry the smell around with you; get rid of the offending chemicals as quickly as possible.*
2. **Take Homeopathic Remedies as needed**. (See Chapter 50: Homeopathic Remedies.) *Treat specific symptoms easily and conveniently with homeopathics.*
   a. Overexertion and physical or emotional trauma: *Arnica* Montana.
   b. Difficulty breathing and fatigue: *Arsenicum album*.
   c. Inflamed mucous membranes, sore throat, and Sinus Congestion: *Belladonna*.
   d. Body aches and exhaustion: *Chamomilla*.
   e. Stiff neck and tension headache: *Gelsemium*.
   f. Swelling in face, sneezing, coughing: *Histaminum hydrochloricum*
   g. Allergic reaction initial stage and anxiety: *Ignatia amara*.
   h. Muscle tension and anxiety: *Magnesium phosphorica*.
   i. Sores in mouth: *Mercurius solubus*.
   j. Nausea and Insomnia caused by worry: *Nux vomica*.
   k. Exposure to petroleum products such as synthetic fragrances and gasoline: petroleum.
   l. Cough and chest congestion: *Phosphorous*.
   m. Sinus pressure and sneezing: *Pulsatilla*.
   n. Hopelessness, feeling overwhelmed, and menstrual cramps: *Sepia*.
   o. Deep-seated fear: *Stramonium*.
3. **Take supplements**. Give your body the fuel it needs to repair and recover.
   a. Activated charcoal will bind to toxins but it will also dehydrate you, so drink extra water. [259]
   b. Magnesium malate is used by the body in stressful situations, reduces the severity of allergic reactions, and relaxes muscles.[260, 261, 262]
   c. DAO (Diamine Oxidase) is an enzyme that can help the body eliminate histamine quickly, which reduces symptoms and allows you to sleep.[263]
   d. B vitamins support the nervous system and the detox system. [264]

e. Vitamin C (ascorbic acid) is an antihistamine and is generally very good for the body.[265, 266, 267, 268, 269]
f. Stinging nettle reduces histamine.[270]
g. Milk thistle improves liver function.[271]
h. Methylfolate and methylcobalamin simultaneously improve detoxing and help cope with stress and anxiety.[272]
i. Salty and fatty foods regulate blood pressure and bind toxins, which are usually fat soluble.[273, 274]
j. Water (Reverse Osmosis remineralized is the best), especially if you take activated charcoal, which can be dehydrating, is used in every bodily function.
k. Baking soda (dissolved in water) reduces immune response and inflammation.[275]
l. Grape juice or tart cherry juice are mast cell stabilizers and anti-inflammatories that reduce body aches, muscle pain, joint pain, and stiffness caused by inflammation.[276, 277, 278, 279]
m. Electrolytes — in t-he form of an electrolyte blend containing potassium, magnesium, and zinc (especially for tremor, weakness, brain fog, low energy, and POTS episodes); or salt (preferably Real Salt, for twitches and spasms); or an "adrenal cocktail" for tremor (see Appendix A: Recipes); or magnesium (for weakness and pain following stress, including season changes) to maintain blood pressure regulation and help cope with stress.[280, 281]
n. Alka Seltzer Gold reduces the initial reaction (it is a mast cell stabilizer), and is especially effective for indigestion.[282]

PREVENT AND REDUCE SYMPTOMS OF ALLERGY/MCAS/MCS AFTER EXPOSURES (Box 1)

1. Wipe skin down with a wet cloth immediately after exposure.
2. Take Homeopathic Remedies as needed.
   a. Overexertion and physical or emotional trauma: *Arnica Montana.*
   b. Difficulty breathing and fatigue: *Arsenicum album.*
   c. inflamed mucous membranes, sore throat, and Sinus Congestion: *Belladonna.*
   d. Body aches and exhaustion: *Chamomilla.*
   e. Stiff neck and tension headache: *Gelsemium*.
   f. Swelling in face, sneezing, coughing: *Histaminum hydrochloricum*.
   g. Allergic reaction initial stage and anxiety: *Ignatia amara*.
   h. Muscle tension and anxiety: *Magnesium phosphorica*.
   i. Sores in mouth: *Mercurius solubus*.
   j. Nausea and Insomnia caused by worry: *Nux vomica.*
   k. Exposure to petroleum products such as synthetic fragrances and gasoline: petroleum.
   l. Cough and chest congestion: *Phosphorous.*
   m. Sinus pressure and sneezing: *Pulsatilla.*
   n. Hopelessness, feeling overwhelmed, and menstrual cramps: *Sepia.*
   o. Deep-seated fear: *Stramonium.*

Ask your doctor before trying anything new.

o. Multivitamins are an easy way to get a lot of vitamins that are needed for all of your different bodily processes. Try to find some made from whole foods instead of synthetic chemicals.

p. TRS (Toxin and Contaminant Removal System) by Coseva creates symptoms sometimes but overall, over time, offers improvement; only a tiny amount is needed. TRS looks and tastes like water, but contains nano-zeolites that can cross the blood/brain barrier and bind to toxins, including heavy metals.[283, 284, 285]

q. Collagen peptides (just a sprinkling, not a whole dosage), while contraindicated for kidney disease, offer your body the protein building blocks it needs to make connective tissues. The people with hEDS/HSD whom I have heard from that take collagen peptides all prefer a very small dose. In my experience, collagen reduces skin yeast flare-ups and skin tenderness (perhaps by helping restore the quality of the collagen in the skin), and also increases energy.[286]

r. Single baby aspirin every 12 hours is a COX inhibitor, which reduces prostaglandin production. However, it can be hard on the stomach, so do not take more than you need; one or two a day is fine for most people. Larger doses can sometimes reduce headache and pains, but the larger doses do not have the same effectiveness for decreasing inflammation because they can activate mast cells. Low-dose aspirin reduces swelling in joints, tongue, salivary glands, and throughout the body.[287]

s. Topical magnesium can reduce cramps or twitches. Magnesium oil is magnesium flakes mixed with filtered water. It does not contain oil but feels oily. I like to mix it up in a glass spray bottle for ease of application. It will sting the skin if you are very deficient in magnesium, in which case a bath with magnesium flakes in it is preferrable. Another alternative is to put a magnesite stone inside your sock, underwear, or bra so that it is against the skin for absorption throughout the day, especially helpful for foot spasms. Magnesium relaxes muscles, heals nerves, reduces inflammation, and helps you cope with stress.[288]

PREVENT AND REDUCE SYMPTOMS OF ALLERGY/MCAS/MCS AFTER EXPOSURES — Continued (Box 2)

3. Take supplements.
   a. Activated charcoal.
   b. Magnesium malate.
   c. DAO.
   d. B vitamins.
   e. Vitamin C (ascorbic acid).
   f. Stinging nettle.
   g. Milk thistle.
   h. Methylfolate and methylcobalamin simultaneously.
   i. Salty and fatty foods.
   j. Water.
   k. Baking soda.
   l. Grape juice or tart cherry juice.
   m. Electrolytes.
   n. Alka Seltzer Gold.
   o. Multivitamins.
   p. TRS (Toxin and Contaminant Removal System) by Coseva.
   q. Collagen peptides.
   r. Single baby aspirin every 12 hours.
   s. Topical magnesium.
   t. Grapefruit juice.

Ask your doctor before trying anything new.

t. Grapefruit juice balances the liver processes for better detoxification of any toxins (like that fragrance that might have triggered you) or hormones (like the excessive histamine the mast cells produced).[289] First check for contraindications with any medications you take.

LINKS FOR PRODUCTS MENTIONED IN THIS CHAPTER

Ozone Generator https://amzn.to/4adAMWd

Magnesium Flakes https://amzn.to/3HrNIvn

Olive Leaf Extract https://amzn.to/3OxpILh

Quercetin https://amzn.to/49oLrgE

Berberine https://amzn.to/3vARi46

Chinese Skullcap https://amzn.to/4aUg9PT

AllergEase Tea https://amzn.to/4aaIQHh

Trace Minerals: ION* Gut Support https://amzn.to/49Dzaoj or Fulvic Acid https://amzn.to/3yOhGZB

Baby Aspirin https://amzn.to/3Snl7Of

Vitamin C https://revitalizewellness.org/products/vitamin-c-as-ascorbic-acid-16oz-fine-powder or https://amzn.to/4a06BBz or https://amzn.to/4bisYmX

Magnesium https://amzn.to/4bawDms or https://amzn.to/44mPmZO

DAO: Histamine Digest https://amzn.to/3WvIqHY or NaturDAO https://amzn.to/3QQKpDi

B Vitamin Complex https://amzn.to/3wmXBsz

Astragalus https://amzn.to/3Qpsaoh or https://amzn.to/4di1Nu8

Milk Thistle https://amzn.to/48LdF4S

Methylfolate https://amzn.to/3U3sSdy

Methylcolbalamin https://amzn.to/422EaRi

Bioplasma https://amzn.to/493krT2

Personal Ionizer https://amzn.to/3OmbfSo

Refined Shea Butter https://amzn.to/4aTnwa1

Specialty Ear Plugs https://amzn.to/42qkGWP or https://amzn.to/3SJoEXp

Arnica Montana https://amzn.to/48ryZwi

Arsenicum album https://amzn.to/3HawrH9

Belladonna https://amzn.to/3NVDR4M

Chamomilla https://amzn.to/4b1KpJ0

Gelsemium https://amzn.to/3tLaTO3

Histaminum hydrochloricum https://amzn.to/3tOerPO

Ignatia Amara https://amzn.to/48QcuRP

Magnesium phosphorica https://amzn.to/3Su6A3u

Mercurius solubus https://amzn.to/3TTMArP

Nux vomica https://amzn.to/3vAOKT3

Petroleum https://amzn.to/3Scgllx

Phosphorous https://amzn.to/47xYESO

Pulsatilla https://amzn.to/3vv0832

Sepia https://amzn.to/3RRVN1t

Stramonium https://amzn.to/428imU9

Activated Charcoal https://amzn.to/3S6Vgc7

Stinging Nettle https://amzn.to/3Unh6Jt

Reverse Osmosis Filter https://amzn.to/43m3qSZ

Electrolytes https://amzn.to/3UlgNk1

Real Salt https://amzn.to/3vAoNDd

Alka Seltzer Gold https://amzn.to/48GafAO

Multivitamins https://amzn.to/3OaHYdw

TRS https://www.ledamedical.com/product-page/copy-of-saccharomyces-boulardii-60-c

Collagen Peptides https://amzn.to/3SqgTp2

Magnesite Stone https://amzn.to/42pdkD5

12

Cerebellar Ataxia, Essential Tremor, & Dystonia

CEREBELLAR ATAXIA, ESSENTIAL TREMOR, and Dystonia are conditions that emanate from the brain and cause undesired, involuntary movement patterns in the body. This may constitute, for example, trembling hands, spasming feet, restricted voice, or nearly-invisibly twitching muscles.

Cerebellar Ataxia

Cerebellar Ataxia is a loss of coordination that manifests as clumsiness, but it is different from the fatigue and weakness that can come along with symptom flares or from overexertion. Ataxia itself is usually not painful, but it feels bizarre and can lead to painful injuries.

There are several types of Ataxia; the one that I and hypermobile people I know have most commonly experienced is dysmetria. Dysmetria affects the body's ability to judge its position in relation to other objects or itself.[290] Doctors initially test for it by asking a patient to touch their nose with their finger; with dysmetria ataxia, their finger won't immediately find their nose.

Combining Ataxia with the potentially decreased proprioception (sense of position and movement of your own body in relation to itself and the space around it) produced by Joint Injuries (due to nerve death, constantly moving joints, and changes in the brain), hypermobile people may become particularly prone to clumsiness and injuries.

There are a number of possible causes of ataxia, including some genetic disorders, alcohol use, structural abnormalities such as Chiari malformation (a defect in which the lowest part of the brain improperly extends down through the opening at the base of the skull), nutritional deficiencies, gluten sensitivity (sickness caused by the protein most famously found in wheat), and changes in blood flow in the brain. There are few blood vessels going in or out of the cerebellum to allow for blood pressure to easily be regulated, so the cerebellum is especially susceptible to increases or decreases in blood flow.[291] Such conditions can be created by, among other things, CCI (Cranio-Cervical Instability) and Migraine.

It has been reported that Cerebellar Ataxia is sometimes caused by inflammation in the brain.[292] Fortunately, in most cases when the inflammation subsides, the Ataxia will subside as well. Thus, Cerebellar Ataxia can be exacerbated by Thoracic Outlet Syndrome or CCI because they prevent the free flow of waste products out of the brain. It stands to reason that other conditions, like MCAS, that cause inflammation throughout the body could also exacerbate Cerebellar Ataxia.

It has also been seen that Migraine manifests with, initially, a decrease of blood flow to the brain, followed by a compensatory increase of blood flow. Either of these conditions could affect the health of the cerebellum. A decrease in blood flow can cause cell death in the cerebellum due to the lack of oxygen. Many Migraine patients report that oxygen therapy reduces their symptoms, and I have had that experience myself.

Any lesions of dead cells in the cerebellum can impact the functioning of the cerebellum. Fortunately, in time, the body will remove the dead cells from the brain, the cerebellum will return to a normal state, and symptoms of Ataxia will subside.

Essential Tremor

Essential Tremor is the most common movement disorder among humans.[293, 294] It is so common that when children play act being elderly people, they mimic the tremor with shaking hands, though tremor can occur in much younger individuals as well.

Tremor of the hands is the most common manifestation of this neurological disorder.[295] It is also found in the voice, head, legs, and tongue and is often associated with gait (walking) abnormalities. It can also manifest with depression, Anxiety, Insomnia, heightened sensitivity to light and sound, and cognitive decline.[296]

Essential Tremor is considered to be a progressive disease, meaning that it gets worse over time. The progression is faster for older patients. Those with young onset can be expected to have the same ultimate outcome of the disease as older patients have because it progresses slowly for those with young onset.[297]

The underlying cause of Essential Tremor is unknown and is likely different among different people. It is often comorbid with Cerebellar Ataxia, Dystonia, and cognitive dysfunction. It is believed to generate in the cerebellum of the brain (which is what Cerebellar Ataxia is named for). In some cases, it is thought that CCI, caused by lax ligaments in the neck, is the ultimate underlying cause of Essential Tremor because it can change the blood pressure in the brain.[298] See Chapter 25: Neck Pain and CCI.

There are pharmaceutical treatments available for Essential Tremor, though they are not effective or not fully effective for a large number of patients.

Dystonia

Dystonia is so similar in some ways to Essential Tremor that it is often misdiagnosed; both diagnoses are made clinically without the benefit of any kind of testing. Neurologists are the doctors most likely to get this diagnosis correct.[299] Dystonia and Essential Tremor can also exist together. As many as 75% of hEDS/HSD patients have Dystonia.[300, 301]

Dystonia can cause shaking, twitching, spasming, pseudo-seizures, and pseudo-paralysis and can accentuate pain, clumsiness, dysautonomia, diminished proprioception, and fatigue.[302] Sometimes, dystonia presents as invisible muscle vibrations that feel like a phone in the pocket on vibrate; facial twitches; sudden flicks of the wrist, shoulder, or other body part; uncontrolled kicking with the leg(s) or hitting with the arm(s); prolonged twisting of the foot at the ankle; jerky hand movements; trembling fingers; rocking of the torso; repetitive movements of the foot while sitting; arching of the body; restless legs at night; and teeth grinding.

Dystonia can often be very painful in the areas where the muscles are seizing. It also commonly leads to falls and injuries. A Dystonic Storm in which the dystonic symptoms are severe and frequent is considered to be life-threatening. It can be the cause of elevated heart rate; rapid, shallow breathing; autonomic instability (inability to control body temperature, blood pressure, etc.); speech problems; swallowing problems; and respiratory failure.[303]

It is thought that Dystonia emanates from the cerebellum of the brain.[304] It is also possible that it is caused or exacerbated by nervous system receptor dysfunction due to the nerves' placement in faulty connective tissues. Dystonia can be treated with medication, botulinum toxin injections, surgery, oxygen therapy, and/or physical and occupational therapy.[305, 306]

My Experience with Cerebellar Ataxia, Essential Tremor, and Dystonia

These conditions are sometimes progressive, but for myself and my sister, they flare up following exposure to triggers and then subside after some time. In fact, as we treated ourselves naturally for hEDS/HSD, these conditions flared much less severely and less frequently.

I usually experienced Cerebellar Ataxia symptoms on days 1-5 of an Allergy/MCAS/MCS reaction or Migraine — it occurred most strongly on the day after the worst day, when the headache pain had just subsided.

Cerebellar Ataxia made me very clumsy. Frequently, Ataxia led to me cutting, burning, or bruising myself, breaking things, and wrecking the car. A perfect example of it is when I intended to drink a glass of water but tipped the glass a few inches in front of my lips and dumped it out on my lap. Often, I reached to take the handle of a tea cup, but instead my hand went to the body of the cup and I knocked it over. Sometimes, I tried to slice a vegetable and instead sliced my finger. I also spilled the vegetables and other things on the floor.

Interestingly, my dog could recognize when I had been triggered — often even before I noticed. On those days, she stood right below me while I was chopping food, well knowing that I would drop some and she'd get a snack. On my good days, this food-loving dog didn't bother to get up from her doggy bed while I was cooking. She became my warning sign that I needed to be careful.

My sister who experienced Cerebellar Ataxia once intended to wipe her mouth with her napkin but instead wiped her forehead. I have a friend with this condition who must walk with a cane because the Ataxia causes frequent falls.

Many of my relatives have had Essential Tremor which got progressively more severe as they aged. Although I do not usually notice it unless I stick out my tongue, I have persistent trembling in my tongue. It may be responsible for me biting my tongue every once in a while, but I would not have noticed it had it not been pointed out to me by an Ayurveda practitioner (an Ayurveda intake session includes analysis of the tongue).

I also experienced trembling hands, whether that was Essential Tremor or Dystonia, as soon as I was exposed to one of my Allergy/MCAS/MCS or Migraine triggers (and also during POTS episodes, though the trembling then is of a slightly different nature).

I found that sometimes when my hand was shaking while I was using it, it was doing so because my fingers were hyperextended and my wrist was overtaxed and unstable. Once I started doing Rice Bucket exercises, my fingers became strong enough that once I noticed the hyperextension, I could round them and keep doing what I was doing with strong fingers and no shaking. (See Chapter 60: Rice Bucket Exercises.) The trembling was sometimes more persistent than that.

I also got Dystonia-style cramps, spasms, and twitches once I had been triggered, and they sometimes lasted for weeks. My feet were very prone to painful cramping but could usually be calmed down with frequent applications of Magnesium Oil Spray (see Appendix A: Recipes). I have had constant rhythmic spasms in my sides that could only be stopped with professional acupuncture. I got eye twitches and random other signs of Dystonia frequently. In addition to Magnesium Oil, meditation with deep breathing, gentle massage, light exercise, and drinking electrolytes could sometimes get the Dystonia symptoms to subside, at least temporarily.

My worst Dystonia symptoms generally occurred as painful neck spasms after exposure to an Allergy/MCAS/MCS trigger. These spasms combined with my CCI usually led to nerve damage, precipitating Occipital or Trigeminal Neuralgia, Migraine, and a variety of symptoms throughout the body related to Vagus Nerve dysfunction.

I have witnessed my sister with severe Dystonia, such as in Dystonic Storms. She had body parts frozen into uncomfortable-looking positions, and she uncontrollably hit herself in the chest. Interestingly, the doctors she reported this to took no notice of it, possibly since they did not witness it in their offices, and never having been given a diagnosis or condition name, she stopped listing it among her symptoms, severe though it was.

Whenever I treated myself prophylactically for these conditions of cerebellum injury as soon as I had been exposed to a trigger, I was usually able to reduce the severity of the symptoms or even prevent them altogether. However, once the symptoms began, I would simply have to wait for them to go away on their own, so quick action was imperative.

The preventative measure that worked best for me for Cerebellar Ataxia, was normobaric oxygen therapy (breathed through the nose) at the onset of a Migraine attack.[307, 308, 309] With the oxygen condenser I was using, it was an imperfect preventative measure; a tank with 100% oxygen flow capabilities might have been more effective. (However, hyperbaric oxygen therapy, in which the whole body is treated in a pressurized chamber, is not recommended due to the many negative results I have heard from people in social media groups.) Oxygen tanks must be prescribed by a doctor, although used oxygen condensers are often attainable. Also, there are oxygen bars selling oxygen instead of alcohol, but they sometimes have scents or fragrances mixed with the oxygen, which would have been detrimental to my healing efforts.

Additionally, as Cerebellar Ataxia is caused by cell (neuron) death in the brain, supplements that support the nervous system may be helpful in resolving the problem more quickly. See Chapter 28: Peripheral Neuropathy for a discussion of neuron/nerve healing and health.

When the oxygen treatment and supplements did not completely prevent Cerebellar Ataxia, I had to move into a coping mode. The side effects of Cerebellar Ataxia are injuries that can be quite dangerous, so it is really important to make safe decisions.

Preventions, Treatments, and Coping Strategies for Cerebellar Ataxia, Dysmetria, Essential Tremor, and Dystonia

Cerebellar disorders are challenging to treat because the symptoms sometimes do not appear until days after the incident that incited the symptoms happened, but the preventative steps need to be taken as soon as the damage happens; later measures will be much less effective. Try to learn to recognize what kinds of injuries and exposures will lead to cerebellar problems so that you can take preventative measures immediately.

Prevent Cerebellar Disorders Following Trigger Exposure

1. **Use oxygen therapy**. *Prevent cell death in the brain.*
2. **Eat basil, oregano, parsley, and/or turmeric**. Note that if you have MCAS, you may need to consume these herbs fresh, not as jarred spices, due to the potential mold contamination. Herbs can support nervous system health.
3. **Take acetylcholine, methylfolate, methylcolbalamin, thiamine, and B6**. Note that although acetylcholine is imperative for proper neuron function, it can exacerbate dystonia symptoms. Also, some people who have not addressed MTHFR problems may have trouble taking methylfolate and methylcolbalamin. *Our bodies need nutrients in order to heal.*

> PREVENT CEREBELLAR DISORDERS FOLLOWING TRIGGER EXPOSURE
>
> 1. Use oxygen therapy.
> 2. Eat basil, oregano, parsley, and/or turmeric.
> 3. Take acetylcholine, methylfolate, methylcolbalamin, thiamine, and B6.
>
> Ask your doctor before trying anything new.

Once damage has occurred to the cerebellum, it will simply take time for it to heal. As it is healing, the symptoms will get worse before they get better. This is something you will do best to accept, as raging and worrying about it will only increase your stress and thereby increase your symptoms. Whereas with most conditions, you might go to great effort to treat the symptoms, with cerebellar conditions, at this point, you need to turn your focus to maintaining your health to the best of your ability and protecting yourself from further injury. Fortunately, whether your symptoms are clumsiness, shaking, or spasms, there are steps you can take to protect yourself.

Cope With Cerebellar Ataxia Clumsiness

1. **Avoid dangerous cooking**. Avoid using knives and ovens. If you must use a knife, use a finger protector when chopping vegetables. Better yet, keep some chopped vegetables in your freezer for times like this. If you must use an oven, wear oven mitts that come all the way up to your elbow. *Have recipes ready that require little preparation so that you can still eat a healthy diet when you are in a flare-up of symptoms.*
2. **Ask family members or friends to help with risky tasks**. I have been lucky to be loved by people who want to help me when I need it. I think they appreciate my independence and strong work ethic when I am well, and I hope that it gives them a sense of fulfillment when they have an opportunity to help. *I pray that you also are loved by people who want to care for you.*

3. **Avoid driving vehicles while experiencing Ataxia.** If you must, drive slowly and carefully, fully alert; though this will not prevent Ataxia, it's still a good idea to be extra cautious during an episode. Make plans with alternative means of transportation in mind. I try not to let hEDS limit my life too much, and I often experienced Ataxia on days when I otherwise felt pretty good. *This meant that I was often motivated to invite a family member or friend who could drive to come with me to events.*
4. **Do not use exercise equipment but instead move slowly and hold onto something for balance when you exercise.** Your exercise needs and abilities will likely vary every day. I have not had good luck following exercise plans designed by personal trainers online. *Ataxia is just one of the many symptoms you need to have in mind when you begin exercising some days because it can increase risk of injury.*
5. **Use braces, canes, and other tools to help protect your joints.** The clumsiness of Ataxia will make you more prone to accidentally hyperextending your joints, so pre-emptively protect them before any damage happens. Prevent your joints from hyperextending, especially the fingers. *Make all of your movements from positions of strength.*
6. **Meditate with deep breathing and become as calm as possible.** *If sitting or lying still only draws your attention to the problem, a very slow walking meditation on a smooth, paved path may be in order.*

COPE WITH CEREBELLAR ATAXIA CLUMSINESS

1. Avoid dangerous cooking.
2. Ask family members or friends to help with risky tasks.
3. Avoid driving vehicles while experiencing Ataxia.
4. Do not use exercise equipment but instead move slowly and hold onto something for balance when you exercise.
5. Use braces, canes, and other tools to help protect your joints.
6. Meditate with deep breathing and become as calm as possible.

Ask your doctor before trying anything new.

LINKS FOR PRODUCTS MENTIONED IN THIS CHAPTER

Oxygen https://amzn.to/3UAirxU
Acetylcholine (Parasym Plus) https://amzn.to/484v0VF
Methylfolate https://amzn.to/3U3sSdy
Methylcolbalamin https://amzn.to/422EaRi
Finger Protector https://amzn.to/3Hlviwv
Oven Mitts https://amzn.to/48YbZoQ

13

Digestive System Problems

HEDS/HSD COMMONLY CAUSES A VARIETY of problems within the digestive system, such as gluten sensitivity, gastroparesis (food does not pass out of the stomach into the intestines as quickly as it should), nausea, indigestion, bloating, constipation, and more. Connective tissue disorders can cause leaky gut, weak muscles in the digestive tract, neurologically mediated digestive problems, and compression of blood vessels that serve the digestive tract.[310]

Many people with hEDS/HSD are sensitive to particular foods, gluten being the most likely culprit. It may be the first place for you to start looking. Also, many people with hEDS/HSD have a hard time with alcohol, even though in small doses it can reduce some of their other symptoms, including gastroparesis.

It can be very challenging to discover what you react to. True allergies or intolerances will be constant, but MCAS triggers will only upset the digestive system when there is already a high level of histamine in the body, which means that some foods will be fine one day and not the next.

Also, foods and food components like gluten can be virtually hidden in places you wouldn't expect. Many people with food sensitivities can taste even minute concentrations of their triggers, but sometimes the concentrations are too small to be tasted but not too small to incite a reaction. Plus, foods and food components' presence in foods can be inconsistent. For example, I would guess that about 50% of ice creams contain coconut oil — but 50% don't. Coconut is also processed into approximately 250 different chemicals for use in food, household products, and toiletries; many of these chemicals, when listed on an ingredients label, do not look like coconut.[311] Another reason why coconut is tricky is that most water filters are made from coconut fiber. We should expect that a water filter is filtering everything out of the water, but trace amounts get through, and that includes trace amounts of the filter itself.

There are numerous diets that have helped people with hEDS.[312] Some people are helped by vegan or vegetarian, while others are helped by paleo or carnivore. A low-histamine diet is the most commonly mentioned one in the MCAS social media groups. If there is a single optimal hEDS diet, it hasn't been determined yet. Some people get great results from drinking apple cider vinegar every day, or from various vitamin and mineral supplements. You may have to try several diets to figure out what is right for you. Keep in mind that it is important not to avoid foods unnecessarily, as this may diminish the spectrum of nutrients you will receive.

There are also a variety of theories about meal timing. Some say 5 small meals a day is best. Others believe in breakfast, lunch, and dinner with no snacking. Intermittent fasting, in all its variations, is very popular right now. Water or juice fasting 1 day per week or on some other schedule has been popular in the past. It is likely that different people need different schedules. In general, I recommend not eating very close to bedtime, but even with that, some people need a little protein snack before bed to keep their blood sugar levels balanced so that they can sleep through the night (especially during pregnancy). To figure out the timing that is best for you, it's a good idea to try a few different schedules and pay attention to how your body feels. Don't simply pay attention to hunger, though — you might feel hungry if you're thirsty, bored, in need of electrolytes, feeling sad, or for a number of other reasons.

My Experience with Digestive System Problems

I have been pretty fortunate in not having severe digestive problems. My family members who have had more severe digestive symptoms are all sensitive to gluten, but I am not. Still, I have suffered from indigestion and bloating frequently, as well as Motion Sickness, and I had Hyperemesis Gravidarum while pregnant. I believe I have also suffered from suboptimal nutrition, as if my body didn't always absorb all of the nutrients I consumed.

I think it is important for you to know that inhaling fragrances would always give me indigestion — we usually expect that an upset stomach comes from something we have eaten, but it can come from other factors, including things we breathe in. Tweaking my neck could also cause a stomachache that lasted as long as the neck pain lasted. I know a few people who get severe stomach aches or diarrhea whenever they get nervous, angry, or uncomfortable. It is helpful to keep a diary of foods, supplements, exercises, and symptoms, to help you figure out what is causing your Digestive System Problems. (You can use the Health Diary I created, which is available for purchase at shannonegale.com.)

My indigestion and bloating improved when I started the probiotic recommended on the Cusack protocol and did all of the recommended treatments for Allergies/MCAS/MCS in Chapter 11: Allergy, MCAS, & MCS.

One of the other factors that significantly helped my digestive state was eating meat. When I was 14 years old, I decided to stop eating meat. I was vegetarian for 21 years; most of that time, I was ovo-lacto vegetarian (I ate eggs and dairy products), but 1 of those years when I was about 24 years old, I was vegan/dairy-free/gluten-free/sugar-free, and the last year, when I was 35, I was pescetarian (I ate eggs, dairy, and fish).

I had become vegetarian because I personally had befriended many animals, including chickens and cows, and I had noticed that they all had personalities. I could not bear to kill them. However, after about 15 years, I started to hurt all over, though I did not seem to have any injuries. And it got worse. I started getting headaches, nausea, and other signs of ill health. I am sure that hEDS was the underlying cause of those symptoms, but the condition was so little known at the time, it was likely impossible for me to find information about it.

So, I prayed, and the answer I got was that I needed to eat meat. At first this was upsetting, but in time I came to understand that it was not natural for me to keep myself out of the circle of life. I also learned that plants have the same pain chemicals that humans have, and although they may not feel pain in the same way we do, their "pain" upon being cut can be scientifically measured. In order to live, I had to hurt something else. I had to decide whether or not I deserved to live more than those plants and animals.

I struggled with this a lot, but when I finally came to my decision, I was enormously empowered. The first meat I ate was bacon, mainly because I knew how to cook it. I have heard from other former vegetarians that it was their "gateway" meat as well. I sat at my patio table to eat it, unsure of the emotional and spiritual implications of this choice. And while I sat there thinking about it, a butterfly flew up and landed on my head. After a few moments, the butterfly alit from my head and flew in a circle over the table, and then it flew back to my head and sat there for a few moments. The butterfly did this three more times before it flew away, just as I was finishing my bacon.

Awestruck, I looked up the spiritual meaning of butterflies, and I read that a butterfly is a messenger from someone who has recently died, coming to tell you that they are OK. That generous pig that gave its life for my nourishment, he was OK.

Within 30 minutes of eating the bacon, my body felt better, and the good feelings lasted until about the time I started getting hungry again. That was my experience with each meal for the next several weeks, and I knew that eating meat was the right choice for my health. After all, my father, who was the most animal-loving human being I have ever known, had never succeeded in being vegetarian for long because it made him feel so bad.

Eventually, I got to a point at which I did not feel bad in between meals and I did not need to eat meat at every single meal, but at a minimum of several times a week. I do make sure that I only eat organic meat, and I prefer to eat meat that was raised on a farm that I have visited and approved of or that was harvested in the wild. Fortunately, in my area, there are a lot of organic and biodynamic farms where animals live happy, comfortable lives, short though they may be. I am exceedingly grateful for my wonderful meat farmer!

Preventions, Treatments, and Coping Strategies for Digestive System Problems

I have seen so many relatives, clients, and friends with Digestive System Problems that it almost seems normal to have these problems. The most confusing aspect about what I have seen is that everyone seems to have different triggers, symptoms, and needs.

Although there are a lot of different options regarding eating, there are some aspects about eating that are likely to be true for everyone:

Reduce Digestive System Problems

1. **Do elimination diets and keep diaries to figure out what you are sensitive to, and then avoid those things no matter what.** There are multiple ways to do elimination diets; most commonly, a suspected problem food is avoided for three weeks, at which time it is tried again to see if you react to it. Note that your sensitivities may change over time; you may need to repeat the elimination diet and diary keeping if you start to get sick frequently again. Many people with hEDS are sensitive to gluten, histamine-containing foods, oxalates, salicylates, garlic, onions, peppers, and mold in food; those are a good place to start, but your sensitivities may

be specialized to you. *If you really get sick from a certain food, you won't feel sad when you have to skip it — you'll just feel glad that you won't be getting sick.*

2. **Avoid your food and environmental allergens**. Surprisingly, sometimes digestive system upset is caused by exposure to something you inhale. *Anything that you have developed a sensitivity to can disrupt your digestive system.*
3. **Live a wholesome lifestyle.** Avoid stress. Sleep well. *Anything that disrupts your body, mind, emotions, or daily rhythm can disrupt your digestive system.*
4. **Take probiotics and eat prebiotic foods.** The Cusack protocol recommends *Lactobacillus rahamnosus GG*, which has been scientifically shown to improve the gut biome and is known not to increase histamine, a hormone that can cause unpleasant symptoms for some people. Every time your stomach is upset, it's probable that your gut biome is out of balance, and if it wasn't already, the upset is probably unbalancing it. *Keep your digestive system healthy with supplementation of quality probiotics.*
5. **Eat whole foods as much as possible**. Cook from scratch. Do not eat junk food or fast food.[313, 314] Avoid synthetic food dyes, preservatives, artificial sweeteners and flavorings, seed oils, hydrogenated and partially hydrogenated oils, etc. If your body is going to have a hard time absorbing nutrients, make sure that everything you eat is nutrient dense. *If your body easily gets upset by what you ingest, make sure that you don't ingest poisons.*
6. **Choose organic foods.**[315] Eat things that were grown on farms and minimally processed. I especially approve of Biodynamic farming methods, so do some research and find out if there is a biodynamic farm in your area — get your meat, vegetables, grains, eggs, and dairy from them. Biodynamic farmers have a spiritual relationship with the earth, and their methods preserve the health of the land while producing nutritious plants and happy animals. This makes their foods better for you.[316] *Foods grown in natural ways on small farms don't contain poisons but do contain greater amounts of nutrients than conventional foods.*
7. **Prepare, store, and serve your food using nontoxic dishes, pots, pans, and utensils**. Teflon, aluminum, plastic, and other poisonous materials can leach chemicals into your food, which isn't going to help a sensitive system feel good.[317, 318, 319] Some silicon products might be okay in some circumstances, but most silicon is mixed with plastic. Wood is an acceptable material to use in the kitchen, if you treat it only with healthy food oils (not mineral oil, seed oils, or any non-natural product) and are very fastidious about making sure that it is cleaned and dried so that it will not harbor bacteria or mold. *Choose stainless steel, glass, and ceramic for preparing and serving pure foods.*
8. **Sit up straight, especially when you eat and for 3 hours afterward**. Make sure there is room for your food to move through your digestive system and for your system to do the work it's meant to do.[320] Especially concentrate on keeping your sternum (chest) lifted. In fact, keep good posture all of the time — I have learned that if I slouch long enough, I'll end up with a tummy ache. Sometimes I find myself slouching because I am cold — my abdominal muscles contract down, a precursor to shivering, so it is also important to keep yourself comfortable and relaxed. This can also happen when I am anxious or stressed; stretching the abdomen and chest by leaning back on a yoga ball can help keep my torso opened up. *Stay upright with good posture so that gravity will help the food move in the direction it should go and your digestive system won't be crowded.*
9. **Don't wear clothes that are tight around the abdomen**.[321] *Anything that compresses your stomach and intestines can upset them.*

10. **Chew your food thoroughly**. It should almost become liquid before you swallow it. If you really have a hard time doing this and you're having a lot of stomach upset, you can puree or blend your food before eating it. It's better to chew it, though, because the saliva will help digest it and chewing is good for jaw health and for keeping the nervous system balanced.[322] *Don't rush your meals.*
11. **Pay attention to your cravings**. If you are eating healthy foods, your body will present you with cravings for the foods that contain the nutrients you need at that time. (If you are eating a lot of junk food or sugar, then your cravings will not be reliable.) *Try to give your body what it knows it needs.*
12. **Eat porridge.** Many traditional cultures feed porridge to people with weak stomachs. Raw foods are more difficult to digest.[323] A porridge is usually rice or another grain well-cooked until it is very, very soft, with well-cooked vegetables and legumes. Bone broth is often used for cooking this meal, and it is mildly seasoned with salt and spices. (Bone broth can be especially beneficial for people with hEDS/HSD, but it can trigger mast cell activation in people with MCAS.) A well-cooked food is essentially partially digested, leaving less work for your stomach to do. *A porridge like this contains a lot of nutrients and can be absolutely delicious.*
13. **Limit foods that are likely to upset the stomach or cause inflammation**, even if they are considered healthy for most people. In today's world, this list is very long: hot sauce, onions, garlic, peppers, fried foods, etc.[324] *Take extra care to eat foods that are gentle on your stomach.*

REDUCE DIGESTIVE SYSTEM PROBLEMS

1. Do elimination diets and keep diaries to figure out what you are sensitive to, and then avoid those things no matter what.
2. Avoid your food and environmental allergens.
3. Live a wholesome lifestyle.
4. Take probiotics and eat prebiotic foods.
5. Eat whole foods as much as possible.
6. Choose organic foods.
7. Prepare, store, and serve your food using nontoxic dishes, pots, pans, and utensils.
8. Sit up straight, especially when you eat and for 3 hours afterward.
9. Don't wear clothes that are tight around the abdomen.
10. Chew your food thoroughly.
11. Pay attention to your cravings.
12. Eat porridge.
13. Limit foods that are likely to upset the stomach or cause inflammation.
14. Drink lots of water and healthy drinks.
15. Filter your water to remove all contaminants.
16. Drink a glass of water half an hour before a meal, but drink very little with your meal.
17. Bless your food.
18. Eat early in the day.
19. Use homeopathic remedies.
20. Drink a small dose of baking soda in water.
21. Use Earthing Therapy Patches on your stomach.
22. Stimulate the Vagus Nerve.
23. Protect your cervical spine.
24. Get Chiropractic or Osteopathic care.
25. Take trace minerals.
26. Try taking DAO 15 minutes before meals.
27. Try eating standing up.

Ask your doctor before trying anything new.

14. **Drink lots of water and healthy drinks.** Don't drink soda, alcohol, or drinks with sweeteners or preservatives. It is best for your digestion to drink warm water — I expected this to be gross, but I really enjoy it! Some of the water you drink should have a good electrolyte blend in it. It is easy to be a little bit dehydrated and not know it, and this can cause a lot of symptoms and trigger Migraine attacks and POTS episodes (see Chapter 29: POTS). *Many drinks other than water are dehydrating or at least not hydrating, so drink a lot of water.*
15. **Filter your water to remove all contaminants.** Distillers or Reverse Osmosis (RO) systems with remineralizers are the best for your drinking and cooking water. *There are so many pharmaceuticals and poisons in tap water, even my plants grow healthier when I water them with RO water.*
16. **Drink a glass of water half an hour before a meal, but drink very little with your meal.** This is to ensure your body has enough fluid to accomplish digestion but the stomach acid does not become diluted and ineffective at its jobs of breaking down food. Room temperature or warm water are better for your digestive system than cold water. I usually drink a glass of water after I put on my apron and right before I start cooking; it's become such a habit that the act of putting on my apron makes me thirsty. I have also found that having water in my stomach reduces the likelihood that I will have an MCAS reaction to either hunger or cooking smells. *You want to time your drinking of water so that your digestive system has the water it needs to digest the food, but your stomach acid will not be diluted.*
17. **Bless your food.** Say grace before eating, whether it is a religious or secular one to give thanks for this food, as well as to the chef who cooked it, the market who sold it, the farmer who grew it, the rain who watered it, the sun who energized it, and the earth who nurtured it. Scientific studies have shown that prayer and mindset change our brains and affect how our bodies respond to foods.[325, 326] There are traditions all around the world of praying before meals that can inspire you to eat with a sense of gratitude and peace. *We may take it for granted these days, but having enough food to eat at every meal is in fact a miracle and a blessing.*
18. **Eat early in the day.** You want all of your food to be digested before bedtime. When you are lying down, stomach acids, if they are profuse, can travel up the esophagus.[327] *Use gravity to help food move down through the digestive system, and sleep better.*
19. **Splurge every now and then, but be aware of what the results will be.** Your favorite childhood treat is probably good for your soul even if it's not the healthiest choice. Eat it or whatever you are really tempted by on occasion, when you have the luxury of not feeling great the next day, and take the time to really savor it. *Enjoy yourself.*
20. **Use homeopathic remedies.** Choose remedies to treat whatever symptoms you have. *Nux vomica*, *Carbo vegetalis*, *Ipecacuanha*, and others can make some difference. See Chapter 50: Homeopathic Remedies. *Homeopathic remedies are a safe way to treat indigestion, nausea, vomiting, diarrhea, and constipation.*
21. **Drink a small dose of baking soda in water.** Baking soda can settle indigestion. One quarter teaspoon of baking soda in about 2 ounces water is a good start, and you can repeat the drink as needed. (Be aware that very large amounts of baking soda are dangerous.[328]) *Baking soda is an inexpensive, quick fix that some people consider to be very good for the body, especially after exposure to an allergen or sensitivity.*[329, 330]
22. **Use Earthing Therapy Patches on your stomach.** I don't know why it works, but an hour of having my stomach plugged into the Earth's electric field often eliminates

my stomach upset. See Chapter 45: Earthing. *Earthing is such an easy way to feel better.*

23. **Stimulate the Vagus Nerve**. If you have done all of these digestive system treatments and techniques, plus probably some others, and you are still having problems, it is likely that your condition — especially if it is gastroparesis — is neurogenic (coming from the nervous system) rather than coming from problems in the physical components of the digestive tract. In this case, healing the brain and nerves and inducing a parasympathetic state is in order. See Chapter 63: Vagus Nerve Stimulation. *Your brain and nerves run all of the processes in your body, so their health impacts all of your health.*
24. **Protect your cervical spine**. Improving posture and strength in your neck is important because sometimes nausea and other digestive problems can be caused by damaged nerves or spinal cord or blood vessel compression that happen in the neck when the cervical vertebrae move around improperly. See Chapter 25: Neck Pain & CCI for more information and exercises to use. *Damaged nerves in the neck can impact any portion or action of the digestive tract, so keep your neck strong with good posture.*
25. **Get Chiropractic or Osteopathic care.** *Aligning the spine can improve gastrointestinal symptoms.*[331]
26. **Take trace minerals**. I have used ION* Intelligence of Nature Gut Support Liquid (just a few drops, not a whole dosage), as well as some varieties of fulvic and humic acids, which taste delicious mixed in hot tea and can give me energy and improve my skin, fingernails, and hair. *Trace minerals reduce inflammation, reduce allergic-type immune responses, maintain gut health, and more.*[332, 333, 334]
27. **Try taking DAO 15 minutes before meals.** If you have MCAS or histamine intolerance, it can cause severe digestive system problems. Sometimes, people with excessive histamine, a problem in removing histamine, or a sensitivity to histamine will become reactive to foods to the point that there are no foods that they can eat without getting sick. *DAO will help your body process out histamine, which can reduce or eliminate reactions to foods.*
28. **Try eating standing up.** Some people with hEDS have a condition called Median Arcuate Ligament Syndrome (MALS), in which the main blood vessel that provides blood to the abdomen is compressed by a ligament. The lack of blood to the stomach and digestive tract means that digestion cannot occur normally. In some cases of abdominal vessel compression, it is believed to be caused when the patient is low weight and there is not enough fat cushioning the ligaments and vessels; in other cases, the cause is either not known or is thought to be the way the person's body is made (these ligaments and vessels are not in exactly the same position in every body).[335] Most of the time, MALS is asymptomatic, but when it causes pain after eating, bowel function disorder, nausea, vomiting, and weight loss, it is usually treated surgically.[336, 337] However, it has also been found that for some people with MALS, the compression is relieved and blood flow is restored when they stand up.[338] The hope then would be that you could gain weight and restore the fat cushioning around the veins and ligaments. Additionally, improving your posture could only help. See Chapter 56: Posture. *If you have MALS, you may find relief if you stand up while eating and until the food is mostly digested.*

LINKS FOR PRODUCTS MENTIONED IN THIS CHAPTER

Reverse Osmosis Water Filter https://amzn.to/43m3qSZ

Probiotic https://amzn.to/3HkFUeX

Electrolytes https://amzn.to/3U4UTRO

Nux vomica https://amzn.to/3vAOKT3
Carbo Vegetalis https://amzn.to/41TiQNP
Ipecacuanha https://amzn.to/3Scgllx
Earthing Therapy Patches https://amzn.to/3VkXac5
Trace Minerals: ION* Gut Support https://amzn.to/49Dzaoj or Fulvic Acid https://amzn.to/3yOhGZB
DAO https://amzn.to/3QQKpDi or Histamine Digest https://amzn.to/3WvIqHY

14
Eye Strain

I HAVE SEEN IT SUGGESTED THAT HEDS causes extra eye strain, though I have not seen very much information about this. There are a number of other ocular manifestations of hEDS that are beyond the scope of this book.[339]

My Experience with Eye Strain

I personally get quite a lot of pain and blurry vision if I look at screens for very long (so I am often typing this book with my eyes closed). However, I find the *Bates Method to Improve Eyesight Without Glasses* to be very effective. I have never yet needed eyeglasses, though I do need a magnifying glass to read small print if I haven't been doing my Bates Method exercises.

I have not had very many clients or friends who were dedicated enough to do the Bates Method, but those who have done it have all had positive results at least to an extent.

Preventions, Treatments, and Coping Strategies for Eye Strain

These ideas are easy to try.

Prevent and Recover from Eye Strain

1. **Avoid looking at screens.** Using cell phones, computers, TVs, etc. too much harms our eyesight and creates eye strain. *Children these days need eyeglasses more frequently and at younger ages due to all of the time they spend looking at screens.*[340, 341]
2. **Take frequent breaks when looking at screens or reading books.** Set a timer if you need a reminder. *You need to move your body more than the average person anyway.*
3. **Exercise the eyes with the Bates Method.** It is especially important to do the Sunning and Palming exercises frequently. There are many other effective exercises in his book *The Bates Method for Better Eyesight Without Glasses.* With the Bates Method, some people can cure their eye health and stop wearing glasses. Some of

this information is offered free at www.seeing.org. *The shape of the eyeball and lens are determined by muscles around the eye, and they can be relaxed and retrained so that you can see well your whole life.*

4. **Go without sunglasses.** At least some of your time outdoors, wear hats with shade brims instead. Your eyes are very perceptive to sunlight; sunlight is very important to your eye and overall health. Sunglasses not only diminish the light that reaches your eye, even more importantly, they filter the light so that you do not receive all parts of the visible and invisible light spectrum. When I began this practice, I found it almost painful because my eyes were so unaccustomed to light, but ever since I made the transition, I have loved being without sunglasses. For me, it is easier to always go without sunglasses except in special circumstances, like during a Migraine attack or when driving on a sunny day with snow. *Lack of exposure to sunlight through the eyes can affect your body's production of melanin, melatonin, and numerous hormones mediated by the thyroid and pituitary gland; it can affect your sleep, appetite, energy, mood, immune system, and more.*[342, 343, 344, 345]

PREVENT AND RECOVER FROM EYE STRAIN

1. Avoid looking at screens.
2. Take frequent breaks when looking at screens or reading books.
3. Exercise the eyes with the Bates Method.
4. Go without sunglasses.

Ask your doctor before trying anything new.

LINKS FOR PRODUCTS MENTIONED IN THIS CHAPTER

The Bates Method for Better Eyesight Without Glasses https://amzn.to/3PXZz98

15

Female Reproductive Concerns – Menstruation, Contraception, Infertility, Hyperemesis Gravidarum, & Subchorionic Hematoma

HYPERMOBILITY AFFECTS WOMEN'S REPRODUCTIVE systems in a number of ways. Women with hEDS/HSD report heavy periods, no periods, and pain during sex more often than do women in the general public. They also contend with a number of other pelvic complaints. (See Chapter 27: Pelvis Complaints.)

Unfortunately, women with hEDS/HSD have a much higher rate of Infertility than the general public. In addition, they have a slightly higher incidence than the general public of childbearing-related difficulties such as Hyperemesis Gravidarum (excessive nausea and vomiting), miscarriage (loss of the pregnancy), preterm delivery (baby is born before 36 weeks of gestation), excessive bleeding associated with delivery (antenatal and postnatal hemorrhage), pre-eclampsia (high blood pressure), exceptionally fast labor (precipitous birth), postpartum psychosis (mental illness following delivery), Post Traumatic Stress Disorder from the delivery experience (difficulty recovering from a terrifying event), and more.[346] It is wise for you to make your obstetrician or midwife aware of these increased risks. Still, the great majority of hEDS pregnancies and deliveries have good outcomes.

Menstruation

The problems that women with hEDS/HSD have with their menstrual cycle vary exceedingly from very heavy bleeding to not bleeding at all. Pain, cramps, nausea, bloating, headache, and other symptoms often accompany periods, for all women.

My Experience with Menstruation

I have experienced what I consider to be fairly normal menstruation throughout my childbearing years. I have occasionally experienced cramping that was so painful that it stopped me from participating in my life for a day, but I was able to eliminate that problem once a Massage Therapist taught me an abdominal self-massage technique, which is described below.

Preventions, Treatments, and Coping Strategies for Menstruation

If you have chemical sensitivities, you probably should not be using regular mainstream menstrual products.

> MENSTRUATION
>
> 1. Use all-natural, organic products.
> 2. Do abdominal self-massage.
> 3. Anticipate menstruation by using a Saliva Ovulation Microscope.
> 4. Use extra caution to protect joints and avoid triggers during menstruation or ovulation, whichever hormone surge is most likely to make you more sensitive.
>
> Ask your doctor before trying anything new.

1. **Use all-natural, organic products in your private areas**: organic disposable pads and tampons, silicone cups (although many of these are made with plastic additives that are unsafe), cotton reusable pads, cotton period underwear, and sea sponges. My favorite are Jade & Pearl Sea Sponges, and the package includes instructions on how to use them (and re-use them). Make sure that the soap you are using is all natural and fragrance-free, and do not use other products (powders, lotions, douches, etc.) in your private areas. *The genital area is even more sensitive than the rest of the body, so it is important to use high-quality, natural products for it.*

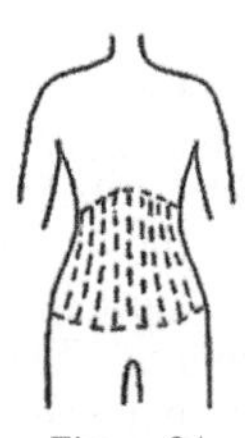

Figure 24: Abdominal Massage

2. **Do abdominal self-massage to prevent cramps.** Lying on your back, consider your abdomen to be divided in lines that stretch from your rib cage to your pelvic bones. Press your fingers down slowly along a section of one of the lines, breathing deeply, and then pressing more deeply as you release your breath. It may be painful, but hold it until the pain releases. You will begin to feel your heartbeat against your fingers, indicating that blood flow to that spot has been restored. Slowly lift up and then move to the next section along the same line and repeat the process of applying pressure. *As you release the tension in your abdomen and get the blood flowing again, you will reduce or eliminate your menstrual cramps.*
3. **Anticipate menstruation by using a Saliva Ovulation Microscope**. If your cycle is irregular, it can be hard to know when your period is coming, which can create anxiety and hassle in trying to have your products ready. Most women get their period 14 days after they ovulate, but your schedule might be different. See more about this tool in the next section, Contraception. *Whatever your schedule is, if you know when you ovulate, you will have a better idea of when you will menstruate.*
4. **Use extra caution to protect joints and avoid triggers during menstruation or ovulation, whichever hormone surge is most likely to make you more**

sensitive. Most women experience changes in their symptoms when hormones fluctuate. Ligaments can be laxer, and you can be more sensitive to your triggers for Allergies/MCAS/MCS and Migraine. *Plan around your menstrual cycle and be gentle with your body when it is doing this reproductive work.*

Contraception

I have read on a number of different websites that women with hEDS often do not respond well to hormonal contraceptives or devices like IUDs (Intrauterine Devices), nor to surgeries for permanent sterilization. Women with MCAS are often bothered by the chemicals that coat condoms, as well. What options are left?

Natural Family Planning is frowned upon because people tend not to adhere to the rules of it, but it is fairly effective when done properly (95% effective when done properly, but only 76% effective with typical use).[347] I have known women who got pregnant while on the pill or using an IUD or a condom, too, so you are always taking chances. If you do not want to get pregnant, the best option is to abstain from intercourse.

If you want to try Natural Family Planning, it should only be when it would be alright if you got pregnant; you should research it thoroughly, and perhaps take a class in it. The most important aspect of Natural Family Planning is getting to know the cycles of your own body, and I believe it would benefit all women to do this, regardless of their reproductive aims and contraceptive choices.

Keep a diary of your symptoms each day of your cycle for a few months and see what patterns emerge. Be sure to record information about your Cervical Mucous (the fluid that is in your vagina); you should notice that it is clear, abundant, slippery, and stretchy at the time of month when you are about to ovulate. Measure your body temperature with a thermometer every morning at the same time, before you get out of bed, to confirm that your CM changes are in line with your temperature changes. A little bit more challenging but interesting is feeling inside to determine the position and texture of your cervix as it changes throughout the month. To help confirm your observations, use ovulation predictor tests that measure the Luteinizing Hormone (LH) in your urine.

Once you are familiar with how your body changes during your cycle, a simpler method of gauging when you ovulate is to use a Saliva Microscope Ovulation Tester. Affordable and easy to use, this is a lipstick-size microscope with a built-in light through which you can see if your spit indicates ovulation. In the morning, regardless of what time you wake up, you use your finger to put a little bit of spit onto the glass of the microscope. (You can put your saliva onto the microscope at any time of day, though it is recommended that you wait two hours after you eat.) Let the saliva dry completely (this takes so long that I usually just wait a couple hours before I go back to check it). Then look at the saliva through the microscope viewer. When you are not near ovulation, you will see a jumble of shapes, but as you near ovulation, you will see a more and more distinct fern pattern; the estrogen in the saliva causes the liquid to dry in a crystal formation.

If you have a normal cycle, you can expect your period to start 14 days after you ovulate (if you are not pregnant). However, your cycle might be slightly different, or you might ovulate more than once during the cycle. If your period starts sooner than 13 or 14 days, it might mean that you have a hormonal imbalance, so this is valuable information.

My Experience with Contraception

When I took a hormonal contraception, after just 3 months, I experienced a mini-stroke (Transient Ischemic Attack). The neurologist who treated me said that I had suffered no long-term effects and should continue to use the hormone pills, but I did not want to risk another mini-stroke or worse.

Strategies for Contraception

Contraception choices are very personal, and everyone's preferences and circumstances are different. New options become available all of the time, as well, so talk with your doctor or a homebirth midwife to learn all of your options.

1. **Get to know your own body's cycles**. Keep track of your Cervical Mucous, Basal Body Temperature, cervix positioning and texture, and Luteinizing Hormone Levels. Also learn what your emotional, energy, flexibility, joint stability, and other changes are throughout the cycle. Use a Saliva Microscope Ovulation Tester to confirm ovulation easily. *It is very empowering to know your own body and to be able to anticipate and understand how it moves through the menstrual cycle.*
2. **Ask your doctor or midwife for guidance**. *Choose the right contraception for yourself.*

> STRATEGIES FOR CONTRACEPTION
>
> 1. Get to know your own body's cycles.
> 2. Ask your doctor or midwife for guidance.
>
> Ask your doctor before trying anything new.

Infertility

Reproductive Infertility is much more common among people with hEDS than the general population (44% versus 10%).[348] There are a number of different possible causes of this that are beyond the scope of this book. There are also a lot of women with hEDS/HSD who are having babies, so there is some hope if you want to become pregnant.

Some fertility-boosting recommendations based on what I have heard from professional colleagues and friends are listed here. If these ideas do not result in conception, consult a professional.

My Experience with Infertility

I have a family member who has struggled with Infertility, and I see the agonizing emotional pain it causes, but I have also witnessed her adopt a child. It turns out that adoption was what God was calling her to do all along. Giving this wonderful child a safe, happy childhood is the most noble and fulfilling act you can imagine.

Preventions, Treatments, and Coping Strategies for Infertility

Everything I have read about trying to conceive that has seemed to me to be smart has essentially indicated that fertility equals good health, so efforts to improve fertility may be good for your body, regardless of the outcome.

Fertility Boosting Ideas

1. **Heal your symptoms of hEDS/HSD and secondary conditions.** *Good health is key to fertility.*[349]
2. **Read *It Starts with the Egg* by Rebecca Fett.** This book gives lifestyle and nutritional supplement recommendations that have been helpful for some women to be able to conceive and that are in line with many of the ideas in this book. *Lifestyle changes and nutritional supplements can make a difference for female fertility.*
3. **Get Chiropractic or Osteopathic care.** See Section VI: Seek Professional Help. *A properly aligned spine enhances fertility.*[350]
4. **Get Acupuncture and Traditional Chinese Medicine treatment.** One of the most popular self-help tenets of this tradition is keeping the womb warm. *This traditional, holistic approach makes a difference for a lot of women.*[351, 352]
5. **Eliminate silent infections.** *Although they may not cause noticeable symptoms the way a flu bug would, hidden viruses, bacteria, and parasites in the body can reduce fertility.*[353]
6. **Baby Dance on the few days leading up to ovulation.** Like the Native Americans' Rain Dancing, Baby Dancing (having sex) honorably let's God know what you want, and of course, actually facilitates conception. *Use the saliva microscope mentioned above in the Contraception section to help you judge your most fertile days, when there are ferns in the microscope.*
7. **Reduce stress.** Not only does stress reduce conception rates, Infertility itself creates feelings of stress, depression, and anxiety in the women who experience it.[354] There are a number of techniques for reducing stress explained in this book, such as Forest Bathing, Vagus Nerve Stimulation, and more. *Reducing stress is an important aspect of improving your health and letting your body know that this is a good time to bring a baby into the world.*
8. **Get a professional Mayan Abdominal Massage.** This can help get the uterus and ovaries into the correct position, as well as bring blood flow to the reproductive organs.[355] *There are videos on YouTube for self-abdominal massage as well.*

FERTILITY BOOSTING IDEAS

1. Heal your symptoms of hEDS/HSD and secondary conditions.
2. Read *It Starts with the Egg.*
3. Get Chiropractic or Osteopathic care.
4. Get Acupuncture and Traditional Chinese Medicine treatment.
5. Eliminate silent infections.
6. Baby Dance on the few days leading up to ovulation.
7. Reduce stress.
8. Get a professional Mayan Abdominal Massage.

Ask your doctor before trying anything new.

Hyperemesis Gravidarum During Pregnancy

Hyperemesis Gravidarum (HG) is a severe form of nausea and vomiting in pregnancy. It occurs in over 25% of pregnant women who have hEDS (but only 3% of the general population).[356] It does not usually result in negative outcomes for the baby or mother, but some of the medications used to treat HG are known to come with a risk of causing birth defects in the baby.

Whereas it is expected for women to get nausea during pregnancy, HG isn't morning sickness or even the kind of morning sickness that hits at other times of day. HG is a constant nausea that causes weight loss and dehydration. It is so severe that it is dangerous for both baby and mom if left untreated, and it is so miserable that it significantly increases the incidence of suicide during pregnancy.

Some medical professionals are unclear about the differences between "morning sickness" and HG — they tend to say that if morning sickness is really bad and/or continues beyond the first trimester, then it is HG. But in fact, the symptoms of the two are different, though they both include nausea and vomiting. HG causes the mother to lose more than 5% of her body weight and frequently causes severe dehydration. It is important to recognize the difference because HG is best treated early before it escalates.

Morning sickness is frequently caused by low blood sugar (pregnancy-induced hypoglycemia), while HG is there regardless of blood sugar levels. Morning sickness is often cured with good posture or physical activity, whereas HG tends to diminish with a reclining position and as little movement as possible. Herbal teas tend to diminish morning sickness, whereas most fluids, and especially warm fluids, can't usually be tolerated with HG.

Doctors and midwives have conflicting opinions about what causes HG. Some believe it is a problem in the gut biome, while others believe the body is in need of a detox, some think it is a neurological condition, others that it is essentially an allergy to pregnancy hormones, or perhaps it is a manifestation of MCAS that was triggered by the fluctuating hormones of pregnancy — and the list goes on.

It is common for women to have HG in subsequent pregnancies, but the few I have known who had it in early pregnancies and not later ones made big changes in their health between pregnancies. If you are planning to get pregnant, it is certainly worthwhile to detox, balance your gut biome, and become as healthy as possible.

My Experience with Hyperemesis Gravidarum

I suffered with HG during my pregnancy, and at first, I was losing weight quickly. My nausea was so severe that if I sat up, I would throw up. It was so severe that if my mother asked me a question, I would respond with a nonsensical string of words. There were even a few days when I had reached my limit of how much I could take, and if it weren't for the prayers and support of my friends, I might have tried to end my life. And all of this was happening during the happiest time of my life — I had always wanted to have a baby more than anything in the world.

At the time, there were no medications that didn't carry a risk of birth defects, so true to my nature, I wanted to find a safer way to cope with my condition. I was in chat groups with women who were struggling with HG, and when they delivered their babies, they then transitioned to chat rooms for moms coping with babies who had birth defects. I was determined not to use medication, and I am glad it worked out for me because my baby was born perfectly healthy and is now a delightful, healthy 10-year-old.

My big turn-around with HG occurred when a friend who had survived cancer and chemotherapy treatments shared with me her tricks for beating nausea. They were not all-natural like all of the other recommendations I am making in this book, but they worked well, whereas the natural recommendations given by the wonderful Traditional Chinese Medicine clinic in my town worked but not well enough. The main recommendations were for fountain sodas and sugar; I normally do not consume much of these except on rare occasions, but sugar has anti-emetic (reduces nausea and vomiting), anti-pain, and anti-anxiety properties.[357, 358, 359] This may be part of why sugar can be addictive.[360, 361] I doubt that sugar would have the same healing properties for someone who has sodas and sugar on a daily basis. During pregnancy, as always, it is a good idea to avoid eating sugar, since it can increase risks of gestational diabetes, preeclampsia, preterm birth, and other pregnancy complications.[362]

Preventions, Treatments, and Coping Strategies for Hyperemesis Gravidarum

As I was reviewing my list of treatments and coping strategies for HG, which was compiled 11 years ago, I realized that most of them are the same as my strategies for MCAS. A quick internet search found a correlation between histamine levels and HG, and doctors suggesting that HG is actually MCAS.[363] Just as there is a great variety in people's MCAS triggers, every woman has different HG triggers.

Reduce Hyperemesis Gravidarum Nausea

1. **Keep the nausea minimized as much as possible.** *This will be easier than trying to decrease the nausea after it has already become serious.*
2. **Keep your MCAS under control**. See Chapter 11: Allergy, MCAS, & MCS. *Avoid triggers.*
3. **Take organic liquid chlorophyll.**[364] Drink it plain or pour it into juice, a smoothie, or apple sauce; if you have nausea, sip tiny little sips of it instead. This is a midwife-recommended supplement that contains the building blocks of blood, which is important at this time when your body is needing to increase the amount of blood. I have known women who had iron deficiency anemia when pregnant and successfully treated it with liquid chlorophyll instead of iron supplements without upsetting their stomachs as iron can do. *By improving blood parameters with chlorophyll, you can reduce your fatigue, dizziness, and nausea.*
4. **Use Homeopathic Remedies.** *Nux vomica* is especially

REDUCE HYPEREMESIS GRAVIDARUM NAUSEA

1. Keep the nausea minimized as much as possible.
2. Keep your MCAS under control.
3. Take organic liquid chlorophyll.
4. Use Homeopathic Remedies such as *Nux vomica.*
5. If drinking liquids exacerbates your nausea, chew pellet ice instead.
6. When nausea is severe, drink one fountain soda and then eat a high-fat, high-protein meal.
7. Eat a small candy to prepare for eating a meal.
8. Wear a Sea Band wrist acupressure band on one wrist and an electric shock wristband on the other wrist.
9. Protect the joints.
10. Take Papaya Enzyme with meals.
11. Chew gum after a meal.
12. Reconsider taking vitamins.
13. Eat high-protein snacks.
14. Massage acupressure points.
15. Use disposable dishes and utensils.

Ask your doctor before trying anything new.

indicated. See Chapter 50: Homeopathic Remedies. *This is a safe, easily tolerated treatment to try.*

5. **If drinking liquids exacerbates your nausea, chew pellet ice instead** (which can be purchased by the bagful inexpensively at Sonic). *It is important to stay hydrated even if you can't drink liquids.*
6. **When nausea is severe, drink one fountain soda and then eat a high fat, high protein meal**. Canned and bottled sodas will not work for this purpose. Only the formulation of fountain sodas will decrease nausea.[365, 366] *This is only recommended once per day or less; drink too many sodas and they will lose their effectiveness.*
7. **Eat a small candy to prepare for eating a meal.** A sweet treat can soothe nausea before eating regular food. *Sugar can settle the stomach.* [367]
8. **Wear a Sea Band wrist acupressure band on one wrist and an electric shock wristband on the other wrist**. *Alternate wrists between the Sea Band and the electric shock wristband, and turn the electricity on and off from time to time so that you don't become insensitive to it.*
9. **Protect your joints**. See Chapter 9: Joint Instability & Pain. *Protecting the posture and joints helps prevent nausea.*
10. **Take Papaya Enzyme with meals**. *This helps with digestion.*
11. **Chew gum after a meal.** (Avoid gum with artificial sweeteners, although xylitol in small amounts may be a good choice for you.) *Chewing gum increases saliva, increases hunger, and promotes bowel function.*[368, 369]
12. **Reconsider taking vitamins.** Many women experience that vitamins increase nausea; sometimes this is specific vitamins in the multi-vitamin pill, or the size of the pill itself.[370, 371] Talk to your doctor or midwife about what your supplementation needs are, if any, and which brands are recommended. *Going without supplemental vitamins may be the best way to reduce nausea, but some studies have found evidence that HG is sometimes caused by deficiency of certain vitamins.*[372]
13. **Eat high protein snacks** to balance blood sugars. Once I was able to begin eating again, some of my favorite snacks that kept the nausea at bay were edamame (frozen, shelled soybeans, not cooked but well salted, and allowed to thaw by my bedside), graham crackers with peanut butter, apple with peanut butter, and yogurt. Keep snacks at your bedside so that your blood sugar can stay balanced at night. *Always have snacks handy.*
14. **Massage acupressure points.**[373, 374] This includes the stomach acupuncture line from the shin to between the 2nd and 3rd toes. Also, massage the palm of the hand in a clockwise motion, which keeps the bowels moving. *Acupressure is an easy treatment you can do for yourself anytime; it is also nice to have a loved one massage you.*
15. **Use disposable dishes and utensils**. Also ask a loved one to do your house chores for you. *Give yourself a break any way you can so that you can focus on your health.*

Subchorionic Hematoma During Pregnancy

Subchorionic Hematoma (SCH) is caused when blood leaks between the uterine wall and the placenta.[375] If this occurs, it is usually during implantation, though the blood can be held in a pocket beneath the placenta for some time and then work its way out and leak from the vagina at a later date. It usually causes spotting but can also cause very heavy bleeding from the vagina. The bleeding may be accompanied by cramps. If the SCH occurs later in the pregnancy, it may be a greater cause for concern.

I have not found research documenting a correlation between SCH and hEDS, but considering what I know of hEDS, it follows logically that it would contribute to the likelihood of developing an SCH, which may develop due to vein fragility.

It is a good idea to see your midwife or OB in case the bleed causes a "spontaneous abortion" (miscarriage or loss of the baby) and other complications occur. However, SCHs usually resolve themselves with no harm to the baby or mother. The only treatment for them is usually bed rest and pelvic rest, though obstetricians and Traditional Chinese Medicine doctors have begun recommending certain nutritional supplements and drugs.

My Experience with SCH

I experienced an SCH early during my pregnancy. When the SCH occurred, I was referred to a high-risk obstetrician, who put me on pelvic rest and advised me either to continue with daily activity as usual (but don't move furniture or carry heavy boxes) or to rest in bed. At the time, he said, the science was mixed regarding the effectiveness of bed rest for this condition; based on a quick review I recently made of the most up-to-date studies on the topic, the scientific opinion remains mixed, though it seems to be leaning toward recommending bed rest.

For me, typical daily activity increased the cramping and bleeding. Also, women with SCH in chat rooms online reported miscarriages following daily activity; whether it would have helped them or not, they wished they had tried bed rest. So, I maintained bed rest, and fortunately, after about 12 weeks, the SCH completely resolved. At that time, I was released from the high-risk obstetrician and cleared to go forward with my home birth plans. My baby is now a healthy, happy, brilliant 10-year-old boy.

Coping Strategies for SCH

1. **Follow your doctor's orders.** Probably, ultrasound imaging will be used to assess the situation. *Pelvic rest, medication, and supplements may be prescribed.*
2. **Rest in bed.** You can get up to use the bathroom, bathe, and get something to eat, but do not exert yourself. *Be gentle with your body while it repairs the connection between the womb and the placenta.*
3. **Pray.** Lying in bed, you will have plenty of time to pray. *Jesus, the healer, and Mary, the mother, or whatever forces or spirits are meaningful to you will be there for you.*

COPING STRATEGIES FOR SCH

1. Follow your doctor's orders.
2. Rest in bed.
3. Pray.

Ask your doctor before trying anything new.

LINKS FOR PRODUCTS MENTIONED IN THIS CHAPTER

Sea Sponges https://amzn.to/3HeKoUr

It Starts With the Egg https://amzn.to/3wPDPWk

Fertility Microscope https://amzn.to/3VhXCrG

Liquid Chlorophyll https://amzn.to/3W11cqp

Sea Bands https://amzn.to/3tT4hND

Electric Shock Bracelet https://amzn.to/48B2ko4

Papaya Enzymes https://amzn.to/3UeJONY

16

Foot Pain — Plantar Fasciitis, Bunion, & Flat Feet

THE MAJORITY OF PEOPLE WITH HEDS/HSD have foot and ankle hypermobility, along with more lower limb pain than in the general public.[376] Some of the most common manifestations of Joint Instability in the foot are Plantar Fasciitis, Bunion, and Flat Feet.

Plantar Fasciitis

Plantar Fasciitis is an inflammation of the plantar fascia of the foot.[377] The plantar fascia is a bundle of fibrous tissues, much like a ligament, that runs from the heel, supports the arch of the foot, and then divides and extends into the toes. Most commonly, Plantar Fasciitis causes pain in the heel that is worst in the mornings, but it can cause perpetual pain throughout the sole of the foot that tends to get worse at the end of the day.

People with hEDS are prone to having inflamed tissues already, plus the hypermobility of the feet and knees make them prone to Plantar Fasciitis. Knee hypermobility can cause tightness in the soleus (the muscle on the back of the calf), which connects to the heel and transfers tightness there. Also, in a case of knee hyperextension, the fascia on the back of the leg will become shortened and pull on the fascia in the foot.[378]

My Experience with Plantar Fasciitis

Plantar Fasciitis can cause stress fractures of the sesamoid, which is what happened to me — one of the small bones under the big toe that act like knee caps for the toe joint broke in half and caused pain for two decades or more. A friend of mine had Plantar Fasciitis so badly that the tissue pulled on the bone of her heel until a little piece of bone broke off; she was in a lot of pain but reversed the condition by wearing a doctor-prescribed boot that kept her foot flexed at all times.

At various times in my life, I have had severe Plantar Fasciitis, and I know it as a pain that can prevent walking. My dedication to dance and gymnastics exacerbated my

Plantar Fasciitis condition, but fortunately, I was able to heal it with the techniques listed below. I now always cross train so that I do not develop the condition again.

I also relieved my husband's Plantar Fasciitis with these techniques, and something interesting I noticed when I massaged his feet was that they were seemingly permanently wrinkled, and the skin was stiff. However, over the weeks of my treatment, the skin softened, the joints became more flexible, and the wrinkles disappeared, along with the painful condition.

The following list of recommendations is appropriate not only for treating Plantar Fasciitis but also for preventing it.

Preventions, Treatments, and Coping Strategies for Plantar Fasciitis

It takes dedication to treat Plantar Fasciitis, but the clients I have worked with have all found immediate relief, and their condition disappeared usually within a month. Better yet, use these tactics to prevent it from ever developing.

Treat Plantar Fasciitis

1. **Roll balls under your feet**. This is probably the most important and quickest way to relieve Plantar Fasciitis. The Melt Method balls are specially designed for this, and they truly work for this purpose better than any of the many other kinds of balls (and frozen water bottles) I have tried. *You can use the Melt Method balls at home, but it is even better to learn how to use them by taking a workshop with a Melt Method practitioner.*
2. **Massage the foot and leg**. When things go wrong in our bodies, the muscles tend to tense up to protect us. *Learn new movement patterns and then cajole your muscles into releasing their tension by massaging them.*
3. **Avoid hyperextending the knees**. Bending the knees backward can put undue force on the plantar fascia, even if it does not hurt the knee. See Chapter 56: Posture. *We always want to avoid hyperextending.*
4. **Keep the muscles of the lower leg balanced between the front (shin) and the back (calf).** Massage the lower leg, then stand up holding something for balance and raise your heels to stand on your toes (do a relevé) for 4 seconds, lower, raise the toes to stand on your heels for 4 seconds, lower, do a knee bend with the feet flat on the floor to stretch the calf and heel. Repeat as many times as feels helpful. *Especially if you point your feet in dance, gymnastics, or other activities including wearing high heels, you may develop overly strong and tight calves with shortened muscles and ligaments, so you need to strengthen your feet to move to a flexed position to counteract that imbalance.*
5. **Elongate the muscles of the calves and thighs**. Never stretch too hard and long, but do gentle stretches that move slowly into a lunge to stretch out the calf. *The tightness that causes Plantar Fasciitis can reach all the way to the hip, so gently release hypertonicity, lengthen muscles, and take the stress off of the ligaments of the leg.*
6. **Do not point your toes when it is not necessary**. Make sure you are not sleeping with your toes pointed — wear a firm boot to bed if you need help making this a

habit. *Plantar fasciitis often occurs when the soft tissues of the soles of the feet and back of the legs become too short, so make a habit of keeping them long.*

7. **Give yourself foot baths.** Use warm water and Ancient Minerals magnesium flakes or Epsom salts. *This should feel so good that you can feel any tension and inflammation dissolve away.*
8. **Moisturize with organic oil** — olive oil, jojoba oil, shea butter, or your favorite oil. Give your feet nutrients to help them repair. Make sure to let your feet dry completely after applying the oil, or put on socks so you don't leave footprints on the floor. *It feels so good.*
9. **Use Earthing Therapy Patches on your feet**. These will help reduce inflammation and pain. When your feet are well enough and the weather outside permits, walk barefoot on the grass, sand, or whatever ground you have available. *The connection with the earth and the challenge of the uneven ground will be very good for your feet.*
10. **Wear barefoot/minimalist shoes**. Be prepared that you may need to build up strength in order to comfortably wear these shoes, so transition as slowly as needed. You can begin by removing the arch supports from the shoes you usually wear. Barefoot/minimalist shoes have wide toe boxes; thin, flexible soles; no arch support; and no lifted heel. Some of my favorite brands can be found at PedTerra.com . I also especially like Vivobarefoot, Carets, Xero, and Merrell, but there are many more to choose from. Although many barefoot shoes are high-priced, they are worth it and tend to be well made, lasting a long time as well as being repairable by a cobbler. *Barefoot/minimalist shoes allow your feet to function the way they are designed to function and to maintain their strength throughout your life, plus they are comfortable.*

TREAT PLANTAR FASCIITIS

1. Roll balls under your feet.
2. Massage the foot and leg.
3. Avoid hyperextending the knees.
4. Keep the muscles of the lower leg balanced on the front (shin) and back (calf).
5. Elongate the muscles of the back of the legs.
6. Do not point the toes when it is not necessary.
7. Give yourself foot baths.
8. Moisturize with organic oils.
9. Use Earthing Therapy Patches on your feet.
10. Wear barefoot/minimalist shoes.

Ask your doctor before trying anything new.

Bunion and Tailor's Bunion

Many people suffer with Bunions, mainly because of the narrow, pointy-toed, and elevated-heel shoes that most people wear.[379, 380] People with hEDS are even more prone to Bunions because our bones slide around so easily. Bunions are very painful and get worse as time goes on; they also become more difficult to treat, so it is best to catch them early and do something about them.

Doctors often offer surgery to "correct" Bunions. Considering that this is a standard treatment, it must be successful much of the time, but I personally have not talked with anyone whose Bunions were improved with surgery. The people I know who have had the surgery have regretted it. Either way, people with hEDS/HSD are more likely to have adverse outcomes from surgery, and I always want to try to heal an ailment with my own power, naturally, before resulting to extreme measures like surgery.[381]

My Experience with Bunions

I had Bunions most of my adult life. Not only did I have lax joints and always wore typical shoes with pointy toes, I also stood with most of my weight on my toes, and worst of all, I danced *en pointe* in ballet. I had a lot of reasons to develop Bunions.

It never bothered me much...until they started to hurt. When the pain became really bad, I looked up online what to do about it, and I found a list of "yoga poses" to heal Bunion. I wish I had taken a "before" picture of my feet because after 10 minutes of doing the exercises, my "after" picture would have been astoundingly different. It was shockingly good news.

Although I got an enormous improvement at once, I wanted full improvement, so I worked hard on the exercises. They are not easy to do; it was a funny experience to sit still in a chair, trying with all of my might to get my pinkie toes to move, sweat pouring off my brow, my breath coming hard with exertion, and not any of my body moving, not even my little toes. Eventually, with the assistance of my hands moving my toes, I was able to train them to move some.

My feet have continued to improve, and I had especially large jumps in improvement when I stopped hyperextending my knees and started putting comfrey oil on my feet. I am happy to report that my feet do not hurt now.

Having seen these good results, I have shared this information with dance students, fellow professional dancers, and clients at my holistic healing center. Everyone who was dedicated enough to do the exercises saw improvement and reduction in pain.

Preventions, Treatments, and Coping Strategies for Bunions

Note that it may be helpful to address a Plantar Fasciitis condition prior to addressing Bunions.

Heal Bunions Without Surgery

1. **Do foot yoga,** including the stretches, massages, and exercises such as the ones on Yoga International's website. They include relaxing hypertonic muscles with self-massage; spreading toes apart; and lifting from the floor toes individually and in twos or threes, in varying patterns. You may notice a large improvement immediately upon following this protocol, but results will continue to occur if you continue the protocol for at least six months or the rest of your life. *My improvement after one session of doing these exercises was truly remarkable.*
   https://yogainternational.com/article/view/9-poses-to-prevent-Bunions-relieve-Bunion-pain/
2. **Stand with proper posture.** Of special note is to keep your weight mostly on the heels. Also, keep your arches lifted, ankles straight, and do not hyperextend your knees. See Chapter 56: Posture. Weight on your toes will encourage them to spread; weight on the inside of the foot will allow the Tailor's Bunion to protrude; hyperextended knees will put too much strain on the heels and soles of the feet. *Use the strength of your entire body to keep yourself lifting out of your feet instead of sinking down into them.*
3. **Balance the muscles of the lower leg**, which can reduce hypertonicity there that can affect the muscles of the foot. Massage the lower leg, then stand up holding something for balance and raise your heels to stand on your toes (do a relevé with legs parallel) for 4 seconds, lower, raise the toes to stand on your heels for 4 seconds, lower, do a knee bend with the feet flat on the floor. Always keep your ankles straight;

hold a tennis ball between your ankles if you need a sensory reminder of their proper position. Repeat as many times as feels helpful. *This should give you nicely sculpted calves as well as more freedom of movement when running and playing.*

> **HEAL BUNIONS WITHOUT SURGERY**
>
> 1. Do foot yoga.
> 2. Stand with proper posture.
> 3. Balance the muscles of the lower leg.
> 4. Walk barefoot on uneven ground.
> 5. Wear barefoot/minimalist shoes.
> 6. Make sure your socks and slippers are not tight.
> 7. Apply magnesium oil.
> 8. Wear toe separators.
>
> Ask your doctor before trying anything new.

4. **Walk barefoot on uneven ground.** Find safe places with various safe ground coverings — grass, pebbles, pine needles, sand, etc. — and walk barefoot as long as you can without tiring your feet. This is the most effective way of increasing flexibility and strength in your feet. A bonus is that it will serve as acupressure treatment, making your entire body healthier. It will also allow you to "earth" or "ground." Coming into contact with the electrical field of the earth has shown measurable improvement in various health measures within twenty minutes, especially reducing inflammation. *It can also be a great stress-reliever and enjoyable way to spend some time.*
5. **Wear barefoot/minimalist shoes.** Be prepared that you may need to build up strength in order to comfortably wear these shoes, so transition as slowly as needed. Shoes should have wide toe boxes; thin, flexible soles; no arch support; and no lifted heel. Some of my favorite brands can be found at PedTerra.com , Vivobarefoot, Carets, Xero, and Merrell, but there are many more to choose from. *Although many barefoot shoes are high-priced, they are worth it and tend to be well made, lasting a long time as well as being repairable by a cobbler.*
6. **Make sure your socks and slippers are not tight.** *Although socks are not likely to squeeze your toes together as much as the typical shoe, any kind of squeezing of the toes can contribute to Bunions.*
7. **Apply magnesium oil.** Apply magnesium oil (a blend of Ancient Minerals magnesium flakes and filtered water) or keep a magnesite stone inside your sock so that the stone is against your skin. *Magnesium will help relax muscles so that the bones can move back into position.*
8. **Wear toe separators.** There are many varieties of toe socks, toe shoes, yoga toes, and other toe-separating devices available. *Squeezing toes together will increase Bunions; separating toes will reduce them.*

Flat Feet

Flat Feet, also known as Fallen Arches, is a condition in which the arch of the foot is lower than it should be. This may be caused by lax ligaments, and it can cause pain and reduced stability and balance when standing.[382] The treatment for Flat Feet is either orthotics (inserts worn in shoes to hold up the arch), which may provide immediate relief, or exercises, which may take a long time to make a difference. Despite this, I recommend exercises so that your feet will recover their strength and health, which affects other aspects of the foot, lower leg, and ultimately the full body's posture, whereas orthotics can potentially stretch out the lax ligaments even further and prevent the muscles from gaining or maintaining strength.

My Experience with Flat Feet

Flat feet do not run in my family, but I have had dance students and healing clients with Flat Feet. They all reported that they hurt a lot.

My clients found relief from the pain by putting earthing electrodes on their feet. Within as little as half an hour, their pain would disappear, even if it was the end of the day when their feet were the most painful. However, I did not see their foot shape improve.

With my dancers, though, it was a different story. Often within a year, my dancers developed arches, and their pain went away for good. Their feet looked prettier after training them through dance, too.

Preventions, Treatments, and Coping Strategies for Flat Feet

It may take over a month before you begin to see improvement, but keep up the work and you should be rewarded.

Heal Flat Feet

1. **Do *tendus*.** This is an exercise in which you start with your feet together, then slide your foot away from your body, keeping the toes on the ground. (First the heel lifts up, then the ball of the foot.) After reaching a full extension or point (*tendu* is French for stretch), then you slide your foot back to your standing foot, lowering first the ball of the foot and then the heel. *There are numerous dance techniques that help build healthy arches; the most important is probably the* tendu.

Move smoothly from the starting position through the next three positions, keeping the toes on the floor

Figure 31: How to do a tendu

2. **Do *dégagés* and *grand battements*.** The *tendu* is the first movement of *dégagé* (French for disengage) in which the toe lifts a couple inches off the floor after it has stretched all the way, and then *grand battement* (large beating movement) starts with a *dégagé* and gets lifted as high as you can take it. Be sure to stretch the legs with a deep knee bend or flexed foot motion afterward. *All of these exercises will help build the arch muscles.*
3. **Do *relevés*.** Another beneficial movement is the *relevé* (rise), which is done by raising your heels off the ground until you are standing only on the balls of the feet and toes with the straight leg extending directly up from the balls of the feet. Then lower and repeat. Always keep your ankles straight; hold a tennis ball between your ankles if you need a sensory reminder of their proper position. Be sure to stretch the

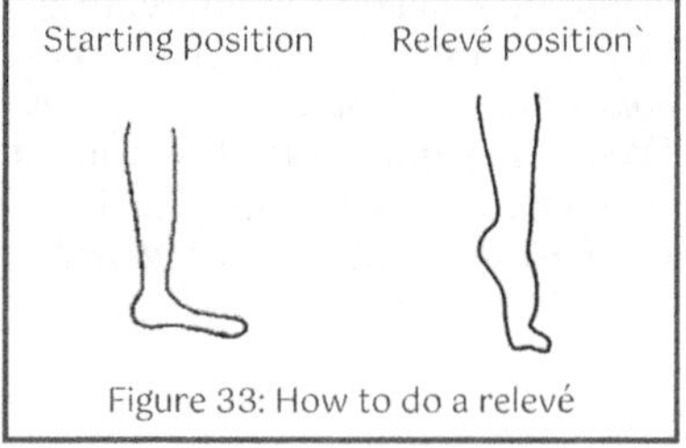

Figure 33: How to do a relevé

> **HEAL FLAT FEET**
>
> 1. Do *tendus.*
> 2. Do *dégagés* and *grand battements.*
> 3. Do *relevés.*
> 4. Do not wear arch supports.
>
> Ask your doctor before trying anything new.

legs with a deep knee bend afterward. Relevés *are like weight lifting for the feet.*

4. **Do not wear arch supports.** Be careful in choosing shoes, which may have built-in arch supports. Most of the time, I recommend barefoot/minimalist shoes. If your arches are always being supported by your shoes, your muscles will never bother to do the supporting and your feet will always be flat when not in shoes. However, when you are transitioning to wearing barefoot/minimalist shoes, sometimes using arch supports for a portion of the day to stretch the feet or give them relief can be helpful. Usually, if your shoes have arch supports in them, you can remove the inserts and go without or put in flat inserts. *Train your feet to support themselves so that they do not need arch supports as inserts or built into your shoes.*

LINKS FOR PRODUCTS MENTIONED IN THIS CHAPTER

Olive Oil https://amzn.to/3VwrYqh

Melt Method Balls https://amzn.to/3u481vV

Magnesium Flakes https://amzn.to/3HrNIvn

Barefoot Shoes www.pedterra.com , www.vivobarefoot.com , www.xeroshoes.com , www.carets.com , or https://www.merrell.com/US/en/barefoot-shoes/

Toe Separating Socks https://amzn.to/3ICd3Dn

Cork Shoe Inserts https://amzn.to/3PYfpAD

Earthing Therapy Patches https://amzn.to/424RmVs

17

Growing Pains

WHEN CHILDREN EXPERIENCE PAIN IN THE arms and legs, especially at bedtime, in the absence of any other diagnosis, it is usually assumed to be Growing Pains...even though scientists say that growing does not hurt and Growing Pains are not associated with growth spurts.[383]

Although there have been few studies looking at the incidence of Growing Pains, it has been noticed that they occur more frequently among children who are hypermobile.[384] Growing pains are also correlated with Migraine, possibly with the same triggers as Migraine.[385]

According to numerous people with hEDS who have commented in social media groups, what doctors call Growing Pains are actually pain from Joint Injury. Their experience is that the pain they felt as a child did not end when they stopped growing; as adults, with their mature knowledge of their bodies, they could feel that the same pain indicated Joint Injury. There may be other causes of Growing Pains, but it is worth trying the Joint Injury treatments, which also might relieve the pains even if they are caused by other conditions.

My Experience with "Growing Pains"

My sweet son gets what we have called Growing Pains because they do often occur when he has had a growth spurt. My suspicion is that he is more likely to injure joints when his body has changed through growth and it is unfamiliar. He also tends to get Growing Pains after doing a lot of strenuous exercise, especially at the beginning of a sports team season, for example.

A lot of the time, ice is my son's preferred treatment; it numbs the pain so that he can sleep. What tends to be most effective for curing the pain so that it won't hurt the next day either is if I give him massages. It also helps for him to have enough blankets to keep him very warm and relaxed and enough pillows to support his body while he sleeps.

Preventions, Treatments, and Coping Strategies for "Growing Pains"

Please do not ignore your child's pain, even if you do not know what caused it.[386]

Ease "Growing Pains"

EASE GROWING PAINS

1. Apply ice.
2. Apply heat.
3. Massage.
4. Apply comfrey oil.
5. Apply magnesium oil.
6. Offer *Arnica montana.*
7. See an Osteopath.
8. Treat possible joint injuries.
9. Get Physical Therapy.

Ask your doctor before trying anything new.

1. **Apply ice.** *If there is inflammation from an injury, ice will reduce it, and ice numbs the pain, though it can slow healing or even cause damage when used too much.*[387]
2. **Apply heat.** *A heating pad on the affected areas or an electric blanket on the whole body can help because it relaxes and soothes muscles.*[388]
3. **Massage.** Myofascial Release Massage is especially helpful. See Chapter 52. *Children usually love to be massaged by their parents, and it can relax and soothe muscles.*
4. **Apply comfrey oil.** *Comfrey oil speeds healing and reduces pain.*[389]
5. **Apply magnesium oil.** *Magnesium oil will help the muscles heal themselves and reduce any cramping or hypertonicity.*[390]
6. **Offer *Arnica montana.*** This remedy can be taken as a sugar pill that melts under the tongue or applied as a cream on the area that hurts. See Chapter 51: Homeopathic Remedies. *The homeopathic remedy, Arnica montana, reduces the pain of bruises, scratches, Joint Injuries, and even emotional upsets.*
7. **See an Osteopath.** Children challenge and injure their bodies jumping off of jungle gyms, falling out of trees, catching their legs on the playground merry-go-round. Frequent visits to the Osteopath can get them back in alignment before a problem develops. Osteopathic treatment is usually gentler than chiropractic techniques, and children respond well to osteopathy, though many children also respond well to chiropracty. When I took my son, I would always get my treatment first because after his treatment, he would feel so good he couldn't sit still anymore; on the other hand, some children can only sit still when they do feel good, so that type of child should get the first turn. *Even very young children will love going to the Osteopath because it makes them feel so good!*
8. **Treat possible joint injuries.** Remember that the joints themselves may not hurt even if they have been injured; the pain may be referred to nearby tissues. See Chapter 9: Joint Instability & Pain. *Your child likely has mildly injured one or more joints and has pain radiating from it.*
9. **Get Physical Therapy.** This is highly recommended by people in social media groups. *It sounds like a good idea to have an expert help train your child in proper movement patterns so that good movement patterns become habitual for the child's entire life.*

LINKS FOR PRODUCTS MENTIONED IN THIS CHAPTER

Comfrey Oil https://amzn.to/3y5ZsSP | *Arnica montana* https://amzn.to/48ryZwi

18
Hand Pain

MOST OF THE PEOPLE I KNOW WITH HEDS/HSD have hand pain, probably because the hands are used so much all day long. Also, they are at the far end of limbs, making it more of a challenge for the body to remove inflammation from them. In addition to Joint Injuries that occur with normal use or happen due to accidents, people with hEDS/HSD are prone to conditions like Dupuytren's Contracture and Trigger Finger.

Joint Injury and Inflammation

It is important to treat Joint Injuries in the hands because they can deteriorate into arthritis that could greatly diminish your quality of life.

My Experience with Hand Pain

For a long time, I experienced pain in all of my finger and thumb joints. Then, when I started sleeping on an earthing sheet at night, the pain went away instantly. This tells me that inflammation is a big factor in hand pain; this is true for Rheumatoid Arthritis, which is an inflammatory state, and for osteoarthritis, in which joints have been damaged by inflammation.

Eventually, some of my hand pain came back, and it wasn't until I started wearing ring splints to reduce the incidences of hyperextension that I noticed that the pain went away for good. It turned out that frequent hyperextension of just a couple of the joints was causing inflammation and pain throughout the entire hand. As the joints began to heal, they became the only sites of pain in my hands, until they were fully healed.

Preventions, Treatments, and Coping Strategies for Hand Pain

The hands are used all day long every day, for tasks large and small; their joints are numerous and small. So, they are prone to injury, but more than that, they are the areas where you may be most likely to feel inflammation in your body from other causes, such as MCAS flares. For these reasons, your hands need some special attention.

Reduce Hand Pain Due to Injury and Inflammation

1. **Do Earthing daily.** *Let the electric field of the earth remove inflammation from your hands.*
2. **Wear ring splints** as necessary. You can buy these on your own, or better yet, have a Physical Therapist fit some for you. *Protect your fingers from being hyperextended accidentally.*
3. **Do Rice Bucket Exercises.** Fill a large bucket with rice, then do exercises of lifting rice and wiggling your fingers in the rice. Also take advantage of the opportunity to strengthen your wrists, which will help take some of the work load off of your fingers. See Chapter 60: Rice Bucket Exercises. *Strengthen your hands in order to prevent hyperextension.*
4. **Do Lymph Drainage Massage** of your hands and arms. See Chapter 51: Lymph Drainage Massage. *It is easy to gently run one hand over the other hand a few times at any point in the day; this will help relieve inflammation and pain.*
5. **Apply comfrey oil.** *Comfrey oil speeds healing and reduces pain.* [391]

> REDUCE HAND PAIN
> 1. Do Earthing daily.
> 2. Wear ring splints.
> 3. Do Rice Bucket Exercises.
> 4. Do Lymph Drainage Massage.
> 5. Apply comfrey oil.
>
> Ask your doctor before trying anything new.

Dupuytren's Contracture

Dupuytren's Contracture is a painful and limiting condition that causes the fingers and hand to curl in upon themselves. It is a result of the fascia in the hand thickening, hardening, and adhering inappropriately.[392] Often, the first signs of Dupuytren's Contracture are the perpetual bending in of the last section of the pinky finger or ring finger, combined with pain in the palm of the hand. Usually, bumps and indentations will be felt in the palm of the hand just below the affected fingers. Ultimately, the entire hand can become involved and be unusable.

My Experience with Dupuytren's Contracture

My mother developed Dupuytren's Contracture, and it was very disappointing because there was a lot of information online about people who have suffered with it for years and have had disappointing results from surgeries. Ultimately, my mother was able to find a Physical Therapist to help her. The PT had never treated it before, but she gave my mother some suggestions, which she followed daily for a year. She no longer has any symptoms.

Preventions, Treatments, and Coping Strategies for Dupuytren's Contracture

The Physical Therapy that my mother did completely eliminated all pain and contractures within months. Even better, the Physical Therapy methods for treating Dupuytren's Contracture are very simple. I have heard that some of these methods are also effective for healing Trigger Finger.

Heal Dupuytren's Contracture

My mother began her treatments before the condition became very severe and was able to have full resolution of the problem within a year; it may be more challenging to get these results with more advanced cases. As with most conditions, it is best to treat it as soon as possible. Do these things every day until symptoms completely subside:

1. **Sretch the fingers back (but not too far) and hold for 30 seconds.** Be careful not to hyperextend them. *Regain the appropriate range of motion.*
2. **Use your other thumb to massage the palm of your hand where the bumps or indentations are, pressing toward the heart for 30 seconds.** Be careful not to hyperextend your thumb while it is massaging. *Gently but firmly encourage the fascia to relax and release its position.*
3. **Apply heat and magnesium oil** as desired. *Heat and magnesium oil will help to nourish and relax the tissues.*[393]
4. **Apply comfrey oil.** *Comfrey oil speeds healing and reduces pain.* [394]

HEAL DUPUYTREN'S CONTRACTURE

1. Stretch the fingers back (but not too far) and hold for 30 seconds.
2. Use the other hand to massage the palm of your hand where the bumps or indentations are, pressing toward the heart for 30 seconds.
3. Apply heat and magnesium oil.
4. Apply comfrey oil.

Ask your doctor before trying anything new.

LINKS FOR PRODUCTS MENTIONED IN THIS CHAPTER

Earthing https://amzn.to/3JZ1LKt

Comfrey Oil https://amzn.to/3y5ZsSP

Magnesium Flakes Magnesium Flakes https://amzn.to/3HrNIvn

19

Knee Pain

THERE ARE MANY POTENTIAL CAUSES OF KNEE pain, including, obviously, hyperextension injuries or a perpetual hyperextended-knee posture. Two other potential causes that are often overlooked are improper posture or function of the foot or hip.[395, 396] (See Chapter 56: Posture.)

The knees are also the most common locations at which people experience crepitus – which is sounds that occur when the joint is moved.[397, 398] The sounds may be cracking, popping, snapping, grinding, sparkling, clicking, crunching, etc. Sometimes, the sounds are completely benign, caused by air bubbles in the joints that pop when pressure is put on them. Sometimes, though, the sounds accompany painful conditions like osteoarthritis. If you hear crepitus in your knees but do not have pain, it is a good idea to put some effort toward improving your knee posture and mechanics and strengthening the muscles that support the knees so that the condition will not progress to pain.

My Experience with Knee Pain

Everyone with whom I have worked in the dance studio or holistic healing center who has complained of knee pain has had hyperextended knees. I have always tried to train them to stand and walk with their knees feeling slightly bent but looking straight. If they felt unstable instead of strong, we worked on activating the quadriceps muscles. The hamstring often needed strengthening and lengthening as well. Those who have been able to accomplish this posture change have been rewarded with the pain going away.

Those who did not want to dedicate themselves to changing their posture continued to have pain; I was able to help them with earthing, essential oils, and foods and supplements to reduce swelling, but I witnessed them becoming more and more sedentary.

As I understand more about hypermobility now and have developed more multifaceted treatment protocols, I am hopeful that people with extremely hyperextended knees and weak leg muscles can find better success in improving their posture.

Preventions, Treatments, and Coping Strategies for Knee Pain

Treating knee injury is just like treating any Joint Injury, but I and my family have developed a special exercise and some specific things to focus on.

Prevent and Heal Knee Pain

1. **Stand with correct posture.** See Chapter 56: Posture. *Your posture from head to toe can make a difference to your knees and put undue pressure on the knee joints.*
2. **Do the seated knee strengthening exercise**: sit in a chair; with thighs remaining still, slowly lift the lower legs until they are straight out, then slowly lower them back down. Do 3 sets of 10 repetitions. *This exercise quickly and easily relieves pain and restores strength and movement to the knees.*
3. **Do Range of Motion exercises for the hips and ankles** so that they are not stiff and affecting the knee. See Chapter 57: Range of Motion Exercises & Dynamic Stretching. *Many knee problems are actually generated in problems in the hips, ankles, or feet.*
4. **Get help from a Physical Therapist.** *These experts will be able to determine the cause of the pain and then implement or recommend the right treatments.*

PREVENT AND TREAT KNEE PAIN

1. Stand with correct posture.
2. Do the seated knee strengthening exercise.
3. Do Range of Motion exercises for the hips and ankles.
4. Get help from a Physical Therapist.

Ask your doctor before trying anything new.

20

Lymph Congestion

THE FIRST SIGNS OF LYMPH CONGESTION THAT you might notice are achiness, swelling, sluggishness, and heightened sensitivity to chemicals, but the symptoms can develop into larger problems.

Lymph is a fluid primarily produced in the liver and digestive system that is part of the immune system.[399] It is responsible for carrying nutrients and oxygen to cells and carrying bacteria, viruses, and other undesired substances and wastes away from cells.[400] The lymph system also maintains the balance of fluids in the body.

Lymph fluid travels through vessels throughout the body, particularly in vessels that thread through layers of the skin.[401] Lymph capillaries and vessels are composed of chains of lymphangions, which are short sections of tubing, 1-2 mm long, with valves on each end. The valves allow the lymph fluid to flow in one direction only. The valves do not open all at the same time but in a regulated or unregulated sequence that can vary greatly.

Lymph fluid is propelled though the lymph system by a number of different mechanisms, including some that are not understood. Pressure differences inside and outside of the lymph channels due to swelling can create movement of lymph; spontaneous contraction of the muscles that are part of the lymph channel walls can instigate lymph flow. Also, breathing, moving, exercising, and outside pressure against the skin can move lymph.[402]

When the lymph system does not operate properly and lymph does not flow sufficiently, it can lead to conditions like neurodegenerative diseases, aging, lymphedema (a swelling of fluids in the soft tissues of the body[403]), obesity, inflammatory bowel disease, and metabolic syndrome (a condition of obesity, low HDL cholesterol, and high blood sugar, blood pressure, and triglycerides that can lead to heart disease, diabetes, and stroke[404]).[405, 406]

Considering that the lymph system acts as the body's waste disposal system, it is likely to be especially important for those of us with Allergy/MCAS/MCS and/or MTHFR to keep the lymph fluid flowing. Unfortunately, our connective tissue disorder can affect the lymph vessels, which are partly made of collagen.[407] When the lymph channels collapse and lymph does not flow freely, you may experience water retention, malaise, swollen lymph nodes, heightened sensitivity to chemicals, and more.

For people who do not have hEDS/HSD, regular movement during the day will move the lymph. When they need a little extra help, gentle rebounding (jumping on a trampoline) or dry brushing of the skin with a specialized brush will do the trick, but we may need extra help.

Fortunately, manual Lymph Drainage Massage is effective and can even help relieve the pain of fibromyalgia.[408, 409] See Chapter 51: Lymph Drainage Massage.

My Experience with Lymph Congestion

For me, Lymph Drainage Massage done by a professional is the best option. The first time I had this treatment done by an expert, I lost two clothing sizes, and those clothing sizes did not come back for years! The second-best option for me is Self-Lymph Drainage Massage, which I frequently use on my hands, face, and neck to reduce pain from mild inflammation.

Also, I always do Lymph Drainage Massage on any family member who is coming down with a sore throat or stuffy nose, and often it prevents the symptom from developing into an actual cold or flu. It is an invaluable tool for relieving earaches.

Preventions, Treatments, and Coping Strategies for Lymph Congestion

Just moving around every day will cause the lymph to flow somewhat, but people with hEDS/HSD often need to take more conscientious efforts to help it along.

Improve Lymph Flow for Better Health

1. **Get a Lymph Drainage Massage** done by a professional or do it yourself. See Chapter 51: Lymph Drainage Massage. *Many Massage Therapists and Physical Therapists can provide excellent Lymph Drainage Massages, but it is also a technique that you can do on yourself easily every day.*
2. **Rebound gently on a trampoline**. You do not even need to jump high enough to get your feet off the trampoline. If you need some stability while jumping, use a support bar. If a mini trampoline is too unstable for you, just do a series of knee bends or small jumps while standing on the floor. *Bouncing not only gets your lymph flowing, it will build muscle and bone.*
3. **Dry Brush before bathing.** Use a brush made for this purpose and brush gently on your skin toward the heart and lymph nodes in the armpits and groin. *Not only will dry brushing improve lymph flow, it will exfoliate the skin.*
4. **Do Abhyanga Oil Massage**. See Chapter 39: Abhyanga Oil Massage. *This technique is helpful for lymph flow, it is relaxing, and it also draws toxins (which are usually oil soluble) out of the body.*
5. **Go for long walks.** Also try to get in a lot of steps all throughout the day. *Our bodies are designed so that when you move, it pumps the lymph system.*

6. **Vibrate the entire body.** Ride in a bouncy moving vehicle, the more vibratory, the better. Many people get good results from standing on a vibration plate or using a chi machine, either at home or at a spa or other public center. *Getting lymph flowing can be fun and easy.*
7. **Do or receive Gua Sha scraping.** This is a Traditional Chinese Medicine technique for moving congestion in the body. I especially love the pain-relieving effects of Gua Sha on the back of my neck when I get neck pain or a headache, and so I keep a jade scraper in my purse. If you scrape all over your body, any areas where there were fluids and blood clogged up, that area of the skin will turn red; it's sometimes amazing to see. Scrape strongly, in any direction. *It feels good.*
8. **Take an herbal blend for lymph support.** *Give your body the nutrients it needs to keep lymph healthy.*
9. **Drink a lot of water.** *The lymph fluids have important jobs to do, so make sure that your body is hydrated enough to make enough lymph fluids.*

IMPROVE LYMPH FLOW

1. Get a Lymph Drainage Massage.
2. Rebound gently on a trampoline.
3. Dry brush before bathing.
4. Do Abhyanga Oil Massage.
5. Go for long walks.
6. Vibrate the entire body.
7. Do or receive Gua Sha scraping.
8. Take an herbal blend for lymph support.
9. Drink a lot of water.

Ask your doctor before trying anything new.

LINKS FOR PRODUCTS MENTIONED IN THIS CHAPTER

Dry Brush https://amzn.to/4bycpnd
Rebounder https://amzn.to/4b14wH2
Vibration Plate https://amzn.to/483V03i
Chi Machine https://amzn.to/3OpCTOf
Gua Sha Tool https://amzn.to/3Hrd9gQ
Lymph Cleanse Herbs https://amzn.to/3JbQTIH

21 Migraine

MILLIONS OF PEOPLE AROUND THE WORLD suffer from Migraine, so it is not surprising that there is no definitive cure for it.[410] However, I used to experience Migraine attacks about 20 days a month or more, but I have not had a single day of Migraine in all the months since I treated myself for it from the framework of treating hEDS/HSD.

It is important to understand that Migraine is not "just" a headache and can even occur without a headache. Migraine often occurs in three or four stages — prodrome, aura, headache, and postdrome, and there are numerous symptoms associated with each stage. It is common to experience the stages in a predictable time frame, but this can vary as well as change over time. Each of the four stages can last for hours, days, or weeks.[411]

Prodrome is the period of time immediately after a trigger has occurred. Sometimes Migraineurs (people who have the Migraine disease) do not notice any symptoms during the prodrome, but if there are recognizable symptoms, they do not usually include headache. Instead, they are usually milder symptoms and can include confusion, irritability, neck pain, nausea, fatigue, and Insomnia.

The second phase, aura, does not occur for every Migraineur, and even those who get aura do not get it every time. It is associated with visual disturbances and is named for the flashes of light that are sometimes "seen" by people who get this. The aura phase can also include numbness and tingling of various body parts; it is a phase when a wave of nerve activity affects the senses.

The most recognizable phase of Migraine, headache, is the next phase. Although it is called headache, there is a long list of possible symptoms. Frequently, people who experience Migraine attacks barely notice the accompanying symptoms because the head pain is so powerful, but they are a valuable clue to the diagnosis. Headache phase symptoms can include brain fog, congestion and runny nose, mouth sores, Insomnia, vomiting, and much more.

The final phase is postdrome, and it is sometimes called a Migraine hangover. The lingering effects of Migraine, the postdrome, can draw out the Migraine experience for several days. In this phase, it is common to feel depression, fatigue, and dullness. It is also possible to experience Cerebellar Ataxia and other neurological symptoms, if the

Migraine attack caused diminished blood flow to the brain severe enough to cause cell death in the cerebellum. See Chapter 12: Cerebellar Ataxia, Essential Tremor, & Dystonia.

For many people with Migraine, if the initial symptoms are recognized and treatment applied very soon after the trigger to the Migraine, it can stop the attack from happening or reduce its severity. Note that people often conflate their prodrome symptoms with Migraine triggers — for example, many people who think that chocolate is a Migraine trigger actually begin to crave and therefore eat chocolate during the prodrome stage when sugar and caffeine can reduce some of the mild but burgeoning symptoms; something other than chocolate had already triggered them.[412]

PRODROME	1 Hour to 4 Days
Irritability, Fatigue, Food Cravings, Mood Swings, Yawning, Insomnia, Digestive System Problems, Brain Fog, Neck Pain, Aphasia, Stiffness, Light & Sound Sensitivity, Blurred Vision, etc.	
AURA	**5 to 60 Minutes**
Visual Disturbances, Body Tingling, etc.	
HEADACHE	**4 Hours to 4 Days**
Head Pain, Nausea, Sinus Congestion, Mood Swings, Neck Pain, Insomnia, Digestive System Problems, Light, Sound, Touch, & Smell Sensitivity, etc.	
POSTDROME	**1 to 2 Days**
Brain Fog, Fatigue, Mood Swings, Body Pain, Clumsiness, etc.	

Figure 39: Phases of a Migraine Attack.[413]

My Experience with Migraine

My sister and I both went many years without being diagnosed with Migraine because the headaches were a more minor and less frequent symptom than many of the miseries we were dealing with. However, we both had noticed that our symptoms went through reliably timed phases that correspond with the four phases of Migraine.

My Migraines have certainly been brought on by POTS and Allergy/MCAS/MCS, but it was especially helpful to recognize my specific Migraine triggers. Some of my Migraine attacks were instigated by CCI (neck instability), but since I have strengthened my neck muscles and learned to avoid my Migraine triggers, now when I tweak my neck or otherwise injure my neck, I often get other kinds of headaches and symptoms instead of Migraine.

I used to get depressed thinking of how many millions of people have been unable to cure their Migraines and that I might live my life among their numbers. My mother would encourage me by reminding me that her father used to get Migraine attacks, but one day he decided he was done with them. With mind over matter, he never had another Migraine attack. I didn't have the same instantaneous success Grandpa had, but luckily, my husband helped me avoid my triggers, and when a trigger happened anyway, he supported me in doing the treatments that would prevent a Migraine attack from progressing.

Perhaps I actually have escaped from being among the millions of Migraine sufferers. Even better, perhaps I will be able to bring some of you along with me with the treatment ideas I have developed.

Prevent Migraine Attacks

There are a number of different suspected and recognized causes of the Migraine syndrome.[414] People who have Postural Orthostatic Tachycardia Syndrome (POTS) and other forms of dysautonomia often experience Migraine attacks brought on by a tachycardia episode. People who have Allergy/MCAS/MCS often experience Migraine brought on by one of those triggers; it has been seen that the dura (the matter surrounding the brain) of Migraineurs has an elevated number of mast cells.[415] Even the Joint Instability and pain of hypermobility can cause Migraine.

There are many pharmaceutical treatments available for Migraine, and some of them work well for some people. I chose not to pursue the medical route because of the undesirable side effects (which could be exacerbated by my chemical sensitivities), and I managed Migraine on my own with good results.

Prevent Migraine Attacks

Because people with hEDS/HSD are prone to Migraine, we should try to reduce our other risk factors. Obviously, living a healthy lifestyle — exercise, don't smoke, etc. — helps somewhat, but try these ideas as well.

1. **Figure out your triggers and avoid them.** Keep a diary of experiences and symptoms to determine what food and environmental conditions precede your Migraine attacks, keeping in mind that the attack may not start for a certain amount of time after exposure to the trigger. The *Hypermobile and Happy Health Diary* at shannonegale.com will make this especially easy. Many common triggers are synthetic fragrances, stress, fluorescent lights, loud noises, dysautonomia, and occipital neuralgia. *Avoiding triggers is the best way to avoid Migraine attacks.*
2. **Minimize the potency of your triggers if you can't avoid them completely.** Wear a personal ionizer if you are going to be around fragrances or other airborne chemicals. If one of your triggers is fluorescent or LED lights (common triggers for Migraineurs due to the lights' nearly imperceptible flickering that is apparent to the sensitive eye and brain), use a flicker-meter app on your phone to determine if you are under lights that flicker beyond your threshold. Excuse yourself from stressful situations. Wear specialized ear plugs to diminish and/or filter noises. *For many of us, we lose out on some of the things we enjoy in life if we insist on never risking exposure to a trigger, so finding special ways to go near our triggers without being exposed to them or with a reduced exposure can give us our lives back.*
3. **Keep your Migraine treatments ready and easily accessible.** They should be on hand any time you might get triggered. No matter how hard we try to avoid triggers, we will sometimes be caught by surprise; have your rescue treatments ready so that you can begin treating yourself immediately. The following pages will give you many ideas of Migraine treatments to use. *Reduce the likelihood or strength of an attack.*
4. **Avoid caffeine and alcohol.** Caffeine can bring on Migraine attacks. It can sometimes be helpful in stopping or reducing the severity of attacks, but

PREVENT MIGRAINE ATTACKS

1. Figure out your triggers and avoid them.
2. Minimize the potency of your triggers if you can't avoid them completely.
3. Keep your Migraine treatments ready and easily accessible.
4. Avoid caffeine and alcohol.
5. Pray.

Ask your doctor before trying anything new.

only if you do not use caffeine on a regular basis. Some people react badly to alcohol as soon as they ingest it, while others won't experience a Migraine attack until the next day, but it is a common trigger and a poison.[416] *Any substance that significantly affects your body will affect your susceptibility to Migraine.*

5. **Pray.** *Studies have shown that meditating on God's goodness can reduce the frequency of Migraine attacks.* [417]

Recognize Migraine Attacks

Since Migraine attacks begin with a prodrome that can last for days before the actual headache begins, it can be difficult to know if you have been triggered. But it is very important to know, because it is during the prodrome that you have a chance to stop the attack before it develops...and the earlier in the prodrome, the better. The ideas listed here have been very helpful for me in recognizing right away that I have been triggered.

Keep in mind that sometimes patients think they have been triggered by something when in fact this thing is a prodrome symptom; they were triggered previously by something else. Some of the commonly conflated trigger/prodrome symptoms are light, sound, stress, and food cravings.[418]

Recognize When You Have Been Triggered for a Migraine

1. **Ask others to help by telling you if they recognize signs that you have been triggered.** Often, you will be distracted in a social situation or with a work project and not notice that you are having symptoms of the prodrome phase. Tell your family, friends, and coworkers what to watch for — perhaps your face gets red and puffy, you get dark circles under your eyes, your hands tremble, or your voice sounds hoarse. Ask those around you to tell you when they notice the signs so that you can begin treating yourself right away. *If you don't know what your signs are, it could be that your loved ones already know some of the visible ones.*
2. **Notice if others are doing annoying things.** Has everyone around you suddenly started to do things wrong? Are you feeling annoyed and frustrated at their ineptitude or lack of consideration? This is a hint to stop and look at yourself — most likely, it is not that they have all suddenly become horrible people, it's more likely that your mood and capability to cope with your environment have been affected by a trigger. Helpful hint here: If it seems like everyone around you is doing things wrong, this is not the time to correct them or berate them for their faults. You can always bring it up in a few days when you're feeling better, if it still matters to you then, and you will handle it in a much more respectful way and get better results. *When you have been triggered, you perceive things differently and have a harder time coping with situations, people, and environments.*
3. **Look in the mirror from time to time.** Is your face puffy? Is your skin red? Do you have dark circles under your eyes? Are your hands shaking? Are you slouching? *When we are coping with a Migraine attack, we do not always recognize what we are feeling but can see it better.*
4. **Notice what difficulties you are having.** Are you dropping things more often? Are you having a hard time making eye contact with other people? Are you having no luck at convincing yourself to get up and do that chore it's time to do? Are you clearing your throat and coughing? Are your eyes watering? Are you forgetting things? Are your words coming out wrong? Are you running into doorways? Are you

getting hyper-focused on specific tasks? Are you finding excuses to remain seated or in bed? Your body is ready to go into a protective state of rest and solitude so that it can recover from the perceived attack that the trigger posed. *Don't beat yourself up about your condition; listen to your body.*

5. **Notice if the environment is providing too much sensation.** Is it too bright? Too loud? Too crowded? Too empty? Smelly? Dirty? Dull? Hot or cold? Windy? Is your chair too hard? After a trigger, it may be more difficult for you to cope with sensations. *Sometimes a change of scenery or fresh air will help, but if you have been triggered, it is likely that the new environment will soon become unpleasant as well, unless it's your bed in your quiet, darkened bedroom.*
6. **Notice if your emotional state has changed**. Are you becoming really down, or angry, or anxious? Does it seem like everyone is against you? Do they all disagree with your decisions? Are they pressuring you to be different than you are? Does no one understand you? Does no one like you? Is it all just hopeless? None of these ideas or feelings are really real — they are part of the disease. Things will look better when you recover. *Don't act on it, don't talk about it, just wait for the symptoms to pass and everything will be easier to deal with.*
7. **Correlate returning or worsening symptoms with the trigger.** Are you having night sweats? Difficulty sleeping? Congestion in your sinuses, ears, or throat? Muscle twitches and spasms? Swelling in your hands? Sores in your mouth? Do you feel like you're buzzing as if you're plugged into an electrical outlet? Did one of your joints spontaneously go out of alignment? Are you having to urinate frequently? Has acne popped up again? Does your neck or jaw or shoulder hurt? Are you having POTS episodes? (See Chapter 29: POTS) *We have gotten used to symptoms coming and going, often with no explanation, but sometimes that explanation could be a Migraine trigger, especially if multiple symptoms are coming on at once.*

RECOGNIZE MIGRAINE ATTACKS

1. Ask others to help by telling you if they see signs that you have been triggered.
2. Notice if others are doing annoying things.
3. Look in the mirror from time to time.
4. Notice what difficulties you are having.
5. Notice if the environment is providing too much sensation.
6. Notice what your emotional state is like.
7. Correlate returning or worsening symptoms with the trigger.

Ask your doctor before trying anything new.

Reduce Migraine Attacks

Once you can recognize that you have been triggered for a Migraine, you can treat it during the window of opportunity to make a difference. Act as quickly as possible. Make sure that you do not try to treat yourself with one of your triggers, though.

Prevent Migraine Attacks As Soon As Possible After Trigger Exposure

As soon as possible:

1. **Drink grapefruit juice.** First check for contraindications with any medications you take; grapefruit can reduce the efficacy of some kinds of pharmaceutical drugs. Most people with histamine intolerance or MTHFR have problems with their liver

detoxification system,[419] and grapefruit juice balances the liver processes for better detoxification of any toxins (like that fragrance that might have triggered you) or hormones (like the excessive histamine the mast cells produced).[420] *Detox to keep your system clean to deal better with triggers.*

2. **Take Homeopathic Remedies** (*Ignatia amara*, *Histaminum hydrochloricum*, *Arsenicum album*, and possibly others). See Chapter 50: Homeopathic Remedies. *Treat specific symptoms.*
3. **Take one baby aspirin**. *This will reduce inflammation and is a mast cell stabilizer.*[421]
4. **Drink 1/4 teaspoon of baking soda in 2 ounces water.** *Baking soda is a mast cell stabilizer, reduces autoimmune conditions, and even improves performance in sport activities.*[422, 423]
5. **Breathe oxygen** (from an oxygen machine or tank or a Boost canister). Migraine may be caused by oxygen deprivation or improper utilization of oxygen, so supplemental oxygen can be helpful. Also, the blood vessels are constricted in the beginning of a Migraine attack and dilated during the middle of it in response to the previous constriction; oxygen can dilate blood vessels and so is helpful in the beginning of an attack and may reduce the body's need to react by over-dilating the blood vessels.[424, 425] *Help get sufficient oxygen to the brain when your body may be having trouble with this.*
6. **Take riboflavin, B12, and folate**. Anyone with an MTHFR SNP will want to take B12 as methylcolbalamin and folate as methylfolate. See Chapter 24: MTHFR. *Riboflavin, Vitamin B12, and folate deficiencies increase Migraine incidence; also, these vitamins are used in greater amounts during stress, so their stores need to be replenished during the stress of a Migraine attack.*[426, 427]
7. **Do the Basic Exercise** of the eyes for Vagus Nerve Stimulation. See Chapter 41: The Basic Exercise. *This will relax the occipital muscles that travel from the eyes, over the head, to the neck, which will also relax the nervous system.*
8. **Do the Red Ball Exercises** for the neck. See Chapter 25: Neck Pain & CCI. *Sometimes Migraine is caused or exacerbated by misalignment in the neck; this exercise will help align the bones of the neck.*
9. **Lie down in the dark for an hour**. Wear a silk eye mask and/or use ear plugs if necessary. Relaxing yourself, eliminating all triggers (smells, light, noise, stress, threatened joints, etc.) may allow your body to return to a normal state. *This is one of the most universally helpful treatments, according to people commenting in the hEDS and Migraine social media groups.*
10. **Do Earthing.** Most effective may be Earthing Therapy Patches applied to the neck. It significantly reduces the severity and length of time of a Migraine attack. I especially appreciate that it reduces the buzzing feeling that I get. I try to earth as long as possible, even overnight when I am sleeping. See Chapter 45: Earthing. *This was one of my must-do techniques when I was experiencing Migraine attacks.*

PREVENT MIGRAINE ATTACKS AFTER BEING TRIGGERED

1. Drink grapefruit juice.
2. Take Homeopathic Remedies.
3. Take one baby aspirin.
4. Drink ¼ teaspoon baking soda in 2 ounces water.
5. Breathe oxygen.
6. Take riboflavin, B12, and folate.
7. Do The Basic Exercise.
8. Do the Red Ball Exercises.
9. Lie down in the dark for an hour.
10. Do Earthing.

Ask your doctor before trying anything new.

After Lying Down, Reduce Migraine Attack Development

1. **Take electrolytes.**[428] *All of our body's processes are reliant on electrolytes (minerals), so this will help your body heal whatever it needs to heal, and especially it will regulate blood pressure and heart rate, which can have a large impact on Migraine.*
2. **Eat fatty, salty food.** Make sure that the fats you choose are healthy fats, not seed oils or hydrogenated or partially hydrogenated oils. Fatty foods help to process toxins — chemicals in the air, in food, or excess hormones in your body — out of your body and give you energy. Salt is a helpful electrolyte, especially if you are having a POTS episode. *Furthermore, fatty foods taste delicious and the act of chewing relaxes the nervous system, so you will feel better and happier, which may reduce the Migraine severity.*[429, 430]
3. **Get a shoulder and back massage**[431] (or give one to yourself with your hands or a vibrating massager — just be careful it is not too rough). *Tight muscles in the shoulders, back, and neck can cause or exacerbate a Migraine, so use massage to relax them.*
4. **Take it easy.** Any amount of stress is likely to increase the Migraine severity. *Give your body an opportunity to heal itself by leaving any tasks for later and just relaxing.*
5. **Continue earthing.** See Chapter 45: Earthing. *Whether with an earthing tool or being in contact with the ground outside, earthing is very helpful.*
6. **Use an herb that is known to reduce pain.** Herbs like peppermint and chamomile can be helpful (chamomile is in the ragweed family, so do not use it if you have an allergy to ragweed). Some other aromatic herbs and Chinese herbs are also recommended for Migraine relief. [432, 433, 434] *Plants have been used to relieve headache pain for millennia.*
7. **If the headache pain or neck pain is very severe, take an adult dose of aspirin.** First check to make sure that aspirin is not contraindicated with any of your other medications or conditions. *Medications like aspirin are not good for you to take frequently (aspirin is especially hard on the stomach), but when you really need pain relief, this and a variety of herbs are fairly mild, safe options.*

REDUCE MIGRAINE ATTACK DEVELOPMENT

1. Take electrolytes.
2. Eat fatty, salty foods.
3. Get shoulder and back massage.
4. Take it easy.
5. Continue Earthing.
6. Use an herb that is known to reduce pain, such as peppermint or chamomile.
7. If the headache pain is very severe, take an adult dose of aspirin.

Ask your doctor before trying anything new.

Reduce The Severity of an Ongoing Migraine Attack

1. **Take a hot shower.** Some people feel worse after a hot shower, but many feel a great relief from the heat and steam. *This treatment often helps me and my sister a lot.*
2. **Use hydrotherapy.** Take a hot foot bath and put an icepack on your neck or head. This treatment improves vagal tone as well as reducing the pain and incidence of Migraine.[435]
3. **Take one baby aspirin.** As long as symptoms persist, you can repeat the single baby aspirin every 12 hours. *This will keep inflammation down.*

REDUCE THE SEVERITY OF A MIGRAINE ATTACK

1. Take a hot shower.
2. Use hydrotherapy.
3. Take one baby aspirin.
4. Drink more electrolytes.
5. Eat chocolate.
6. Stay relaxed in the dark.
7. Apply heat or cold.
8. Use a Zok device in the ear.
9. Do gua sha scraping of the neck.
10. Do self-acupressure.
11. Do self-Reiki.
12. Use a Near Infrared and Red Light Therapy box.
13. Get fresh air.
14. Endeavor to keep good posture.
15. Take a nap.

Ask your doctor before trying anything new.

4. **Drink more electrolytes** and/or warm sweetened tea. *Warm drinks are soothing, and electrolytes are necessary for healing.*
5. **Eat chocolate.** The caffeine, sugar, and deliciousness in chocolate can reduce Migraine. *Caffeine increases heart rate and constricts blood vessels, while sugar is a pain reducer.*[436, 437, 438]
6. **Stay relaxed in the dark.** *Continue to reduce exposure to triggers and sensory overload until you are healed.*
7. **Apply heat or cold.** Try a heating pad on the back of the neck or a cool washcloth on the forehead. Some people have gotten great results from putting their feet in cold water. *Temperature variations can reduce headache pain.*
8. **Use a Zok device in the ear**. *This may balance pressure and drain congestion to relieve headache pain.*
9. **Do gua sha scraping of the neck**. Gua Sha increases blood flow and relaxes muscles. See Chapter 20: Lymph Congestion. *This is a wonderful, easy technique for reducing neck pain during a Migraine.*
10. **Do self-acupressure** according to the figure here. If your finger hurts when holding a point, wear a ring splint or use a tool to hold the pressure point. *Self-acupressure is free, easy, and always available.*
11. **Do self-Reiki.** Reiki also is free, easy, and always available once you have learned it. See Section VI: Seek Professional Help. *It is very effective at reducing anxiety and pain.*

Back of head on each side
Fleshy part of hand between thumb and pointer
Top of foot
Inside edge of each eyebrow and the cheek right beside each side of the nose

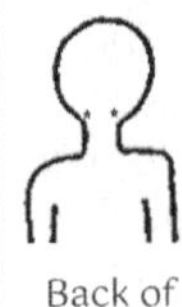

Figure 45: Acupressure points to relieve headache.

12. **Use a Near Infrared and Red Light Therapy box.**[439] *Only use this when you are not feeling photo sensitive; it is very health-giving.*
13. **Get fresh air** (depending on the sun). *Oxygen, changing temperature, and the gentle caress of the breeze are all helpful in reducing a Migraine attack.*
14. **Endeavor to keep good posture.** *Poor posture and misalignment in the neck, back, shoulders, and chest can pull on joints, tense muscles, and compress veins and nerves, all of which will exacerbate a headache, while good posture lets your body do the healing it wants to do so that the Migraine attack can pass quickly.*
15. **Take a nap.** Sleep is known to be both a trigger and a cure for Migraine.[440] *Perhaps you will feel better when you wake up, but if not, at least you'll have been unconscious for some of the Migraine attack.*

LINKS FOR PRODUCTS MENTIONED IN THIS CHAPTER

Personal Ionizer https://amzn.to/3OmbfSo

Specialty Ear Plugs https://amzn.to/42qkGWP or https://amzn.to/3SJoEXp

Ignatia amara https://amzn.to/48QcuRP

Histaminum hydrochloricum https://amzn.to/3tOerPO

Arsenicum album https://amzn.to/3uaqCX7

Aspirin https://amzn.to/3Snl7Of

Boost Oxygen https://amzn.to/3UdO9kR

Riboflavin https://amzn.to/3vE7hi3

B12 https://amzn.to/422EaRi

Folate https://amzn.to/3U3sSdy

Red Ball https://amzn.to/4bgpYXU

Eye Mask https://amzn.to/3UEnBIY

Earthing Therapy Patches https://amzn.to/424RmVs

Electrolytes https://amzn.to/3UlgNk1

Vibrating Massager https://amzn.to/3U5y4xm

Zok Device https://amzn.to/3HnmRAO

Gua Sha Tool https://amzn.to/3Hrd9gQ

Near Infrared and Red Light Therapy Box https://amzn.to/3S8vLXG

22

Motion Sickness

IT IS SUGGESTED THAT MOTION SICKNESS is common among hEDS patients because movement challenges and injures joints.[441] The body's reaction to this threat is nausea, and it is quite effective at preventing harm since it convinces a person to avoid riding on moving vehicles, planes, boats, etc.

It is also possible for Motion Sickness to be caused by Benign Paroxysmal Positional Vertigo (BPPV).[442] This is a condition in which the tiny bones in the ear canal (whose rolling around in the canal alerts the body to movement) become displaced. They may become displaced due to a hit to the head, congestion in the ears, or tilting and rolling of the head. Fortunately, they can be put back into position with the Epley Maneuver, and if BPPV is your problem, your Motion Sickness will instantly disappear.

You can have an ENT (Ear, Nose, and Throat Doctor) or Physical Therapist do the Epley Maneuver on you, or you can learn to do it yourself. It is simple and noninvasive. A professional will watch your eyes and other movements to determine that the maneuver is being done correctly, but it is still worth trying it at home if you aren't going to the doctor soon. There are many videos on YouTube describing it, both in the version that a professional would do and in some altered versions for doing it on your own.

My Experience with Motion Sickness

Unfortunately, even with a professional's help, the Epley Maneuver did not solve my Motion Sickness problem. There were times when I could not even sit in a rocking chair without becoming nauseated. I was also known to get nauseated when sitting still watching a movie or TV show filmed with a moving camera. There were many times I missed out — like when I was in the boat's bathroom throwing up when my family saw a magnificent, but elusive, whale.

However, I eventually discovered treatments that cured my Motion Sickness, and I can happily travel again without needing to use any of the treatments, aside from an occasional revisit with the Motion Sickness Glasses. I will note that I tried two other purported Motion Sickness cures that only made me worse: ginger candy or tea and essential oils. They are not on my list, but you can try them if you think they will work for you.

Preventions, Treatments, and Coping Strategies for Motion Sickness

After a lifetime of suffering with Motion Sickness, when I was finally successful in curing it, it was because I did all of these techniques at once during one long journey. It took a lot of effort at the time, but within a day, I was cured.

Eliminate Motion Sickness

1. **Keep your eyes on the road, water, or sky in front of you**. It is common for people who don't have Motion Sickness to tell people who are suffering from it to keep their eyes on the horizon, but that is not nearly as effective. *Make sure your brain knows what ground, waves, or clouds you are about to pass over.*
2. **Wear Motion Sickness Glasses** when riding in a moving vehicle. *The movement of the blue water in these Occupational Therapy glasses trains your brain to understand the movement you are feeling; I imagine that this helps your body know how to brace your joints correctly.*
3. **Wear Sea Bands**. This is a common and easy treatment; when treating Motion Sickness, you can wear a Sea Band on one wrist and an electric shock bracelet on the other wrist. *These tight bracelets activate an acupressure point in your wrist to diminish nausea.*
4. **Wear an electric shock bracelet**. It was most effective for me to alternate which wrist the bracelet was on every hour or so. *The adjustable shock is a strong acupressure treatment.*
5. **Sit in a supported position**. Use pillows or other supports to keep your body from knocking around with each movement of the vehicle. Don't forget to control the movement of your head with supports. Wrap a blanket tightly around you. Sit in a nice, straight position. *You do not want to risk bruises or Joint Injuries.*
6. **Sleep.** If you sleep while on a moving vehicle, first make sure that your body is fully supported and safely secure so that you will not injure a joint while sleeping. *When Motion Sickness will not subside, you may be able to fall asleep and not sense the nausea while sleeping.*
7. **Drive.** *If you are the one in control of the car, you are much less likely to get nauseated.*
8. **Put the breeze in your face.** Open the window, get on the prow of the ship, turn on a personal fan. This is not usually the most effective treatment, but the wind is sometimes helpful. *A change in temperature can be helpful, too.*
9. **Use Homeopathic Remedies.** Some of the best for this condition are *Nux vomica*, *Tabacum*, *Ipecacuanha*, and *Cocculus indicus*. See Chapter 50:

CURE MOTION SICKNESS

1. Keep your eyes on the road or water in front of you.
2. Wear Motion Sickness Glasses.
3. Wear Sea Bands.
4. Wear an electric shock bracelet.
5. Sit in a supported position.
6. Sleep.
7. Drive.
8. Put the breeze in your face.
9. Use Homeopathic Remedies such as *Nux vomica, Tabacum, Ipecacuanha,* and *Cocculus indicus*
10. Eat peppermint candy.

Ask your doctor before trying anything new.

Homeopathic Remedies. *This is an easy way to communicate to your system that it is OK to stay calm.*

10. **Eat peppermint candy.** Both the sugar and the peppermint are *somewhat* antiemetic (reduce nausea and vomiting).[443, 444] *Candy makes you feel a little happier even when you have nausea.*

LINKS FOR PRODUCTS MENTIONED IN THIS CHAPTER

Motion Sickness Glasses https://amzn.to/3tyy0vq
Sea Bands https://amzn.to/3tT4hND
Electric Shock Bracelet https://amzn.to/48B2ko4
Nux vomica https://amzn.to/48pZv9l
Tabacum https://amzn.to/3RN56je
Ipecacuanha https://amzn.to/3HueQu1
Cocculus indicus https://amzn.to/48jxvUW

23

Mouth Health: Teeth Care & Mouth Posture

ON THIS TOPIC, WE HAVE SOME GOOD NEWS: people with hEDS/HSD are not thought to have more problems with tooth health than the general population, except that they may have more plaque (a film composed mostly of bacteria that coats teeth and develops into tartar if not removed by toothbrushing or cleaning).[445, 446]

However, studies have shown that people with hEDS are more displeased with their mouth health than are people in the general public. This may be partly due to anxiety and also due to the fact that people with hEDS are already coping with so many health issues that any other health issue is even more stressful. More importantly, the oral mucosa (inside of the mouth) is more fragile in people with hEDS/HSD, which means you might frequently have mouth sores or injuries to contend with in addition to cavities and other tooth problems.[447]

Teeth

Periodontitis, inflammation in the tooth-supporting tissues that causes a deterioration of these tissues and ultimately results in tooth loss, is the most common chronic inflammatory disease in humans.[448] Even though it is not more prevalent in people with hEDS/HSD, it is likely that many of us will experience it, considering that as many as 83% of people have periodontitis at some point.

There are many types of collagen found in the tooth-supporting tissues, so it is especially important for people with hEDS/HSD to treat them gently. For this reason, I like the Bass toothbrushes, which are smaller and made with fewer and softer bristles than regular toothbrushes, as well as a shorter handle, which means that you can't press quite as hard while brushing. These toothbrushes will still clean your teeth, but they will do less damage to the gums that support the teeth.

Also, it is important to understand that teeth are living body parts.[449] Lymph channels run through the teeth, carrying nutrients to them and removing undesired substances from the mouth. Theoretically, if you provide the needed nutrients to the teeth through diet and mineral-rich tooth powder, they will keep themselves alive and healthy.[450]

For this reason, it is a good idea to use a tooth powder that contains the minerals your teeth need, instead of a typical toothpaste. [451] Many toothpastes contain undesirable ingredients, such as glycerin, which essentially leaves teeth coated with sugar, and fluoride, which is a neurotoxin.[452, 453] The tooth powder will also whiten teeth, and it is easy and inexpensive to make, or you can find a variety of choices in health food stores.

My Experience with Teeth

My father had cavities at every dentist visit, so I suggested he try remineralizing tooth powder. After that, he had many fewer cavities, and the dentist told him to keep doing what he was doing. Some of my family members loved the remineralizing tooth powder right from the start when we switched from regular toothpaste, but those who didn't soon adjusted and grew to like it.

Preventions, Treatments, and Coping Strategies for Teeth

Once you get your adult teeth, you never get new ones. Take good care of them so that you'll be comfortable, attractive, and able to eat well your whole life.

Tooth and Gum Care

1. **Brush your teeth twice per day**. Disrupt the bacteria in your mouth once every 12 hours to allow your body to keep it from forming into plaque and tartar.[454] With the brush at a 45-degree angle to the gum line, brush side to side in a small section, about the size of the toothbrush head, for 5 seconds. Repeat until you have brushed the fronts and backs of all teeth. Then, brush the surfaces of the molars, and finish by brushing your tongue. Run your tongue over your teeth to make sure that you haven't missed any spots; attend to them if you have. *You can also find videos at www.orawellness.com to see the proper way to brush with a Bass Toothbrush and why.*
2. **Use a Bass toothbrush**. These toothbrushes with soft bristles, small numbers of bristles, and short handles, prevent you from brushing too hard and damaging the gums. The Ora Wellness website also contains articles and videos about using the Bass toothbrush properly. *Get your teeth clean without causing damage to the softer tissues.*
3. **Use remineralizing tooth powder.** Many regular toothpastes have bad-for-you ingredients, but remineralizing tooth powder has the minerals your teeth need.[455] Buy this premade, or to save money and tailor it to your preferences and needs, make your own with the recipe in Appendix A. This tooth powder will also whiten your teeth naturally. *Once you are used to it, tooth powder, flavored to your preference, is a pleasure to use.*
4. **Brush the front top of the tongue.** Some people prefer to use a tongue scraper, but I prefer using my toothbrush. If you brush too far back on your tongue, you may scrape off some helpful bacteria that are, surprisingly, potentially important for heart health. In fact, brushing the tongue is not necessary for preventing gingivitis and tooth decay, but it does prevent bad breath.[456] *Gently take care of your tongue.*
5. **Floss your teeth daily.** I prefer to use a water flosser because it is gentler on the gums than string floss,[457] but I also keep some natural floss picks on hand —some in

the house, and some travel ones in my purse. *Avoid inflammation in the gums by keeping the food cleaned out from between the teeth.*

6. **Do oil pulling occasionally and as needed.**[458, 459] Swish a tablespoon of organic sesame oil or olive oil in your mouth for 20 minutes and then spit it into the trash, not the sink. Follow this by rinsing with water. *Oil pulling can pull out the beginnings of infections and provide nutrition to the teeth.*
7. **Do not use mouthwash on a regular basis.** Most mouthwashes aim to kill all of the bacteria in your mouth, but the health of your mouth and in fact your entire body rely on the good bacteria (and other organisms) in your mouth (the oral microbiome).[460, 461] Some new mouthwashes are being developed with probiotics or bee propolis, so if you have a specific need for mouthwash, you may find an appropriate option. Still, most mouthwashes have unhealthy ingredients in addition to their potential to unbalance the oral microbiome. *You can use a mouthwash with healthy ingredients on occasion, when you feel it is needed.*
8. **Follow the diet in *Cure Tooth Decay*** by Ramiel Nagel. *Although remineralizing tooth powder is helpful, most of the nutrients that form the structure of your teeth must come from the food you eat.*
9. **Moisturize the lips with organic refined shea butter**, as needed. It is important not to use commercial lip treatments that commonly contain poisons. *Natural moisturization is best for people who are sensitive.*
10. **Do not get amalgam fillings** for cavities (the silver ones) because they contain mercury, which can cause problems in individuals who are hypersensitive to mercury (which is up to 4% of the population,[462] and I would imagine that people with hEDS might be more likely than the general population to be hypersensitive). If you have amalgam fillings, it would be best to have them removed by a biologic dentist who will take extreme precautions to prevent you from getting any of the mercury into your body. (After having an amalgam filling removed, you will need to chelate either with the Andy Cutler method or TRS.) Many biologic dentists will let you muscle test or otherwise test the filling options to see which will work best for your body if you need a filling.[463] *Your teeth and anything that is put in them will be in your body for a long time, and the fillings will decay ever so slowly; make sure you only put health-giving components in your body.*

> TOOTH AND GUM CARE
> 1. Brush your teeth twice per day.
> 2. Use a Bass toothbrush.
> 3. Use remineralizing tooth powder.
> 4. Brush the front top of the tongue.
> 5. Floss your teeth daily.
> 6. Do oil pulling occasionally and as needed.
> 7. Do not use mouthwash on a regular basis.
> 8. Follow the diet in *Cure Tooth Decay*.
> 9. Moisturize lips with organic refined shea butter.
> 10. Do not get amalgam fillings.
>
> Ask your doctor before trying anything new.

Mouth Posture

One of the most unusual things about the hEDS/HSD mouth is that it is more mobile than most people's mouths. Because of this, it is common for people with hEDS/HSD to develop a high, narrow palate and crowded teeth. However, orthodontic braces, which are the course of action for the majority of people, are usually not the best option for us. Once you use braces, your teeth are even more likely to move around, and they often return to the pre-braces position or an even more crooked alignment.[464]

The better option for most hEDS/HSD patients with misaligned teeth or jaw may be orthotropics. Instead of simply moving teeth, orthotropics reshapes the mouth in a beneficial way that allows the teeth to align properly. Whereas braces can lead to a misshapen face and many side effects, orthotropics improves the shape of the face for better function and appearance.[465, 466]

Orthotropics was invented by John Mew and has been spreading across the world in recent decades. The validity and efficacy of orthotropics, as a new field in opposition to orthodontics, is hotly debated, but he has many followers who have benefited from orthotropics.[467]

Orthotropic interventions (like the Biobloc[468]) are usually used on children and teens, but people with connective tissue disorders are more likely than others to be able to reshape the mouth at an adult age. However, there are two treatment options that are subtler and less expensive that can be tried before going for orthotropic treatment.

Craniosacral Therapy is a very gentle, hands-on therapy that can help the body align the bones correctly. With the help of a Craniosacral Therapist, you may be able to release tension in the jaw and widen the palate a little bit, giving the teeth room to straighten.[469, 470] See Section VI: Seek Professional Help.

Correct resting tongue posture and tongue position during swallowing can also make a difference in the jaw and palate positioning. Some people call correct tongue posture (with the tongue spread against the roof of the mouth) "mewing," after John Mew who popularized the importance of correct tongue posture.

John Mew and his son, Mike Mew, have released videos that give detailed information about how to do the posture correctly and why: "Tips and Exercises to Correct the Position of Tongue by Prof John Mew." There are many more helpful and interesting videos on their YouTube channel, Orthotropics.

https://www.YouTube.com/watch?v=MPZBVmzAO1M

https://www.youtube.com/@Orthotropics

Tongue posture is extremely important for numerous health concerns, like sleep apnea, snoring, posture stability, strength, and attractiveness.[471, 472] You may need to correct yourself 5,000 times a day for a week, but eventually you will develop a habit of keeping your tongue in the correct position and you may never need to think about it again.

Some people have difficulty maintaining proper tongue posture because they have tongue and buccal ties (excessive or tight frenulum holding the soft tissues of the mouth in restricted positions). These ties are frequently associated with EDS.[473] They are sometimes inherited and sometimes develop as a result of stress or *in utero* as a result of the mother's folate deficiency (or excessive folic acid). Tight frenula can lead to problems with speaking and eating, excessive cavities and other dental health problems, sleep apnea and other sleep problems, TMJ pain, and more.[474]

The frenula are mostly made up of fascia and oral mucosa. As discussed in Chapter 52: Myofascial Release Massage, people with hEDS develop thicker fascia with more adhesions than the general public. However, the condition of the fascia is not permanent; it can be released with various massage techniques. For this reason combined with our inherent flexibility, I believe that most people with connective tissue disorders rarely need to have tongue or buccal ties cut — more gentle techniques can be tried first. However, when cutting a tie is necessary, it should only be handled by a recommended provider who specializes in this, as some dentists who do the procedures use the wrong techniques and get poor results. The removal of the ties should be preceded and followed by other types of therapy as well, such as speech therapy, Craniosacral Therapy, and Occupational Therapy.[475, 476]

For those with hEDS/HSD, I recommend trying Craniosacral Therapy, Occupational Therapy, stress reduction, meditation, and massage before resorting to tie revision by a professional. Even stretching the tie on your own with your fingers and tongue movements might be successful since you are extra stretchy.

In addition to improving tongue position, your mouth may benefit from increasing jaw strength. As the Mews explain, our cultures eat tough, chewy, or crunchy foods much less frequently than our ancestors did; with the soft foods available now, our jaws do not get the everyday workouts they need. Chewing gum, tree resin, or a product like a Myo Munchee can increase strength in the muscles of the jaw, which then can keep the bones in place better.

Also, lip position matters for tooth positioning. Many of us who have been chronically ill have also begun to chronically frown, grimace, pout, or sneer. The tightening of the lips in these facial expressions will work against your tongue's efforts to widen the palate and spread the teeth. Try to develop a "resting bliss face," as I like to call it (as opposed to a "resting bitch face" which was a popular phrase on social media not too long ago). The gentle pressure of your slightly smiling lips will help shape your jaw and teeth into an attractive position. It will also send a message to your body that you are happy and ready to heal. And, it might help things go more smoothly in any social or family interactions.

One final aspect of mouth posture to be aware of is the importance of babies' suckling. When babies are breastfed, the muscular action of withdrawing milk from the breast improves the development of their jaw. They should not be spoon fed until around 1 year old, although they can experiment with foods beginning around 6 months, for optimal jaw development.[477]

My Experience with Mouth Posture

I had braces as a teenager, and despite wearing a permanent retainer for many years afterward and then wearing a removable retainer every night, my teeth moved. It was very painful and looked bad, so the orthodontist gave me braces again, this time for free. The second time, I kept the permanent retainer even longer, but yet again, once it was off, my teeth moved again.

I have seen friends get braces and end up very unhappy with their faces, in exactly the ways that the Drs. Mew warn about. I, however, have finally had improvement since learning about mewing.

When I was a teenager, a guest speaker at our school told us that when people are nervous, they jam the tip of their tongue against the back of their teeth. According to the speaker, they supposedly do this to protect their teeth from being knocked out if they get hit in the face. She advocated for us to let our tongue rest at the bottom and back of our mouth, so I went from one bad position (tongue-to-teeth) to an even worse one (tongue on the floor of the mouth).

When I learned about mewing and started holding my tongue on the roof of my mouth, I experienced some reduction in stress and anxiety, and I started getting better sleep; over the years, my palate noticeably expanded, so that it is lower and broader than ever before, and my teeth are straighter than any time except when I had orthodontic metal glued to them.

Preventions, Treatments, and Coping Strategies for Mouth Posture

Good mouth posture has many impacts on our health, including adding strength to the tensegrity of the neck and improving stability when standing and exercising.

Create Healthy Mouth Posture

1. **Practice mewing** or correct tongue position. Whenever you are not eating or talking, place the tongue suctioned against the entire roof of the mouth with the top and bottom teeth barely touching and the lips closed. This will help keep the palate wide and low, as it should be. *Proper tongue posture makes you stronger, healthier, and more attractive.*
2. **Chew a lot.** Eat foods that have not been processed to the point that they are soft. Also chew on gum, tree resin, or a Myo Munchee to build the strength in your jaw so that the muscles can hold it in the correct position. *A strong jaw is not only protective of health, it is also attractive.*
3. **Do Buteyko Mouth Taping during sleep** if you usually sleep with your mouth open. *Many important health factors depend on you sleeping with your mouth closed.*[478]
4. **Eliminate tongue and buccal ties.** Try stretching, massage, relaxation, Craniosacral Therapy, Speech Therapy, and Occupational Therapy to relax the tight frenula. If these therapies are not successful, seek out a skilled provider to cut the ties properly. *Oral ties limit the movement of the tongue, lips, and cheeks, causing problems with tongue posture and speech, as well as potentially creating many other symptoms.*
5. **Keep your "resting bliss face" on.** The pressure of the lips against the teeth helps to form them into the correct shape when you smile slightly, but frowns will malform them. *Improve your mouth posture, look more attractive, increase your health, and look friendlier to the people who see you.*
6. **Relieve hypertonicity in jaw muscles**. Injuries and stress can cause our facial muscles to tighten up in ways that pull our jaw out of alignment. See also Chapter 36: TMJ. *Use meditation, massage, Craniosacral Therapy, and other relaxing techniques to keep the muscles healthy.*
7. **Use good sitting posture at the dining table.** Sitting up straight and not talking while chewing improves jaw positioning, especially for young children whose facial structure is developing.[479] *All of the body is connected.*

CREATE HEALTHY MOUTH POSTURE

1. Practice mewing.
2. Chew a lot.
3. Do Buteyko Mouth Taping during sleep.
4. Eliminate tongue and buccal ties.
5. Keep your "resting bliss face" on.
6. Relieve hypertonicity in jaw muscles.
7. Use good sitting posture at the dining table.

Ask your doctor before trying anything new.

LINKS FOR PRODUCTS MENTIONED IN THIS CHAPTER

Bass Toothbrush https://store.orawellness.com/products/bass-toothbrush?variant=31237245841

Tongue Scraper https://amzn.to/4cMp5bv

Water Flosser https://amzn.to/3RTLidI

Floss Picks https://amzn.to/3JfcyQ9

Travel Floss Picks https://amzn.to/4cQmOfg

Olive Oil https://amzn.to/3VwrYqh

Cure Tooth Decay https://amzn.to/3NWMKuW

Refined Shea Butter https://amzn.to/4aTnwa1

Myo Munchee https://myomunchee.com/

24 MTHFR

MTHFR IS A GENE THAT MAKES AN ENZYME also called MTHFR (Methylenetetrahydrofolate Reductase), which metabolizes folate so that it can be used in a number of very important processes in the body, including some detoxification processes. Colloquially, the term MTHFR is used to indicate a condition in which a person has one or more SNPs of the MTHFR gene (single-nucleotide polymorphism, which means changes in the gene).

MTHFR is not caused by hEDS and does not cause hEDS (probably), but approximately 40% of the general population has it, and some clinics have found that a much larger percentage of people with hEDS have it.[480] MTHFR especially impacts hypermobility because it can cause abnormalities in the collagen matrix of connective tissues. It also causes a thickening of the fascia, which causes pain; people with hEDS tend to have unusually thick and painful fascia.[481] Clearly, these conditions and other MTHFR symptoms will make hEDS/HSD symptoms more pronounced.

MTHFR can also significantly decrease the body's detox pathways' effectiveness and is thought to cause a plethora of possible symptoms such as chronic fatigue, ADHD, hormone imbalances, digestive problems, allergies, pain, and so much more.[482, 483, 484] The detox pathways are the organs and systems that the body uses to remove and excrete unwanted chemicals.[485] These chemicals may be metabolic wastes (products that cells make as part of being alive), hormones that are no longer needed (without proper detoxification, hormonal imbalances can be created or exacerbated – for those with MCAS, note that histamine is a hormone), or noxious chemicals that originated outside of the body (such as fragrances, other household chemicals, and synthetic food additives).

In order to remove these chemicals, the body must break them down through multiple phases along the detox pathways. Each of these phases requires specific nutrients that are components of the foods we eat. A varied, complex diet of whole foods (not processed foods), especially plants, is the most supportive diet for the operation of the detox pathways. However, people who have MTHFR may need supplementation of additional quantities of these food components in order to maintain optimal detoxing.

Additionally, maintaining a toxin-free lifestyle can reduce the burden on the detox pathways, resulting in fewer symptoms.

My Experience with MTHFR

A recent clinical study showed that patients with hEDS lost their symptoms when they took folate, which is the main treatment for MTHFR.[486] Based on my experience of having followed the MTHFR treatment protocols but still having hEDS/HSD symptoms, I believe that they are two separate conditions, but they do affect each other.

Nevertheless, following the MTHFR protocol was valuable and reduced my chemical sensitivities somewhat. It seemed that my body became more capable of detoxing noxious chemicals and hormones. I continue to take the two most important supplements of the protocol: methylcolbalamin and methylfolate. I also continue to avoid toxins and especially laughing gas (nitrous oxide).

Preventions, Treatments, and Coping Strategies for MTHFR

These steps are probably necessary only if you have one of the MTHFR SNPs, which you can discover through a genetic test. However, these steps should be health promoting for anyone.

Compensate for MTHFR

1. **Get medical help and study Dr. Ben Lynch's recommendations** for MTHFR. Naturopathic doctors are likely to be able to help you with MTHFR. Dr. Lynch has written a book called *Dirty Genes: A Breakthrough Program to Treat the Root Cause of Illness and Optimize Your Health*, which I have not read but which has been a bestseller. Based on his recommendations, you will likely begin with avoiding folic acid and supplementing with methylcobalamin and then adding in methylfolate. *There are a number of different gene changes that impact what protocol you should follow.* https://mthfr.net/mthfr-c677t-mutation-basic-protocol/2012/02/24/
2. **Detox your lifestyle** so that you reduce the workload on your body's detox system. Eliminate synthetic fragrances, food dyes, food preservatives, plastic food storage containers, Teflon-coated pots and pans, synthetic fabrics, cleaning products containing toxic chemicals, etc. Eat whole foods that are not processed. Some of my favorite products are listed in Appendix B — Annotated List of Recommendations. See also Chapter 44: Detox. *Although it is challenging to change which products and foods you use, and although there are a lot of products that are advertised as toxin-free that are really expensive, when you really get to the simple, natural ingredients that are good for you, they are inexpensive and luxurious at the same time.*
3. **Detox your body.** There are many detox methods to try depending on your body's specific needs. I recommend milk thistle extract supplementation for liver support. Get your lymph flowing using the techniques mentioned in Chapter 51: Lymph Drainage Massage. Have silver amalgam fillings extracted by a biologic dentist who specializes in doing this safely. Most of the chapters of this book include information about nontoxic products. Doing a detox can cause what is known as a Healing Crisis or Herxheimer Reaction, in which getting better causes a temporary increase in symptoms. *It would be ideal if you could find a naturopathic doctor to help you with this so that you have only good results.*

4. **Consider chelating** with either TRS by Coseva or the Andy Cutler Chelation method. Chelating is using supplements to help the body remove poisonous heavy metals from the cells and flush them out of the body. Chelating can sometimes make people feel worse because the heavy metals can redistribute instead of fully being flushed out and create new symptoms. *Make sure you choose a safe method.*

COMPENSATE FOR MTHFR

1. Get medical help and study Dr. Lynch's recommendations.
2. Detox your lifestyle.
3. Detox your body.
4. Consider chelating.

Ask your doctor before trying anything new.

LINKS FOR PRODUCTS MENTIONED IN THIS CHAPTER

Dirty Genes https://amzn.to/3TSkV9m
Methylfolate https://amzn.to/3U3sSdy
Methylcolbalamin https://amzn.to/422EaRi
Milk Thistle https://amzn.to/48LdF4S

25

Neck Pain & CCI

NECK PAIN IS COMMON FOR A LOT OF PEOPLE, but especially those with hypermobility. Among people who have hEDS/HSD, two of the concerning causes of neck pain are Cranio Cervical Instability (CCI) and Atlantoaxial Instability (AAI). CCI is diagnosed when the topmost bone of the neck (the first cervical vertebra) interacts with the skull (cranium) with excessive movement due to ligament laxity, moving around in ways that it is not designed to move. AAI is excessive movement between the first and second cervical vertebrae (the two topmost neck bones) due to ligament laxity.[487, 488]

Frequently, both conditions are present together, and so in common usage, the term CCI encompasses AAI as well. Although these conditions are rare, they happen frequently in hEDS/HSD patients because our ligaments are not strong enough to hold the bones in place, especially since few sports and workout routines include exercises to strengthen the neck muscles sufficiently to stabilize our neck joints.

When the joints of the neck are unstable, it is potentially an even more serious problem than when other joints are unstable because the spinal cord passes down through the middle of them and the cranial nerves pass on the outside of them. All of the nerve signals to the body can be affected if these nerves and/or the fluid that surrounds and protects them are compressed. The Vagus Nerve, which innervates most of the organs and regulates the Sympathetic Nervous System, is among those affected, so compressions or strains in the neck can cause a person to be persistently in the fight-or-flight state and never in the rest-and-digest state.

There are also other causes of neck pain, such as Military Neck and/or Forward Head Posture and Upper Crossed Syndrome (all of these are posture problems); these conditions can be partially caused by CCI or exist on their own. Neck pain can be brought on by traumatic events like being hit in the head, getting whiplash in a car accident, experiencing a stressful social incident, or sleeping in a bad position. Many online Physical Therapists report that tension in the neck can be a result of instability in the pelvis. Other hEDS/HSD secondary conditions such as TOS, Migraine, TMJ, and others can be the underlying cause of neck pain as well. On the other hand, neck instability can be the underlying cause of other conditions, such as Migraine, Occipital or Trigeminal Neuralgia, Lhermitte's Sign, POTS, Cerebellar Ataxia, Motion Sickness, Dysphagia (difficulty and/or pain when swallowing), Digestive System Problems, and other painful conditions.

Some people, like Dr. Ross Houser of Caring Medical, believe that CCI is responsible for most of the symptoms that hEDS patients suffer from. Dr. Houser has produced a lot of interesting YouTube videos in which he promotes prolotherapy to reduce or eliminate CCI. I have not yet found it necessary to try this medical treatment, but it sounds promising because in addition to the good results reported on Dr. Houser's YouTube channel, it is minimally invasive and can use the body's own cells rather than chemicals to affect healing of the ligaments treated. Prolotherapy is performed in a number of different hospitals, but I have not found robust information about it from any source other than Dr. Houser.

https://www.youtube.com/@CaringmedicalProlotherapy

With as many symptoms as neck instability can cause, including perpetual activation of the Sympathetic Nervous System and the cascade of symptoms that follows that, I have come to believe that improving neck alignment and increasing neck strength is the most important thing we can do for our hypermobile bodies. We need our necks to be able to handle all of their daily requirements plus the unexpected bumps or shakes. And, when we do tweak our necks or get injured, we need to focus our efforts on regaining our neck alignment and mobility.

My Experience with Neck Pain

The worst of my hEDS/HSD symptoms radiated from my neck ever since I was a child. I did not understand then that the agonizing electric shock pains I got when I turned my neck just so (Lhermitte's Sign) were signs of a condition. I did not understand that many (but not all) of my headaches and body pains were coming from my cervical vertebrae being out of alignment. In fact, it was only very recently that I began to understand and finally get relief.

The best thing I did for my neck was the Red Ball Exercises. The second-best thing I did for my neck was to improve my posture, and third was to sleep on my back with my pillow tucked under my neck for proper support; when I need extra support for my neck, I also sleep with a rolled-up towel under it on top of my pillow.

When I "tweaked" my neck or injured it in any way, my protocol of treating it usually went in this order: Red Ball Exercises; sprayed with Magnesium Oil; took one baby aspirin; took a spray of methylcolbalamin; chewed a methylfolate tablet; when the magnesium oil had dried, applied evening primrose oil; sat in a hard chair so I could be very upright, or if the pain was really bad, lied down with a pillow or rolled towel under my neck. Often, this would be enough to eliminate symptoms. If it continued to be painful or cause other symptoms, then I did the Basic Exercise; took homeopathic medicines; lay on a heating pad; did a very gentle self-massage of surrounding areas, especially my face and back; applied comfrey oil; did gentle Range of Motion exercises — if this was too painful, then I needed the assistance of an Osteopath. Almost always, I also included treatments for Peripheral Neuralgia, since that was likely to have occurred: B vitamins, acetylcholine (as long as Dystonia was not present), evening primrose oil, Homeopathic Remedies, Earthing, etc.

One of the most surprising symptoms I got with neck injury was Digestive System Problems: upset stomach, indigestion, bloating, and diarrhea. When this happened, my stomachache was worst when I was hungry. The food choices I made did not impact the stomachache, but if I overate, that made it worse. I also often got congestion when I hurt my neck, which for a long time led me to think that Allergy/MCAS/MCS were always the problem when in fact sometimes it was CCI...or that the neck injury was the MCAS trigger. Whenever the neck pain resolved, so did the digestive problems and congestion.

As my neck got stronger, it needed less attention, but every effort I put into caring for my neck was worth it.

Preventions, Treatments, and Coping Strategies for Neck Pain

It is important to get your neck muscles strong before you start releasing very much of the hypertonicity, or else your condition could get so much worse you can't work on improving it. Once your neck is strong and mobile, you will be able to drop some of these treatments and only bring them out again when a traumatic injury occurs.

Prevent and Treat Neck Pain

1. **Maintain correct head posture.** Pull the ears up; do not let the neck hinge upon itself and do not jut out the chin. Notice that when you are stressed out about anything, be it a financial problem, a social situation, a cold day outside, etc., you may have a tendency to jut out the chin. Also notice that when you bend forward, you may allow the cervical spine to get jammed together. Keep it long all of the time. If you have slumping shoulders, lift your chest and sternum – this will pull the shoulders back, and if you lift the chest enough, it will help pull the head back into position so that you can concentrate on lifting the head rather than pulling it back. Head posture is societal, meaning that it varies from culture to culture, and it is learned when we are babies, so changing head posture is extremely difficult. It will take years of dedication and possibly help from professionals such as Physical Therapists, Chiropractors, and Osteopaths, but it will be worth it. See Chapter 56: Posture. *This is the most important step for eliminating neck pain, but it will also allow your diaphragm to work properly for good deep breathing.*
2. **If your neck gets tired, lie down to rest**. Usually when my neck was tired, I would hinge it and kind of rest my cranium (skull) on top of my spine with my chin jutted forward. The hinged position is very bad for your neck and can damage the nerves. *In order to prevent injury, lie down with a rolled towel or supportive pillow under your neck and rest until you can hold your neck upright.*
3. **Do the Basic Exercise** from *Accessing the Healing Power of the Vagus Nerve* by Stanley Rosenberg. This is an eye exercise that takes two minutes, so it is very easy to incorporate whenever you feel that you need it. Some people prefer to do the exercise with their eyes closed. Keep your head still, and look with your eyes all of the way to the right for one minute and then all of the way to the left for one minute. The eyes are connected via the occipital nerves to the neck, so they are able to turn off stress and release tension and pain throughout the head, neck, and body. This exercise can also reduce or eliminate sound sensitivity. *It is common to need to do the Basic Exercise following a difficult social encounter or time spent in a sensory-rich environment.*
4. **Maintain correct tongue posture.** See Chapter 23: Mouth Health. The position and tension of the tongue affects the tensegrity of the neck. *Tensegrity refers to the balance of tension and relaxation among the muscles, ligaments, tendons, and fascia, and it is critical for stability.*[489, 490]

5. **Do range-of-movement exercises very slowly.**[491] Gently, slowly turn the head side to side, up and down, and tilt the ears down on each side. Do not move the head forward and back, and do not roll your head while looking up as some trainers might teach; this is not safe if you have CCI (rolling while looking down is probably OK). Do not tip the head back too far, as people with hEDS tend not to have a sense of when to stop and end up pinching nerves in the neck. Moving very, very slowly will allow your nervous system to recognize where your body is in space and find its own correct alignment. Then, moving slowly, but not quite as slowly, going smoothly through the neck's natural range of motion will stretch and activate muscles without challenging the joints. *It is extremely important to keep the neck muscles in good condition.*
6. **Do Red Ball Exercises** to strengthen the neck. Some neck strengthening exercises are dangerous for people with hypermobility, so proceed with caution. This routine was developed by Sterling Cooley of the Vagus Nerve Stimulation and Repair Program. It is often effective at realigning the cervical spine, in addition to strengthening it. It will take one minute to do the exercises, and you should start doing them just once a day, but you can slowly build up to doing them frequently throughout the day. Place a rubber ball, inflated to only 90%, against a wall at head height. Then, press the head gently into the ball 15 times, keeping the neck straight and head stable the whole time. Do this for all 4 sides of the head. *Strengthening the muscles of the neck is key to eliminating CCI and keeping the entire body healthy.*
7. **When lying down, use a pillow or a rolled-up towel to support the curve of the neck.** A specialty pillow might work best for you, but I prefer my down and cotton pillow with a rolled cotton towel, plus it didn't cost anything extra. *Especially when asleep, support tools will help keep the cervical curve even when your muscles are tired.*
8. **Do the suboccipital muscles stretch** from Motivational Doc on YouTube: "TRY THIS...Feel How Your Eyes Connect to the Neck! (Neck Pain, Headaches, Dizziness) - Dr Mandell." Wait to do this stretch until after you have strengthened your neck with the Red Ball Exercises and Range of Motion exercises; if you do it too soon, you may become more unstable than before. This is an exercise that uses eye and head position to stretch the muscles that connect between the eyes and the neck — you look all the way down and press your head down, then look up and lift the head. It is always extremely important to be careful and go slowly when stretching, especially when stretching the neck. There are many neck stretches recommended in YouTube videos, and this is the only one that I recommend you do, but you may need to start with fewer reps than Dr. Mandell recommends. *This stretch can release neck tension, which will make it much easier to achieve correct head posture.*
   https://www.YouTube.com/watch?v=gj0luiN422Q&list=LL&index=26
9. **Do neck stretches** to release hypertonicity.[492] Wait until you have strengthened your neck; if you release tension when you don't have strength, your neck will become even more unstable than before. Be very careful, and do not stretch your neck daily. Stretch it only briefly when you cannot release hypertonicity another way. Do not stretch it if you have a nerve injury that was caused by overstretching the nerve; this will slow the repair. Begin with a gentle stretch: lie down in bed, put your hands behind your head, and with the strength of your neck, push your head back into your hands, then release. The next level of stretching the neck is best done in the front seat of an automobile. With your head against the head rest, tuck your chin a bit and push your head back into the head rest (your hands are not involved in this stretch). After a few seconds, release. You can then turn your head

slightly to each side and press against the headrest again. Do this in various positions to release the various muscles in the neck. Do it gently, slowly, and for a short amount of time. It is especially important not to stretch the back of the neck too much, as anyone with Military Neck or Forward Head Posture may already have too-long ligaments in the back of the neck.[493] Once you have stretched a time or two and your muscles are less tense, you may do best to refrain from stretching the neck any more. *Releasing hypertonicity in the neck will relieve pain and allow the muscles to work appropriately and the bones of the neck to move into better alignment.*

10. **Use heat.**[494] Apply a heating pad at the end of a stressful day so that your muscles can relax before sleep. Heat will relax hypertonic (overly tense) muscles so that the cervical spine can settle into the correct position. However, do not fall asleep with a heating pad that doesn't have an automatic-off feature; extremely excessive use of heat can damage skin cells, resulting in discoloration and eventually, potentially, cancer.[495, 496] *Heat will feel soothing.*
11. **Massage.**[497, 498] Self-massage or massage from a friend or a therapist are all helpful. Do not press hard on any area where there may be a nerve injury; the nerve will be vulnerable and can be further damaged. Gently press and rub on any knots that are found. Always massage gently. Sometimes massaging the shoulders, chest, and back are even more helpful to the neck than rubbing the neck itself. A good scalp and ear massage can be beneficial as well. *Human touch is a magical tool for making us feel better.*
12. **Do Myofascial Release Massage.** Make sure that you have first built up a lot of strength in your neck. Before you try to release the fascia, the Red Ball Exercises should be easy to do, and you should rarely have any cervical spine misalignment; if you release the fascia when the neck muscles are weak, you will have far too much movement and will cause yourself pain and other symptoms. See Chapter 52: Myofascial Release Massage. Repeat the gentle manipulation on all the areas of the neck, upper shoulders, and jaw. *Releasing the fascia of the neck, shoulders, and jaw will allow the neck to regain its full range of motion and move into a new, more appropriate posture.*

PREVENT AND TREAT NECK PAIN

1. Maintain correct head posture.
2. If your neck gets tired, lie down to rest.
3. Do The Basic Exercise.
4. Maintain correct tongue posture.
5. Do Range of Motion exercises very slowly.
6. Do Red Ball Exercises.
7. When lying down, use a rolled-up towel or specialty pillow to support the curve of the neck.
8. Do the suboccipital muscle stretch.
9. Do neck stretches.
10. Use heat.
11. Massage.
12. Do Myofascial Release Massage.
13. Cope with stress by keeping good posture.
14. Apply comfrey oil.
15. Use Homeopathic Remedies.
16. Treat any nerve damage.
17. Do advanced neck strengthening exercises.

Ask your doctor before trying anything new.

13. **Cope with stress by keeping good posture**. It is best if you can avoid stress, but this is not always possible. When you are anxious, your body may respond by

clenching the abdominal muscles, rolling the shoulders in to the front, and letting the sternum and rib cage collapse down. This torso positioning makes it especially difficult to maintain correct head posture, so aim to keep the sternum lifted and the chest opened. *Even when you feel threatened, stand tall and proud to let your body know that you are not giving up — you have many more good days to be here for.*

14. **Apply magnesium oil.** *Magnesium is a safe way of relieving tension, and it helps nerves heal.*[499]
15. **Apply comfrey oil.** *Comfrey will help repair tissue damage and relieve pain.*[500]
16. **Use homeopathic remedies.** *Gelsemium* has been especially helpful for me. *Homeopathic remedies can communicate to your neck the ways it needs to heal.*
17. **Treat any nerve damage.** Take B vitamins (especially methylcolbalamin and methylfolate), nerve-supporting culinary herbs, and a single baby aspirin. See Chapter 28: Peripheral Neuropathy for more information. *The nerves in the neck are especially vulnerable to damage because of the large amount of movement possible among the cervical vertebrae and the small clearances for nerves, so supporting the health of the nervous system can reduce pain in the neck.*
18. **Do advanced neck strengthening exercises.** See Chapter 56: Posture for more advanced exercises. *Continue increasing the challenge of the exercises to increase the strength of the neck and protect the valuable nerves here.*

LINKS FOR PRODUCTS MENTIONED IN THIS CHAPTER

Accessing the Healing Power of the Vagus Nerve https://amzn.to/3S1xRJ8
Red Ball https://amzn.to/4bgpYXU
Comfrey Oil https://amzn.to/3TDV4D9
Magnesium Bath Flakes https://amzn.to/3HrNIvn
Gelsemium https://amzn.to/3tLaTO3
Methylfolate https://amzn.to/3U3sSdy
Methylcolbalamin https://amzn.to/422EaRi
Aspirin https://amzn.to/3Snl7Of

26

Osteopenia & Osteoporosis

OSTEOPENIA IS A CONDITION OF LOW BONE DENSITY, and osteoporosis is a condition in which the structure or strength of bones has decreased due to diminished bone density or mass. On their own, these conditions do not cause pain and often go unnoticed until a fall or other accident causes a fracture. In addition to increasing the risk of fracture, low bone density can cause pain in the spine as the vertebrae collapse.[501]

Bone density loss frequently occurs as people age, but the risk of it is even greater among those with connective tissue disorders.[502] We should all be aware of the risk and make efforts from a young age to build up strong bones.

Fortunately, bone density can be increased, osteoporosis can be prevented, and osteopenia can be halted or reversed with jumping or bouncing and resistance training (Strength Training with weights, body weight, or resistance bands).[503, 504]

Jumping or bouncing is effective at building bone density throughout the entire body, including in bones that are in areas that are difficult to affect with resistance training. However, resistance training increases bone density even more effectively than does jumping, for the areas that the training addresses.[505] It is best to do both kinds of exercise in order to get the strongest bones possible throughout the body.

These kinds of exercise are much better for you than the pharmaceutical drugs for osteopenia and osteoporosis that have harmful side effects. In fact, jumping has the beneficial side effects of getting lymph flowing and building muscle and cardiac and pulmonary stamina. Resistance training has similar beneficial side effects, including reducing fall risks that can lead to bone fractures in people with osteoporosis.

Because low bone density increases the risk of injury during exercise, it is useful for people with osteopenia or osteoporosis to have the help of a Physical Therapist or qualified Personal Trainer when initiating an exercise program that includes jumping and/or resistance training. Fortunately, under supervised conditions, these exercises are unlikely to be dangerous even for people with low bone density. In fact, even for these patients, high-intensity workouts are safe and can be more effective than low-intensity workouts.[506] People with Joint Instability should be similarly cautious.

My Experience with Osteoporosis

My mother was diagnosed with Osteopenia, and her doctor put her on a medication to stop bone loss. However, after a few months, my mother had the intuition that the medication was not good for her, and when she looked up the side effects of it, she saw that she was right. Someone she knew well developed Osteonecrosis of the Jaw (progressive bone destruction) as a side effect of the medication for osteoporosis. My mother investigated further and learned that jumping could be as effective as the medication.

So, my mother went to her doctor and asked if it would be OK for her to stop the medication and try jumping. The doctor replied that she had recommended the medication because she didn't think anyone would actually jump. "I don't believe you'll jump enough to stop your bone loss, but if you want to try it for a few months, we can test your bone density again after you have tried it to see if it is successful."

The doctor told her that she could halt the medication if she would jump for at least 10 minutes a day, which was impossible for my mother at first. But, she did the best she could and increased her jumping over time. Even so, she only got up to about 2 minutes a day of jumping.

The results on her next bone density test were surprising. Not only had she stopped the bone loss, but unlike the results she had gotten from the medication, her bone loss had now begun to reverse.

She abandoned the dangerous medication and continued to jump – she now completes 100 jumps on the floor and 100 jumps on a mini-trampoline each day. She also added Strength Training to her regimen and continues to do well. I pray that doctors will learn to trust their patients and encourage exercise when appropriate.

Preventions, Treatments, and Coping Strategies for Osteoporosis

Finding the motivation to do the work to build up bone density can be challenging because low bone density does not cause unpleasant symptoms. The effort can make a big difference in your future, though. Fortunately, you will probably get enjoyment and other positive and more immediate health outcomes from your efforts.

Prevent and Reverse Osteopenia and Osteoporosis

1. **Jump** on a trampoline or on the floor for as long each day as possible. [507] Jump at least 20 times, twice a day. Carefully assess your ability before you begin — jumping should not be done if you have any injuries or problems with balance. Holding onto a balance bar can help. Jumping on a trampoline requires more balance than jumping on the floor and the unevenness of it can challenge joints, but the harder impact of jumping on the floor can be harder on the joints. Bouncing without leaving contact with the trampoline surface is also effective when jumping is too dangerous. *When you jump, your body is stimulated to build up the density of its bones in response; there are many other positive health effects as well, such as increased lung capacity, increased muscle mass, and improved lymph flow.*

> **PREVENT AND REVERSE OSTEOPENIA AND OSTEOPOROSIS**
>
> 1. Jump.
> 2. Do resistance training.
> 3. Take collagen peptides.
> 4. Take vitamins and minerals.
> 5. Get sunlight.
> 6. Maintain a healthy gut microbiome by taking *L- rhamnosus GG.*
> 7. Reduce inflammation.
>
> Ask your doctor before trying anything new.

2. **Do resistance training.**[508] Strength Training the legs will make a significant improvement in the bone density of the hips, which are an especially vulnerable area for people with osteoporosis. When lifting weights with the arms, make sure that some of your exercises reach over the head. I recommend going slowly so that the joints are not put in danger, but work with as heavy a weight as you can for as long as it feels good — once you begin to feel weak, you should stop and rest. High intensity effort without using a timer or counting repetitions is the best way for many hEDS/HSD people to exercise. See Chapter 62: Strength Training. *Building strength in your muscles will also build the strength of the bones.*
3. **Take collagen peptides.**[509, 510, 511] As we age, our bodies need more help making collagen, regardless of whether we have a connective tissue disorder or not. Of course, as hEDS patients so frequently point out, the collagen we ingest will be broken down in our digestive tracts and the protein building blocks will be used to make faulty collagen in the way that our hypermobile bodies have always made it. However, having a deficiency of collagen is even worse if the collagen is faulty than if it is normal. It is extra important that people with hEDS/HSD have all of the nutrients necessary for collagen production. The people I know who have hEDS and take collagen peptides report that it gives them energy but that they prefer to take a very small dose, and this has been my experience as well. *Collagen peptides contain all of the proteins that will be used for building bones and are shown to increase bone mineral density.*
4. **Take vitamins and minerals.**[512] *Sufficient levels of calcium, magnesium, boron, Vitamin D, Vitamin K, and potassium can delay age-related bone loss.*
5. **Get sunlight.** [513] Five hours or more a day is optimal. *The Vitamin D in sunlight is very supportive of bone health.*
6. **Maintain a healthy gut microbiome by taking *L- rhamnosus GG*.** [514] Take a probiotic that will not activate mast cells, and eat a prebiotic diet high in fiber. *A healthy gut microbiome is highly associated with good bone health, perhaps because you are able to absorb the vitamins and minerals you need to continue building bone.*
7. **Reduce inflammation.**[515] Many of the symptoms and secondary conditions of hEDS/HSD produce inflammation; throughout this book, I have mentioned numerous ways to help reduce inflammation. Be diligent about keeping your inflammation down. See especially Chapter 11: Allergy, MCAS, & MCS and Chapter 20: Lymph Congestion. *Bone loss can be caused by inflammation, so keep your system as calm and healthy as possible.*

LINKS FOR PRODUCTS MENTIONED IN THIS CHAPTER

Mini Trampoline https://amzn.to/4b14wH2

Collagen Peptides https://amzn.to/3SqgTp2

Probiotic https://amzn.to/3HkFUeX

27

Pelvis Complaints

IT IS WELL DOCUMENTED THAT PEOPLE WITH HEDS suffer from a variety of complaints in the hip and pelvic region.[516, 517] Weak or inflexible ligaments lead to mechanical problems, delicate tissues lead to tears in the vaginal and anal walls, as well as prolapses (when organs fall from their normal position), improper action of pelvic muscles leads to improper function of the organs of the pelvis, and inflammation from Joint Injuries, Digestive System Problems, and Allergy/MCAS/MCS lead to irritation in pelvic organs.

Hypermobile people often report subluxations (significant but incomplete dislocations) in the hips. Painful conditions like Hip Torsion, in which the hip is twisted or rotated to the front or back, or Hip Upslip, in which the pelvic bone (ilium) moves upward along the sacroiliac joint in relation to the sacrum (the bone just above the tailbone), are common and can be chronic.

Pelvic Floor Dysfunction is common among people with hEDS. The pelvic floor is the muscles, fascia, and ligaments that stretch between the pubic bone in the front to the tailbone in the back; they support the organs of the pelvis and assist with the functions of the organs. In Pelvic Floor Dysfunction, some muscles and the fascia may be weak while others may be hypertonic (excessively tense).[518] This frequently causes pain in the pelvis and lower back, as well as a variety of difficulties with going to the bathroom and having sex. Pelvic Floor Dysfunction can also contribute to pelvic organ prolapse.

People with hEDS are much more likely to have pelvic organ prolapse and at younger ages than the general population. Perhaps as many as 75% of women with hEDS experience prolapses such as:

- rectocele (the rectum bulges into the back wall of the vagina, causing problems with emptying the bowels).[519]
- cystocele (the bladder bulges into the front wall of the vagina, causing urinary symptoms).
- urethrocele (the urethra through which urine flows droops, causing urinary symptoms, pain during intercourse, or vaginal bleeding).
- enterocele (the small intestines bulge into the back wall of the vagina, causing constipation or diarrhea).
- uterine prolapse (the uterus drops down into the vagina, potentially causing back pain, heavy bleeding, and pain with sex).

- vaginal vault prolapse (the top part of the vagina drops into the vaginal canal, causing pelvic pain).
- rectal prolapse (the rectum drops down through the anus, causing pain, incontinence, constipation, or diarrhea).[520, 521, 522, 523]

Additionally, these prolapse conditions can result in symptoms like pain, discomfort, difficulty with sex, difficulty when going to the bathroom, incontinence, urinary frequency, urinary urgency, fecal incontinence, urinary tract infection, constipation, dysmenorrhea (lack of a menstrual period), menorrhagia (excessive menstrual bleeding), interstitial cystitis (bladder pain, urinary frequency, and urgency), and more.

Most pelvis complaints can be treated with Physical Therapy from a pelvic specialist. My brilliant pelvic specialty Physical Therapist told me that incontinence is not something that should naturally happen as we age; she had successfully cured a 90-year-old woman of incontinence; she had also successfully treated countless other pelvic conditions. However, I have also been to a different Physical Therapist who told me that she was a pelvic specialist but who clearly did not have the knowledge and experience to achieve the same success rates. If your PT is not getting you the results you hope for, try another one. Ask around for recommendations from friends who have had pelvic PT, or ask Chiropractors, Osteopaths, Pilates Teachers, dancers, etc. — people who work with clients with these conditions will likely know who is getting good results.

My PT also told me that in our society, the things that happen in the pelvis — elimination and reproduction — are taboo subjects, so we spend very little time talking or thinking in healthy and robust ways about this part of our body. This has led to our brains and nervous systems having fewer connections to the pelvis than are meant to be there, and so pelvic pain and dysfunction are common in our society.

My Experience with Pelvis Complaints

By the time I had my son, I had been having untreated pelvic problems for many years; I was as yet unaware of the potential for Physical Therapy to help. When I gave birth, my pubic symphysis (the joint in the pubic bone which separates during childbirth) closed up wrong, though I didn't know it at the time, and it led to very severe pelvic misalignments. When I talked to my obstetricians and midwives about the pain I was experiencing in my hips, thighs, and lower back, they all thought the pain would go away on its own and did nothing about it. It was another two years before I learned about Physical Therapists that specialize in the pelvis.

By that time, my pain extended throughout my entire body, as it had become severe in the pelvis and referred from there, and additionally it had caused compensatory misalignments in my back and other body parts. I was having such urinary frequency and urgency that I had to rush to the bathroom every 15 minutes while awake and several times every night when I should have been sleeping. Sometimes, the skin on my thighs would burn due to nerve damage from my condition (Peripheral Neuropathy).

The worst symptom, though, was the feeling that there was no earth below me. It felt like I had nothing solid to stand on. Clearly, I was walking with my feet on the ground, but with my pelvis so unstable, it felt like the ground was made of pudding.

The muscles in my pelvis were all hypertonic, and I required years of bi- or tri-weekly myofascial release and other treatments and exercises to get the pain down to a manageable level. My pelvis and especially my coccyx were so hypermobile that I would have to be re-evaluated each session to see what adjustments needed to be made. As my body settled into the healing process, the diagnosis that was most frequent was Hip Upslip.

My Physical Therapist said that there were five probable contributing causes of my pelvic instability, the most severe of which was my sensitivity to chemicals (MCAS), which caused inflammation in the tissues of my pelvis. The others were professional-level ballet dancing without cross training, prior sexual assault, natural hypermobility, and injury during childbirth and episiotomy.

Getting Physical Therapy on the pelvis is not the most delightful of activities. Much of the work was done inside the vagina, but I was blessed with very kind, gentle, and understanding Physical Therapists. I was even more blessed by the encouragement and solidarity of my mother and best friend, both of whom also came to the PT office and got their pelvic complaints fixed. Having them going through the same uncomfortable treatments was very reassuring. I was also blessed that PT was covered by my insurance for several years.

I worked really, really hard to straighten out my pelvic problems, and I was successful. I remember the first day that I was able to scrub the dishes in the sink again. (Did you realize that you can't accomplish the scrubbing motion if you don't have stability in your pelvis?) Washing dishes is one of my least favorite chores, but what a relief that I could take care of myself once more. I also clearly remember the first time I could open a car door without pain or a commercial building door, or push a shopping cart, or stand on one foot to put on a sock, or walk up or down the stairs. It was still many more years before I could sit on the floor or on a chair that wasn't cushioned, but all of these improvements came, eventually, following hard work and dedication.

After healing my pelvic problems but a couple years before I discovered that my problem is hEDS/HSD, I was talking to someone who had received an Ehlers-Danlos Syndrome diagnosis. It turned out that his worst symptom was a Hip Upslip. He was bemoaning the fact that it would never heal. I said, "I had that same problem! I healed it with Physical Therapy." He looked at me and said, very seriously, "I can never heal because I have EDS. My doctor said that it is not worth trying."

I pray that my book can help change the minds of the doctors and patients who currently think that there is nothing to be done for the problems caused by hypermobility. Of course we may have experienced damage that cannot be undone, but we are also capable of healing so much. And, with the awareness that this book brings, I pray that we can prevent most of the damage and live comfortably.

Preventions, Treatments, and Coping Strategies for Pelvis Complaints

The pelvis is the foundation of the spinal column and the location of reproduction, digestion, and elimination systems. It is very important to keep it as healthy has possible.

Treat Pelvis Complaints

1. **Get pelvic specialty Physical Therapy**. I do not recommend that you try to heal your own pelvic dysfunction without help from an expert. This is a part of the body that is very complex and can have a lot of different problems and different needs. *A PT will be able to release hypertonic muscles and fascia, help reduce inflammation, evaluate if the muscles are working correctly, and give you very personalized exercise routines.*

2. **Avoid harming your joints further.** Try not to do anything that hurts. See Chapter 9: Joint Pain. Hip pain is especially troublesome when it comes to cleaning your house. Hire a cleaning service until you get better, and when you need to sweep up a mess on the floor, use a Vietnamese Grass Broom. *Use any hacks you can think of to keep your pelvis safe.*
3. **Try some of the go-to maneuvers for the pelvis**. If you are not able to see a Physical Therapist and need help right now, there are some maneuvers that I, my friends, and people on social media have safely used. *Ask your PT if these are right for you before trying them, and then use the appropriate ones to take control of your pelvic comfort.*
    a. Mobilize before you stabilize: Before you do any other maneuver, do these 3 steps. Lie on your back, hug your legs to your chest, then put your feet on the ground and raise your hips into a bridge position while shoulders stay on the ground, and then stretch your legs out straight.
    b. Knee-to-heels: Lie on your back with your knees bent and feet flat on the floor or bed. Slowly drop your right knee down toward your left heel, then bring it back to its starting place. Repeat with your left knee. I was always told to do 20 sets and to go very, very slowly. I was advised to do this exercise before getting out of bed every morning.
    c. Knee swings: Standing next to a chair, place your knee on the chair and, keeping your knee in position, swing your foot side to side so that your thigh within your hip turns out and in. This can be done without a chair by standing on one leg and twisting the other leg with the ball of the foot on the ground like you are softly smushing something with your toes.
    d. Doorway squeeze: Lie in a doorway with one knee on each side of one of the walls, and squeeze the wall with your knees. Hold for 5 seconds and repeat 5 times.
    e. Belt press: Lie on your back with your knees bent and feet flat on the floor or bed. Secure a belt around your knees, and press your knees apart against the resistance of the belt. Hold for 5 seconds and repeat 5 times.
    f. Sacrum squeeze: To strengthen the sacrum to prevent sacroiliac pain, lie on your stomach with the bent knees out to the sides. Squeeze your heels together. Hold for 5 seconds and repeat 5 times.
    g. Kegel exercises: Tighten the pelvic floor muscles that you use to stop the flow of urine, then release them all the way. The relaxation half of the exercise is as important as the tightening half. Physical Therapists can use tools or their hands to make sure that you are doing Kegel exercises correctly. These should only be done when you do not have excessive inflammation or hypertonicity in the pelvis. Physical Therapists can also give you a variety of patterns and positions for doing Kegel exercises to get the most out of them.
    h. If your pelvis is rotated or lifted or otherwise out of alignment, ask your Physical Therapist to teach you the correct maneuver so that you can realign it yourself in between appointments.

TREAT PELVIS COMPLAINTS

1. Get pelvic specialty Physical Therapy.
2. Avoid harming your joints further.
3. Try some of the go-to maneuvers for the pelvis.

Ask your doctor before trying anything new.

LINKS FOR PRODUCTS MENTIONED IN THIS CHAPTER

Vietnamese Grass Broom https://amzn.to/43k26A4

28

Peripheral Neuropathy

PERIPHERAL NEUROPATHY IS SENSATIONS caused by damage to nerves of the Peripheral Nervous System (all of the nerves outside of the spinal cord and brain).[524, 525] The sensations can be pain, itching, burning, pins-and-needles, numbness, electric-like shocks, weakness, and trembling. Peripheral Neuropathy can be caused by exposure to poisonous chemicals, infections, alcohol overuse, hormonal imbalances, vitamin deficiencies, deficiency or excess of calcium, lack of blood flow, inflammation, allergic reactions, traumatic injuries, diabetes, or, most commonly among people with hEDS/HSD, Joint Injuries.[526, 527, 528, 529, 530, 531]

When a Joint Injury occurs, it can pinch (compress) or stretch (strain) the nerves that run through the joint, or the blood vessel that serves a nerve can be compressed so that the nerve becomes starved for oxygen. There is usually pain at the site of the injury immediately, but what are sometimes more noticeable are the symptoms that occur along the nerve's route. For example, a pinched or stretched nerve in the neck can manifest as tingling, numbness, weakness, cramping, sun sensitivity, or pain in the hand and fingers or even the feet, as well as headache, face pain, itching, or twitches.

One of the most common locations for Peripheral Neuropathy symptoms is in the toes because the longest nerve cell (neuron) arm (axon) in the human body runs from the base of the spine to the big toe, which gives plenty of opportunity for damage.[532] Another common site of nerve damage is the wrist, which causes Carpal Tunnel Syndrome.[533] For people with hEDS/HSD one of the most common manifestations is in the forearms, but this indicates nerve damage in the neck.[534, 535]

Nerve damage can occur in any joint in the body, but it is especially a problem when it happens in the neck because of the important nerves in that location. There are three nerves in the neck that are frequently harmed in this way among people who have CCI (Cranio-Cervical Instability): the Trigeminal Nerve, Occipital Nerve, and Vagus Nerve. All three of these nerves are often implicated in Migraine and other types of headaches.[536, 537, 538]

The Trigeminal Nerves run from the back of the neck, over the ears, and into the face at the eyes, nose, mouth, and jaw.[539] Damage to or inflammation around these nerves creates Trigeminal Neuralgia. I read about a woman with this condition whose itching was so intense, she scratched through her skull and had to be locked into a helmet so that she could recover.[540] Neuropathic itching in the face and head are particularly dangerous because humans naturally touch their faces and heads frequently, making it very difficult to resist scratching. Trigeminal Neuralgia is known to be one of the most painful conditions humans can experience. It can also cause grimacing and lead to TMJ Disorder.

The Occipital Nerves run from the back of the neck, over the top of the head, to the eyebrow.[541] They innervate the occipital muscles which run in the same pattern as the nerves. It is surprising and remarkable that you can feel the occipital muscles move if you push your thumbs into the tissue at the back of the head right where it meets the neck, then without moving your head or neck, turn your eyes side to side. Damage to these nerves is called Occipital Neuralgia.

The Vagus Nerve is the wandering nerve and is involved in many organs and processes throughout the body. See Chapter 63: Vagus Nerve Stimulation. Damage to the Vagus Nerve can cause POTS, gastrointestinal problems, and hypervigilance.

So long as the damage to the nerve is continuing, Peripheral Neuropathy symptoms will continue. After the damage has been stopped, it simply takes time for the nerve to heal. If a nerve is pinched or strained only momentarily, the nerve may heal within a few days; if the pinch or strain lasted longer or was more severe, the symptoms may continue for months.

When the nerve is healing, a series of changing symptoms may occur. As soon as the injury has been sustained, the neuron (nerve cell) sends out new nerve fibers along the axon (long arm of the nerve cell that reaches to body parts). At this time, minor symptoms will be noticed. Then, 1-2 days after the injury, the components of the axon that have been damaged will be dismantled and removed during what is called Wallerian degeneration; at the same time, the nucleus of the neuron will move out of the center of the cell body to a safer location on the edge of the cell body, and the chemicals that are normally inside the neuron will be sent away. It is during that time of degeneration that the worst symptoms will be noticed. Next, the axon will rebuild itself, bit by bit. Finally, the nucleus will return to the center of the neuron, and the chemicals will be pulled back into the cell. It may take days or months for this healing process to occur and for symptoms to be alleviated.[542]

In all cases of nerve injuries, one of the most important things you can do to help nerves heal is to keep moving and using all of the affected body parts.[543] The nerves will only grow back where they know they are needed. If you allow a body part to rest for too long, the nerve will not reach to where it used to be and you can develop limited sensation and/or motility in that part.

However, you must be careful not to damage the nerves further. Stretching the joint or near the joint where the injury occurred can further damage the nerve or interrupt the healing process; for example, the axon may rebuild itself into the wrong place.[544] Also, massaging the area of the damage can cause more damage while the nerve is still in a vulnerable state. If the Joint Injury created hypertonic muscles in the area, try doing massage at more distant sites; do only very, very gentle Myofascial Release Massage or Lymph Drainage Massage; or wait until symptoms subside before you massage the area. In fact, if it is possible to relieve pressure from the joint, which is the opposite of stretching, it may be helpful to do that. For example, if the left side of the neck sustained a nerve injury, instead of tilting the head to the right to stretch out that painful left side, tilt the head to the left to give it a little tension release.[545]

Acetylcholine is a very important neurotransmitter that is required throughout the nervous system.[546] Supplementing with this nutrient can help the nerves continue to operate while healing is being undertaken. (However, if you experience Dystonia, acetylcholine supplementation can exacerbate the symptoms because your already-overactive nervous system will become even more active.)

Vitamins that are extremely important for nerve repair and health are B1 (thiamine), B6, B9 (folate), and B12; in fact, a deficiency in B12 can cause Peripheral Neuropathy on its own.[547, 548, 549] Thiamine can be found in whole grains, dairy products, and red meat. B6 can be found in fish, beef, starchy vegetables, and fruit. Folate can be found in beans, asparagus, beets, and beef liver.[550] B12 can be found in fish, beef, poultry, and dairy products.

Vitamin B12 and folate work synergistically together for nerve health, and should be taken together. The best forms to use are methylfolate and methylcolbalamin. These may be the most important supplements to take when healing from Peripheral Neuropathy. Additionally, magnesium is necessary for nerve repair and is used excessively by the body during states of stress; it is effectively supplemented by spraying magnesium oil onto the areas where the symptoms are felt.[551, 552]

Many herbs are known to support nerve health and help damaged nerves heal faster as well.[553] Some of those that are most commonly found in American cuisine are basil, oregano (which is also a mast cell stabilizer), and parsley.[554] Also, curcumin, a substance in turmeric, has been found to be especially helpful for healing nerve injuries, especially when ingested immediately after the injury.[555, 556, 557]

Another herb that has been shown to enhance nerve regeneration and diminish the symptoms of Peripheral Neuropathy is evening primrose oil. It can be taken internally, but I appreciate the immediate effects of applying it to the skin both at the site of the nerve injury and at the site(s) of the neuropathic symptoms.[558, 559]

Nerves heal fairly quickly and well. They want to heal, I believe. Protect the nerves from further damage, and give them time to recover from any injury. Also protect the parts that are experiencing the Peripheral Neuropathy sensations; try not to injure them in response to the inextinguishable itching or pain. At the same time, keep moving and using all of the affected parts.

My Experience of Peripheral Neuropathy

I experienced Peripheral Neuropathy mostly as itching on the inside of my left ankle and on my left big toe. Sometimes it felt like itching or pain on my right big toe or as an intense burning sensation on the skin of my thighs (parasthesia). My skin sometimes became very sensitive to anything touching it, even my soft, lightweight skirt blown by the gentle breeze of someone walking past me. Upon inspection, there was never anything on my skin where the itching or burning pain was occurring.

When my neck was injured, as from an accident, sleeping on it wrong, turning my head funny, tension from stressful situations, or dystonia incited by MCAS reactions, I almost always experienced either Occipital or Trigeminal Neuralgia. This included pain and itching on my face, head, and neck and usually incited a headache or Migraine attack. As my neck muscles grew stronger, I became more capable of protecting the nerves in the neck even when something threatened or harmed my neck.

Previously, when I had not strengthened my neck, I could expect to have these neuralgia symptoms almost perpetually. It was extremely difficult to live like that. I found it very helpful to understand that the itching or pain I was experiencing was not caused by a problem in the affected body part but by damage to a nerve elsewhere.

Often when my pelvis became misaligned, certain movements of my legs could result in painful cramping in my feet and toes due to compressed nerves in the hip joints.

Realigning the pelvis could offer immediate relief, but the cramping would return a day or so later, when the nerves were going through the healing process, and at that time, there was little relief to be found, but it came from magnesium oil, evening primrose oil, intense relaxation, and heroic patience.

Peripheral Neuropathy can manifest as more severe symptoms on more body parts than I have experienced. For example, for my sister it has caused itching and photosensitivity on her forearms so severe that she sometimes scratched her skin until it bled.

Preventions, Treatments, and Coping Strategies for Peripheral Neuropathy

It is best to prevent neuropathy and neuralgia because once nerve damage happens, it takes time to heal. However, there are some ways to help it heal faster.

Treat and Cope with Peripheral Neuropathy

1. **Relieve pressure on the site of the nerve injury.** Do not stretch or massage it.[560] Take measures to prevent it from being injured again. *Give your nerve a chance to heal.*
2. **Prevent yourself from scratching** your skin to the point of injury. If you have itching, wear clothing over the itchy area, trim your fingernails short, etc. [561] *It is important to prevent further injury to the skin or nerves.*
3. **Apply evening primrose oil to the skin at the sites of the injury and symptoms.** *EPO will speed the healing of the nerves and calm the symptoms.* [562, 563]
4. **Take acetylcholine, methylfolate, methylcolbalamin, thiamine, and B6.** [564, 565] Note that although acetylcholine is imperative for proper neuron function, it can exacerbate dystonia symptoms. Also, some people who have not addressed MTHFR problems may have trouble taking methylfolate and methylcolbalamin. *Our bodies need nutrients in order to heal.*
5. **Apply ice to the location of the symptom.** *When there is no way to immediately cure the root cause of the discomfort, numb it with an ice pack; but be careful not to cause additional nerve damage with too much cold.*[566]
6. **Apply magnesium oil to the location of the symptom.** If you have muscle tension and pain at the location of the injury, you can apply magnesium oil there, too. *This treatment has worked for me and someone I know.*
7. **Apply heat to the location of the injury.** Use the heat for only 20-30 minutes at a time to reduce the risk of harming the skin. *Heat is soothing, and the temperature gives the nerves a different job to do.*[567]
8. **Drink grape juice.** *The high concentration of resveratrol is anti-inflammatory and neuroprotective.*[568, 569]
9. **Eat culinary herbs that support nerve health,** especially basil, oregano, parsley, and/or turmeric.[570, 571, 572, 573] If you have MCAS, eat these culinary herbs fresh; jarred spices may contain mold. *Let food be the first medicine.*

10. **Use Homeopathic Remedies.** One that is labelled for nerve pain is *Hypericum perforatum*. See Chapter 50: Homeopathic Remedies. *Homeopathic Remedies safely communicate with our bodies, teaching them how to heal.*
11. **Do light exercise that does not endanger the site of the injury but uses the sites of symptoms.** Especially make sure to move the affected body parts.[574] However, do not stretch or compress the area where the nerve was damaged. *Increased blood flow will make healing happen faster, and it will distract you from the discomfort.*
12. **Do Earthing.** See Chapter 45: Earthing. *Keep the electric system of your body in the best state possible so that the electric wires of the body — the nerves — can be as healthy as possible.*
13. **Use Near Infrared and Red Light Therapy.** See Chapter 53: Near Infrared and Red Light Therapy. *Near Infrared Light helps the body heal faster.*
14. **Avoid any neurotoxic medications, chemicals, or foods.** Even without a pre-existing injury, these substances can create Peripheral Neuropathy.[575] Get used to researching chemicals before consuming them. *Give your body the best chance to heal Peripheral Neuropathy.*
15. **Get Reiki.** See Section VI: Seek Professional Help. *Reiki is a very soothing treatment.*
16. **Pray, use Affirmations, and try Forest Bathing.** When symptoms cannot be alleviated while healing is taking its time, distraction helps, but what helps even more is a positive attitude. See Chapter 55: Positive Prayer, Chapter 40: Affirmations, and Chapter 48: Forest Bathing. *It works!*

TREAT AND COPE WITH PERIPHERAL NEUROPATHY

1. Relieve pressure on the site of the injury.
2. Prevent yourself from scratching.
3. Apply evening primrose oil to the skin at the sites of the injury and symptoms.
4. Take acetylcholine, methylfolate, methylcolbalamin, thiamine, and B6.
5. Apply ice to the location of the symptom.
6. Apply magnesium oil to the location of the symptom.
7. Apply heat to the location of the injury.
8. Drink grape juice.
9. Eat culinary herbs that support nerve health.
10. Use Homeopathic Remedies.
11. Do light exercise that does not endanger the site of the injury but uses the sites of symptoms.
12. Do Earthing.
13. Use Near Infrared and Red Light Therapy.
14. Get Reiki.
15. Avoid any neurotoxic medications, chemicals, or foods.
16. Pray, use Affirmations, and try Forest Bathing.

Ask your doctor before trying anything new.

LINKS FOR PRODUCTS MENTIONED IN THIS CHAPTER

Acetylcholine (Parasym Plus) https://amzn.to/4cpH3jQ

Evening primrose oil https://amzn.to/3QnGbCH

Methylfolate https://amzn.to/3U3sSdy

Methylcolbalamin https://amzn.to/422EaRi

Thiamine https://amzn.to/3WjNHT6

B6 https://amzn.to/3QoP8vP

Magnesium flakes https://amzn.to/3HrNIvn

Hypericum perforatum https://amzn.to/4cbQTWa

NIR and Red Light Therapy box https://amzn.to/3S8vLXG

29 POTS

POTS STANDS FOR POSTURAL ORTHOSTATIC Tachycardia Syndrome and is well known among people with hEDS/HSD because 80% of them have it.[576] However, there are also a lot of people who have POTS but do not have hEDS — among POTS patients, only 55% have either hEDS or generalized hypermobility.[577]

Postural means positional, Orthostatic means standing upright, Tachycardia means a fast heart rate, and Syndrome means a varied group of symptoms. This condition is sometimes called Chronic Orthostatic Intolerance.[578] POTS is a dysautonomia (a malfunction in the Autonomic Nervous System, which controls the unconscious activities of the body including heartbeat) in which there is an increase in heart rate of at least 30 beats per minute within 10 minutes of standing up after lying down for at least 30 minutes. There is disagreement among doctors as to whether there is a corresponding drop in blood pressure, and if there is, whether it is causative or responsive.[579, 580]

A POTS episode can create feelings of anxiety, shakiness, heart palpitations, and severe pain in the heart, as well as long-lasting symptoms of oxygen deprivation such as dizziness, nausea, brain fog, pain in the muscles, shaking, weakness, coat-hanger headache (pain in the shoulders, neck, and head), tingling and numbness in the upper body (especially the lips), and Migraine. POTS episodes can be instigated by standing up quickly, bending over, exercise, MCAS flares, and stress. Menstrual periods and illnesses tend to make people more prone to these episodes while the conditions last.[581, 582] Many people with POTS are unable to work, attend school, or participate in recreational activities.

I believe that POTS in people with hEDS/HSD can be caused by a number of different conditions working together:

- Stretchy blood vessels that do not constrict (get narrower) and dilate (get wider) properly. Blood vessels are made of collagen and are supported by collagen in the fascia that surrounds them. When they need to constrict to help the blood move to the heart, they cannot always do it.
- Dysautonomia (a malfunction of the autonomic nervous system, which controls the unconscious processes in your body, such as your heartbeat, breathing, and digestion). The nervous system may operate improperly as a

result of overly excited nerves (for example, if MCAS has them on constant alert) or nerves that have been damaged by hypermobile joints such as in CCI.

- Compression of veins in the soleus (calf muscles) coupled with ineffective pumping of the soleus (these muscles are known as the second heart because they are partly responsible for pumping blood from the lower extremities back up into the upper body). The soleus can become hypertonic and essentially be partially paralyzed if you have a posture with hyperextended knees.
- Dehydration (a condition in which there is not enough fluid in the blood for the body to maintain the blood pressure). The imperfect connective tissues of the gastrointestinal system lead to an insufficient amount of minerals being absorbed; minerals are an important component of the body's fluid and are essential for the fluid balance to be maintained.
- Lymph insufficiency (the lymph system is a series of vessels made of collagen that move fluid throughout the body). If the lymph system cannot maintain the balance of fluids in the body, it may contribute to dehydration or edema, which can affect blood pressure.
- Mast cell activation (an inflammatory immune response). An immune response can increase heart rate and/or decrease blood pressure.
- Lack of stamina (the ability to exercise without raising the heartrate excessively). Many people with hEDS are permanently or periodically bed-bound or chair-bound due to Joint Injuries, Migraine, and other conditions; this can lead to a loss of stamina that leaves the heart "out of shape" to do the work it is intended to do and also impacts the balance of hormones (renin, angiotensin, and aldosterone) that regulate blood plasma volume and hemodynamic homeostasis (the regulation of blood circulation to meet the needs of the body).
- Other biological differences that scientists have found present in some people with POTS but that are not apparent to the patient and require more investigation before they can be well understood. These differences may include small hearts, small stroke volume, low blood volume, low nitric oxide, unusual sympathetic nerve activity, elevated levels of epinephrine and/or norepinephrine, small fiber neuropathy in nerves that regulate the constriction of blood vessels, blunted adrenal response to the hormones that regulate hemodynamic homeostasis, and more. [583, 584, 585]

POTS is very similar to another condition called Vasovagal Syncope (and Exercise-Induced Syncope, Postural Syncope, and Postprandial Syncope). Vasovagal means having to do with the Vagus Nerve, and Syncope means to faint (or pass out). Vasovagal Syncope and POTS are so similar that they are sometimes conflated (wrongly diagnosed as each other).[586] In addition to fainting or near fainting, Vasovagal Syncope can cause sweating, dizziness, nausea, brain fog, pain in the muscles, shaking, and headache (just like POTS).

The Vasovagal Syncope response is the same mechanism that makes possums play dead and fainting goats faint. It is a version of the freeze response to danger (of Fight/Flight/Freeze/Friend/Fornicate fame). The blood drops into the lower extremities, and the loss of blood flow to the brain causes you to lose consciousness. If you are lying seemingly dead on the ground, you are less likely to get into a life-threatening fight, and you are less likely to be attractive prey to most hunting animals. Also, in the case of an injury, this reaction may prevent excessive blood loss.

However, sometimes the Vasovagal Syncope blood pressure drop is less severe or the heart speeds up enough to compensate for the low blood pressure, and fainting does not occur. In this case, presyncope occurs, which is a condition with symptoms much like POTS symptoms. Fainting is much more dangerous — some people have been seriously injured or have died from hitting their heads or other body parts when they fell — but if the fall does not injure them, then when they awaken a few minutes later, they will be in a euphoric state that feels very blissful and pleasurable, like floating.

POTS is considered to be a dysautonomia, while Vasovagal Syncope is considered to be a sign of a healthy, robust autonomic system.[587] Oddly, however, it is possible to have both conditions comorbid to each other (existing at the same time). POTS results in an elevated heart rate without lowered blood pressure (except in some people the blood pressure drops), whereas Vasovagal Syncope results in lowered blood pressure without an elevated heart rate (except in some people, especially those who experience presyncope, the heart rate elevates). POTS is chronic, while Vasovagal Syncope is episodic.

Among people with hEDS/HSD, POTS is the more common diagnosis. Regardless of their differences and the possibility of inaccurate diagnosis, the two conditions have the same treatments. I am suspicious that they could be different manifestations of the same condition.

My Experience with POTS

I was first diagnosed with Vasovagal Syncope following an immunization for travel about eleven years ago, though I understood immediately that I had always had this condition. The doctor told me that it is a biological response, not a psychological response: "You cannot meditate yourself out of having a Vasovagal Syncope response."

Ever since that diagnosis, I have always made sure to be lying down with my knees bent up before any kind of needle work is done in a hospital or clinic. Considering that some people with hEDS/HSD experience MCAS reactions to stress and pain, it may be wise for anyone with POTS also to lie down throughout any painful procedures.

Eventually, I also developed POTS symptoms, including severe pain in my heart, racing and pounding heart, sudden severe nausea, fainting, pain throughout my body, weakness, shaking, brain fog, clammy skin, sweating, dizziness, chills, pale or yellow skin tone, ringing in the ears, and headache, all of which could last for a day or more following the episode. Sometimes I got all of these symptoms at once and was stopped in my tracks; other times, the symptoms would come on one at a time, building slowly. Either way, I was in a full episode before I realized what was happening. Once I began to recognize the symptoms when they were mild, I learned to stop the episode before it progressed.

With an understanding of POTS, I was able to begin exercising lying down until I built up the tolerance to be able to exercise seated. Then, I graduated to exercising standing, though it was a long time before I could do any exercise bent forward without instigating a POTS episode. Sometimes, I used a tiny dose of caffeine to increase my tolerance of exercise, but eventually that was no longer necessary. I was also careful not to overdo my exercise efforts when I was on my period.

This process of building exercise tolerance and stamina took about a year and a half. When I could only exercise on the floor, it felt like almost no progress was occurring, but now when I'm running around the pickleball court, I can hardly believe what a short time it took to progress this far. Thank goodness my husband pushed me to keep trying every time I thought I might as well give up.

Although I essentially eliminated my POTS as a response to exercise, I still very rarely got POTS episodes in response to other triggers, especially MCAS, stress, and viral illness, even though I continued to take preventative measures such as taking electrolytes, rising from bed slowly, and maintaining an upright posture throughout the day.

Preventions, Treatments, and Coping Strategies for POTS

Preventing POTS episodes is preferable to trying to treat the symptoms after they have started. Not only is it unpleasant once the symptoms start, it is harder to stop them progressing.

Prevent POTS Episodes

1. **Take electrolytes daily.**[588] I drink one glass of water with Hydrant Hydrate in it every day, and this keeps my dysautonomia at bay except when I have a fever or start my period. *Electrolytes are extremely important for maintaining proper blood pressure.*
2. **Get out of bed slowly.**[589] I try to spend 15-45 minutes in bed after waking up before standing up. If I go to the bathroom, I come back and lie down flat for several minutes. (This is a good opportunity to do some knee-to-heel exercises to lubricate the hips so that they will be strong and comfortable when I do eventually stand up. See Chapter 27: Pelvis Complaints.) Then, I slowly add pillows and increase my incline by degrees, spending several minutes in each position, until I'm sitting up all the way. (During this time, I drink a glass of water that I had put on my bedside table before going to sleep at night, so that I have good hydration and blood volume). Then I sit with my feet hanging down to the floor for a minute. (This is a perfect opportunity to do some seated Range of Motion exercises, especially for the ankles, knees, and neck; it eliminates the stiffness and pain that I would otherwise feel upon first walking after waking. See Chapter 19: Knee Pain and Chapter 57: Range of Motion Exercises.) When I finally stand up, I do it slowly. I have to give my body lots of time to build up the blood pressure to pump the blood into my upper body when I'm upright. *Not only is it pleasant to spend some time in bed after you wake up, it will build up your blood pressure before you stand and keep you relaxed.*
3. **Stand up slowly.** Every time you stand up, use the muscles in your legs to lift yourself slowly with your back straight. *Do not rush from a lying or seated position; give your body time to adjust to your new elevation.*
4. **Don't bend over.**[590] Squat down or ask for someone's help when reaching for something that is on the floor or down low. Supine (lying on your back) exercise routines are ideal during times that you are prone to a POTS episode. *In addition to reducing POTS episodes, squatting instead of bending over can build up muscular strength in the legs and prevent back injury.*
5. **Avoid climbing stairs or hills**, or if going up, go slowly and do not carry anything heavy. Make sure that you maintain your posture and do not lean forward, as you may be inclined to do when climbing. As you improve your posture and increase your exertion stamina, you will be able to climb more and more.[591] *Go up hills and stairs at a pace that allows for you to remain standing tall and strong.*
6. **Avoid standing still** for long, or if standing, cross the feet so the legs put pressure on each other. Better yet, find ways not to stand still — continue moving, crouch down, or sit.[592] *Do movements and get in positions that ensure that the blood can be pumped up to the vital organs and not pool in the lower extremities.*

7. **Avoid stressful situations.**[593] If there is a stressful situation, sit or lie down. POTS episodes can be caused by a loss of blood pressure first and an increase in heart rate to compensate, but an increase in heart rate from stress can confuse the nervous system and instigate a dysautonomic reaction. *When someone warns you that they have something to tell you and, "You'd better sit down," do it.*
8. **Wear compression stockings**,[594] though I find them uncomfortable; there are partly-natural-fiber options available in case you are sensitive to synthetic fabrics. *Outside pressure on the lower legs can help keep the blood from pooling in them.*
9. **Avoid caffeine** on a regular basis because it increases heart rate and makes you more susceptible to POTS attacks. However, during an episode, caffeine might help resolve it because caffeine constricts the veins.[595] *Respect caffeine as a treatment to be used only as needed for constricting veins so that the blood can more easily be pumped to the upper organs.*
10. **Do not overeat.**[596] Stand up slowly from the table after eating. *Be gentle with your body, and give it time to adjust blood pressure.*
11. **Drink plenty of water and eat sufficient salt.**[597] Eat enough salt to keep your blood volume where it should be. Do not eat too much salt, but be prepared to eat extra if needed during an episode. I believe that other minerals are more important than sodium — magnesium, phosphorous, and zinc, which you can get in electrolyte blends — but sodium does get fast results when used during an episode. *Use only a moderate amount of salt with food so that it can be a more effective treatment.*
12. **Maintain proper head and neck posture.** CCI can contribute to POTS if it is causing damage to the Vagus Nerve, which is the pacemaker of the heart, and can create an elevated Sympathetic Nervous System activation.[598, 599] So, make every effort to stabilize the cervical spine. Pay special attention to keeping the back of the neck stretched and pulled back whenever leaning forward or climbing stairs or hills. See Chapter 56: Posture. *Be careful not to allow your head posture to pinch nerves in the neck that are responsible for regulating blood pressure and heart rate.*
13. **Do not hyperextend your knees** while standing or walking. See Chapter 56: Posture. When you hyperextend your knees, your soleus (the muscle that stretches from the back of your knee to your heel) will become hypertonic (tense) and will not be able to do its job as the "second heart," pumping blood back up into the upper body from the lower extremities.[600, 601] *Give your body every chance it has to keep the blood pumping the way it should.*

PREVENT POTS EPISODES

1. Take electrolytes daily.
2. Get out of bed slowly.
3. Stand up slowly.
4. Don't bend over.
5. Avoid climbing hills or stairs.
6. Avoid standing still.
7. Avoid stressful situations.
8. Wear compression socks or stockings.
9. Avoid caffeine.
10. Do not overeat.
11. Drink plenty of water and eat sufficient salt.
12. Maintain proper head and neck posture.
13. Do not hyperextend your knees.
14. Follow the Cusack Protocol.
15. Exercise.
16. Build postural orthostatic tolerance.
17. Take extra precautions when you are having your menstrual period.

Ask your doctor before trying anything new.

14. **Follow the Cusack Protocol.** If it works for you like it did for me, your connective tissue will become healthier and firmer. See Chapter 42: The Cusack Protocol. *Firm, strong veins can better regulate blood pressure and heart rate.*
15. **Exercise.**[602] If your POTS is sensitive, start by exercising while lying on the ground. Follow some of Jeannie di Bon's YouTube videos for some good ideas. I also liked to do my floor Physical Therapy exercises when my POTS was sensitive. Start with gentle exercises that won't get your heart rate up, but over time, build up to more difficult activities, even if you are still lying on the ground. Then, as your stamina increases, start doing seated exercises, then moving on to standing exercises. Do not try doing exercises that bend forward or backward until you have really built up your orthostatic tolerance. *Many doctors report having seen patients kick their POTS diagnosis by faithfully following an exercise routine.*
16. **Build postural orthostatic tolerance**. If you begin with all of the cautions listed here in order to reduce the frequency of POTS episodes, you will soon get to a calm state in which you can begin to build your tolerance for positional changes. Make sure that you always keep your chest lifted and your neck long and lifted, especially when bending over or climbing hills or stairs. See Chapter 25: Neck Pain & CCI and Chapter 56: Posture. In order to practice bending over without inciting an episode, take a deep breath, exhale completely and hold your breath out, slowly bend over and even more slowly straighten, then breathe in again. Repeat this just a couple times a day to start with, and on strong days, increase the number of repetitions.
17. **Take extra precautions when you are having your menstrual period**. POTS episodes can be triggered much more easily during your period. If there are things on this list that you do not always have to do, you might want to add them in when you are on your period. Go slowly, and don't get mad at yourself if you get POTS episodes anyway (I sometimes got them when lying in bed when I was on my period), just move onto the recovery techniques. *Treat your body gently when it is going through the hard and miraculous work of menstruating.*

Recover Quickly from POTS Episodes

1. **Pay attention to POTS warning signs.** Do you get dizzy, nauseated, nervous, weak, or clumsy? Sometimes these signs will start subtly before you feel the racing of the heart. Don't try to keep going and ignore these warning signs. Act quickly. *If you can stop a POTS episode before it gets bad, by lying down and drinking electrolytes, you may not end up feeling bad.*
2. **Drink electrolytes.** I always choose Hydrant Hydrate electrolytes (with sodium, potassium, magnesium, and zinc). Try these or another form of electrolytes, or eat salt, which is also an electrolyte. *Electrolytes regulate blood pressure.*[603]
3. **Lie down with feet up**, the higher the better, but even just up on a pillow is sufficient. *Most of the unpleasant symptoms that POTS causes are symptoms of oxygen deprivation to the organs, brain, and muscles of the upper body, so use gravity to help the blood flow to the upper body.*[604]
4. **Put feet and lower legs in cold water**, or put cold wash cloths on the lower extremities. *Cold will constrict the blood vessels, which will increase blood pressure and prevent blood from pooling.*[605]

5. **Drink caffeine** in acute situations. [606] Caffeine constricts blood vessels, which will help regulate your blood pressure, but it also increases heart rate, so you must use it cautiously. Hydrant Hydrate now offers an electrolyte blend with caffeine, which makes it easy to get everything you need, but it is a larger dose than you may need. My favorite source of caffeine is not widely available and no longer perfectly natural, and it is best in glass bottles but expensive if you have to order it online because you don't live in Kentucky, but it does the trick with 22 mg of caffeine — Ale 8 One. *A healthy drink with caffeine can stop a POTS episode quickly.*
6. **Do the Valsalva Maneuver or cough.**[607] Take a deep breath, close your mouth and pinch your nose, try to breathe out, straining against your throat to increase pressure in the chest. Then release the nose and breathe out as normal. Forcing yourself to cough also may work in the same way. *This exercise is especially useful if you have had an increase in POTS episodes due to having corrected your posture in such a way that it diminished the pressure in your chest.*

RECOVER QUICKLY FROM POTS EPISODES

1. Pay attention to POTS warning signs.
2. Drink electrolytes.
3. Lie down with feet up.
4. Put feet and lower legs in cold water.
5. Drink caffeine.
6. Do the Valsalva Maneuver or cough.

Ask your doctor before trying anything new.

LINKS FOR PRODUCTS MENTIONED IN THIS CHAPTER

Electrolytes https://amzn.to/3UlgNk1
Compression socks https://amzn.to/4bhcqvy
Ale 8 One https://amzn.to/4b5yoCf
Electrolytes with Caffeine https://amzn.to/3wcdIcm

30

Rib Cage Pain – Rib Subluxations, Costochondritis, & SRS

RIB SUBLUXATIONS, COSTOCHONDRITIS, AND Slipping Rib Syndrome (SRS) are all conditions of the rib cage in which the tissue that connects the rib bones to the sternum or spine gets stretched and inflamed, causing pain and sometimes difficulty breathing and/or moving. Frequently, the intercostal muscles (between the ribs) and the fascia become rigid and painful; blood vessels and nerves can become involved, as well. All of these conditions are connected with hEDS/HSD.[608, 609, 610]

A Rib Subluxation is a partial dislocation of a rib from its position either at the sternum or backbone. One or more ribs can sublux at the same time. Rib subluxation is supposed to be one of the most painful problems that hEDS/HSD people commonly deal with.

Costochondritis is an inflammation of the cartilage that connects the ribs to the sternum. This is often caused by the ribs pulling at the cartilage, and it causes pain that is often thought by the patient to be a heart attack.[611]

Slipping Rib Syndrome (SRS) is inflammation and possibly even separation of the cartilage and/or ligaments that reach from the "false" ribs to the sternum. (False ribs are numbers 8, 9, and 10; they are above the floating ribs and connect to the true ribs, which in turn connect to the sternum). SRS can cause pain, breathing difficulties, loss of motility, and gastrointestinal symptoms.[612]

The cartilage, ligaments, and muscles that hold the ribs in place are designed to let the rib cage move in many directions when we breathe, reach, bend, or arch our torsos. Of course, in people with hypermobility, the cartilage, ligaments, and muscles may allow the rib cage to move too much, causing Joint Injuries. As with most Joint Injuries, the body responds by freezing the muscles and fascia around the joints so that they will not move anymore.[613] This protects the joint, but it hurts...and it causes more problems.

Once the rib cage's mobility is reduced, the risk of Joint Injury actually increases. The rib cage is going to expand and move when you breathe, reach, or bend, but rigidity in the area means that a joint will have to get pulled on in order to make the movement. When the joints in the front get pulled on, the resulting inflammation is Costochondritis. When a rib gets pulled on so much that it partially dislocates, it is called Rib Subluxation. When the lower ribs get pulled on, the resulting damage to the cartilage is Slipping Rib Syndrome.

Not only will Joint Injuries in the rib cage create rigidity that potentially leads to more Joint Injuries in the rib cage, rigidity in the rib cage can also be caused or exacerbated by Allergy/MCAS/MCS reactions. When an allergen or airborne trigger is inhaled, the intercostal muscles (the muscles between each of the ribs) retract and tighten up. If this happens frequently enough, it can become pathological (habitual or compulsive though maladaptive). In this case, the muscles surrounding the ribs may be essentially frozen.

My Experience with Rib Subluxation

The first time I was diagnosed with a Rib Subluxation, my doctor exclaimed, "I cannot believe you are walking around and smiling with this happening in your back! Most people would have gone straight to the emergency room. They would have thought they were dying!" Rib subluxation is known to be a 10 on the 10-point pain scale, and yet we who are hypermobile often learn to live with it.

I lived with 4 nearly constantly subluxing ribs for over 8 years. I had the subluxations treated by a Chiropractor, a Massage Therapist, a Pilates instructor, and an Osteopath but they were never able to offer a long-lasting solution. Usually, they made enough improvement that the pain diminished somewhat, but it didn't last for long. If I got tired, my back would really hurt because the rib would slip further out of position; if I got really tired, my arms and legs would hurt, too, from the referred pain of the greater and greater subluxation. The more exhausted I got, the worse the dislocation became and the more referred pain I experienced.

Although the professionals had not been able to cure my Rib Subluxations, eventually with the help of my husband, I was able to cure them. As I was curing the subluxations in my back, I discovered that I had pain all throughout my rib cage, especially along the sternum in the front. The fascia was extraordinarily tight, and releasing it required a lot of dedication. The relief was worth it, though, and I breathe more easily now as well.

Once my ribs were almost healed and rarely popping out, I plateaued at a place where I still had a niggling amount of pain and had to be very cautious in my movements so that I wouldn't dislocate the ribs again. I was applying comfrey oil twice a day to keep the pain down. Then, I went and played pickleball with the family for the first time. Some kind of magic happened on that little pickleball court because by the end of the hour of good-natured play, my back felt strong and the pain was gone. After a week, it started to come back, but another hour on the pickleball court and I was strong and pain-free again. Although a game like this would have been too much for me early in my healing process, and although I had not been able to find the precise strength-training exercise I needed at this point, this game was a really fun way to complete my healing. See Chapter 61: Sports and Hobbies.

Preventions, Treatments, and Coping Strategies for Rib Subluxation, Costochondritis, and SRS

When you treat your Rib Subluxation, Costochondritis, or Slipping Rib Syndrome, have some patience. The tissues have been damaged and need time to heal before they stop hurting. If they have not stopped hurting after a couple weeks, then it means that you need to do more release of the fascia and muscles elsewhere in the rib cage; for example, if you have pain in the back, you may need to work on the front and sides.

Return Strength and Flexibility to the Rib Cage to Reduce Pain

1. **Do Jeannie di Bon's Pilates exercises.** She has several videos geared specifically to correcting Rib Subluxation. Much of what she has you do is very simple — my husband sometimes thinks I'm sleeping when I'm doing this workout. If taught fascia and tense muscles are restricting the movement of the ribs, the tendons might give before the muscles and fascia do, and that creates a lot of pain. *These are the gentlest but also most effective exercises I have found for releasing taught fascia and hypertonic muscles.* https://www.youtube.com/@JeannieDiBonHypermobility
2. **Apply heat to the area.** Do not use the heat for an extremely long time; it can seriously damage the skin. *Heat is very relaxing and healing, and it reduces pain.*[614, 615]
3. **Gently massage the entire rib cage.** Massage the back, front, and sides, not just where you notice the pain. *Massage will relax the muscles that have frozen up around any threatened or injured joints, as well as increasing healing blood flow to the area.*[616]
4. **Release the fascia of the rib cage.** Even if your pain is in the back, the most restrictive tightness that is causing pain might be in the front, and vice versa. Work on small areas and do gentle micromovement massaging first and then light, slow, directional fascial release. See Chapter 52: Myofascial Release Massage. *The fascia bind the rib muscles into place and must be released so that your ribs can move and stop pulling on each other.*
5. **Pop the rib(s) back into position, if necessary.** What worked best for me was for my husband to press on each subluxed rib with his thumb (it is easiest for him if I am holding my best posture and my shoulders are rotated externally, so he has me keep my bent elbows by my side and rotate my hands out to the side so that my forearms are parallel to the ground, sticking out to the side). The Chiropractor and Osteopath were able to use various methods to pop the ribs into place, but it is better if you can find a maneuver you can do yourself as frequently as needed. Sometimes I was able to pop ribs back into place using a tennis ball inside a sock which I held and leaned against on the wall or floor, or by pressing my hand against the kitchen counter in a certain way, or by pulling my arms behind my back and squeezing my shoulder blades together. Do it as many times a day as you need to. Keep the rib in place as much of the time as possible so that the ligament can tighten back up — plus it feels so much better. The pain will not instantly disappear since the connective tissue is damaged, but it might instantly diminish. *You'll be able to breathe again.*
6. **Do pull overs and rows.** For pull overs, use a workout band or exercise machine mounted above the head; with straight arms, start with the arms lifted higher than

RETURN STRENGTH AND FLEXIBILITY TO THE RIB CAGE TO REDUCE PAIN

1. Do Jeannie di Bon's Pilates exercises.
2. Apply heat to the area.
3. Gently massage the entire rib cage.
4. Release the fascia of the rib cage.
5. Pop the rib(s) back into position.
6. Do pull overs and rows.
7. Exercise the serratus anterior muscles.
8. Apply comfrey oil.
9. Do the Cusack Protocol.
10. Keep awareness of the injured area.
11. Sleep in safe, supported positions.

Ask your doctor before trying anything new.

the shoulders and pull down until the hands are by the thighs. For rows, you can sit down and put a resistance band around your feet or a table leg, then pull on the band, with your elbows travelling backwards. Repeat until you begin to feel it become more difficult. Do not fatigue your muscles. *If you want the rib to stop moving out of position, you must strengthen the muscles that holds it in place.*

7. **Do exercises for the serratus anterior muscles.** Depending on the strength of your shoulders and propensity for POTS, you might try dumbbell pullovers, high bear crawls, scapular pushups, dip shrugs, and scapular plane lateral raises.[617] *You want all of your muscles to support and move the rib cage as it is meant to move.*
8. **Apply comfrey oil.** When I am actively healing, I apply it 2-3 times a day. *Comfrey will help the connective tissues heal as quickly as possible, and it will almost instantly provide pain relief.*[618]
9. **Follow the Cusack Protocol.** If this works for you, it will tighten up the loosened ligaments so the ribs won't pop out as readily. See Chapter 42: The Cusack Protocol. *The supplements cost a little money, but this is the easiest way of making a difference in the health of your ligaments.*
10. **Keep awareness of the injured area.** We tend to ignore the injured areas so that we can get on with life, but once healing of this area begins, you need to be aware of it at all times. If you feel a slight tugging or pulling on it or a whisper of pain, then stop doing what you are doing. You will get stronger in time, but do not challenge the area until the strength has been developed. Once the muscles unfreeze and the ligaments begin to heal, you will be able to feel a slight tugging when the rib joint is threatened. Immediately stop what you are doing. If you feel the rib pop out or simply start to hurt, immediately try to get it put back into place. *The longer the rib is out of place, the longer it will take to heal and the longer you will be in pain and experiencing breathlessness.*
11. **Sleep in safe, supported positions.** Use pillows as needed to support your body, and sleep on your back as much as possible. Once my Rib Subluxations were mostly healed, the rare times when a rib did pop out were usually when I was asleep. See more information about sleep position in Chapter 9: Joint Instability & Pain. *You cannot keep awareness of your ribs while you sleep, so you must try your best to get yourself into a supported position that will not pull the ribs out of position.*

LINKS FOR PRODUCTS MENTIONED IN THIS CHAPTER

Comfrey Oil https://amzn.to/3TDV4D9
Resistance Bands with Handles ttps://amzn.to/3OawB5k

31
Scoliosis

SCOLIOSIS IS A SIDEWAYS CURVATURE of the spine. It is more common among hEDS/HSD patients than in the general population and is one of the most common diagnoses for hEDS/HSD people.[619] Laxity in the tendons that hold the vertebrae in line, along with weakness in the muscles that support the spine are usually the cause of Scoliosis, though it is possible for the spine to grow unevenly.

Signs of Scoliosis include a shoulder or hip that is higher than the other, perpetual leaning to one side, and the head not being centered over the body. For many children who have Scoliosis, it is not an uncomfortable condition, but pain, along with problems like difficulty breathing, can develop over time. Doctors treat Scoliosis with Physical Therapy, braces, and surgery.

My Experience with Scoliosis

One of my friends had severe Scoliosis, underwent surgery, and was very happy with the result. In fact, after the surgery, although it reduced the range of motion of her legs and back, she was able to become a professional dancer in my company.

When my sister was diagnosed with mild Scoliosis as a child, her doctor suggested trying to avoid braces and surgery; instead, he prescribed for her to swim. My sister joined the FAST (Fairmore Area Swim Team), and even though she wished she could instead join an imaginary team she called SLOW (Swimming Leisurely Over Water), she stuck with it even though she didn't love it until her 17-degree curvature had mostly resolved. She no longer has Scoliosis, even though she stopped swimming regularly after her curvature improved. (Inspired by my sister and her witty humor, my mother, Kathy Johnson Gale, has written a novel for ages 8-14 about a girl's experience dealing with Scoliosis and hEDS. When it becomes available, I will put a link to it on my website shannonegale.com .)

Preventions, Treatments, and Coping Strategies for Scoliosis

I find swimming to be an excellent exercise for many conditions associated with hEDS/HSD, but there are some precautions that you may need to take, as well as some other treatments you may want to add to your arsenal.

Swimming to Treat Scoliosis

1. **Stay upright in the pool if you have POTS, doing aerobics or treading water** until you improve your stamina and orthostatic tolerance. When you do swim facing down, come up from that position slowly and keep moving your legs to help keep the blood pumping up from the lower extremities. See Chapter 29: POTS. Swimming is a great physical challenge when you are first starting, so only swim in shallow water, where you can easily stop if you become exhausted or your heart begins to race. Swim across the short end of the pool to start with, and build up your stamina over time. *Go slowly and pay attention to your body's needs as you build up your strength and stamina.*
2. **Avoid or protect against chlorine if you have MCAS**. If you can find a salt-water pool, it will have less chlorine and may be safer for you. Some people with sensitivities do well to swim in the ocean or a lake, but the cleanliness of the water will make a difference. When you do swim in a chlorine pool, take some Iodine internally to counteract the chlorine you may absorb.[620] Also, spray Vitamin C on your skin before and after swimming; the Vitamin C very quickly neutralizes chlorine. See Appendix A: Recipes. Also, if you are in a public location, avoid people who are spraying sunblock; use a natural sunblock on yourself if it is needed. *Staying free of noxious chemicals will make your swimming experience feel natural and enjoyable.*
3. **Alternate different swim strokes and activities**. Go in any order you like, but vary your strokes with each lap so that different muscles get turns working and no one set of muscles fatigues before you've gotten in a good workout. The strokes I like to do are the crawl, breast stroke, right side stroke, left side stroke, and back stroke. Sometimes, I also do a "mermaid swim" under the water, and when I am especially strong, I try the butterfly. It is also nice to take some time floating on your back to relax in an activated way. Treading water is good exercise in an upright position, and a lot of people enjoy water aerobics. Join a class in your town, or look up YouTube videos that teach you how to swim or do water aerobics. Perfecting good swim technique can be a very enjoyable and satisfying endeavor, it makes you faster and look better, and it could be lifesaving, too. *Using a variety of movements in the pool will strengthen all muscles that you need to support a straight spine in a balanced way, and it can be interesting and fun to do.*
4. **Drink water with electrolytes before swimming.** *You may not feel thirsty while you are in the water, but you need electrolytes and water to keep your muscles working and your blood volume balanced when exercising.*
5. **Practice deep breathing before beginning a swimming routine.** For me, the hardest part of swimming is taking deep enough breaths and exhaling rhythmically without feeling like I am suffocating. *Developing strength and capacity in your lungs before you get into the water will allow you to do the swimming you want to do.*
6. **Rinse and moisturize after swimming.** Ideally, as soon as you leave the water, you should wash with a natural soap and water, spray on some more of the Vitamin C Chlorine Neutralizing Spray, and moisturize with a natural product like jojoba oil to keep the skin barrier strong.[621] Dry skin can be "leakier" than moisturized skin. *Keep your skin free of chemicals and full of moisture to stay healthy.*

7. **Massage after swimming.** *Whether from a professional, a loved one, or yourself, a gentle massage later in the day will help keep tired muscles healthy and reduce fascia adhesions and tightening.*
8. **Do Myofascial Release Massage once you have built up strength.** See Chapter 52: Myofascial Release Massage. You do not want to do this until your muscles are strong enough to support your joints, but it will help you break out of suboptimal movement and posture habits. *Releasing the fascia will give you a greater range of motion to make swimming easier and more comfortable, and it will give your spine the opportunity to move into a better alignment.*

SWIM TO TREAT SCOLIOSIS

1. Stay upright in the pool if you have POTS, doing aerobics or treading water.
2. Avoid or protect against chlorine if you have MCAS.
3. Alternate different swim strokes and activities.
4. Drink water with electrolytes before swimming.
5. Practice deep breathing before beginning a swimming routine.
6. Rinse and moisturize after swimming.
7. Massage after swimming.
8. Do Myofascial Release Massage once you have built up strength.

Ask your doctor before trying anything new.

LINKS FOR PRODUCTS MENTIONED IN THIS CHAPTER

Sunblock https://amzn.to/3TAtUNw

Electrolytes https://amzn.to/3UlgNk1

Ascorbic Acid powder (for making Vitamin C Spray) https://revitalizewellness.org/products/vitamin-c-as-ascorbic-acid-16oz-fine-powder

Jojoba Oil https://amzn.to/3VkZUEY

32
Sensitive Skin

PEOPLE WITH CONNECTIVE TISSUE DISORDERS can have weak, fragile, and "leaky" skin, which makes it more sensitive than other people's skin, so it needs more cautious care.[622]

My Experience with Sensitive Skin

My grandma and I both get flaky, itchy skin on our scalps on the right side at the back of the head just above the hairline whenever we are stressed. It can take quite a while for it to go away. I think that calming the system with Vagus Nerve Stimulation helps it go away faster, as does applying a boron solution. I put water and a little bit of Borax into a small spray bottle and then shake it. Then, I spray it on the affected area and let it air dry. See Appendix A: Recipes.

Sometimes when I have gone into rooms that were filled with fragrance, I have used a mask and ionizer and still gotten sick. I finally figured out that it was because I was absorbing the chemicals through my skin. So, I began to cover my skin with clothing or coat it in shea butter, and I got sick from contact with airborne toxins much less frequently from then on.

Most of the friends, clients, and relatives who I have seen with open sores, eczema, psoriasis, or dermatitis had little luck curing their skin conditions with topical treatments. In order to stop the breakouts, they had to find out what their triggers were, and they were usually foods.

I have rarely had skin trouble, though I suffered with acne as a teenager and young adult. Once I discovered the Oil Cleansing Method, I no longer had such trouble with acne. However, on occasion, when I suffered an illness, severe allergic reaction, or significant emotional and physical healing leap, I would get body acne. I have learned that an Epsom salt bath following any potential body acne trigger will prevent body acne from appearing.

I have also dealt with tinea versicolor on my trunk. This is pink or white patches caused by a yeast (fungus) that normally lives on the skin but can grow out of control during times of illness or stress. Fortunately, it does not itch or hurt, but it is unsightly. The best cure for it is the same boron solution I mentioned above. If I am in a stressful time of life, I may need to spray my skin three times a day for up to a week before the spots disappear completely, but once the stress or illness has passed, it does not usually take such dedication to eliminate the rash.

Preventions, Treatments, and Coping Strategies for Sensitive Skin

Be gentle with your fragile, hypermobile skin, and keep it nourished so that it can be as strong as possible.

Prevent and Treat Skin Conditions

1. **Keep the skin clean.** This is especially important for children, whose faces will get blemishes if food is left on them. Use only gentle, all-natural soap, like Arizona Sungold's Liquid Shampoo or just use warm water and no soap. Dry thoroughly with a cotton towel. *Remember that people with hEDS have "leaky skin"; you need to protect it from absorbing anything it shouldn't absorb.*
2. **Wash your face with the Oil Cleansing Method.** See Chapter 54: Oil Cleansing Method. *This cleansing method is a luxurious way to start your day.*
3. **Use only gentle, all-natural moisturizers.** Organic olive oil, used sparingly, is a wonderful health-giving moisturizer that is anti-inflammatory and antiseptic. Organic filtered shea butter is also a good moisturizer that protects the skin from absorbing toxins in the air and serves as a nice base for makeup. *Only put things on your skin that you would eat.*
4. **Use only all-natural makeup, or none at all.** I rarely wear makeup, but when I do, it is usually the pressed powder products from Mineral Fusion. Makeup is really designed to make a person look healthy. Healthy is beautiful; beauty is health. *When you are healthy, you are beautiful without makeup.*
5. **Prevent body acne by taking baths with Epsom salts.**[623] *Epsom salts help draw toxins out of the skin and kill the harmful bacteria that might be on the skin.*
6. **Take Vitamin C.** *It can improve the firmness and integrity of skin.*[624]
7. **Do not wear sunglasses all of the time.** If your eyes do not recognize the amount of sunlight to which you are being exposed, your skin will not make enough melanin to protect itself from burning. *Wear a hat and stay in the shade when the sun is really bright, but don't fool your eyes with sunglasses; they need the light and the information in order to keep your skin healthy.*
8. **Eat watermelon when you are going to be in the sun.** *Watermelon and other summery foods that are full of water, antioxidants, and vitamins can help prevent sunburn.*[625]

PREVENT SKIN CONDITIONS

1. Keep the skin clean.
2. Wash your face with the Oil Cleansing Method.
3. Use only gentle, all-natural moisturizers.
4. Use only all-natural makeup or none at all.
5. Prevent body acne by taking baths with Epsom salts.
6. Take Vitamin C.
7. Do not wear sunglasses all of the time.
8. Eat watermelon when you are going to be in the sun.

Ask your doctor before trying anything new.

LINKS FOR PRODUCTS MENTIONED IN THIS CHAPTER

Soap http://azsungoldsoaps.com/mobile/order/liquid/products_shampoo.html

Olive Oil https://amzn.to/3VwrYqh

Makeup https://amzn.to/47FlZlQ

Shea Butter https://mountainroseherbs.com/refined-shea-butter

Vitamin C with bioflavanoids https://amzn.to/4bisYmX

Epsom Salts https://amzn.to/3S4Y1KQ

33

Shoulder Pain

THE SHOULDER IS THE MOST COMMONLY injured joint for people with hEDS. Not only are the soft tissues of the shoulder lax, but the structure of the shoulder is usually different in someone with hEDS compared to the general public.[626] Diagnosis can be especially difficult because the problems that are occurring in the shoulders of hypermobile people often do not show up on diagnostic scans.[627]

Sadly, hEDS patients tend not to have good outcomes from surgery of the shoulder. For severe tears, surgery may be necessary, but when possible, the best avenue to pursue for healing shoulder pain is Physical Therapy with a therapist who is very familiar with hypermobility.

Shoulder pain can limit mobility of the arm and impact daily life significantly. The shoulder joint might also pinch nerves, causing neuropathic pain in the arms and hands (pain caused by damage to nerves). In fact, for many people, the pain is not felt in the shoulder but instead in the upper arm, where the muscle and fascia are pulled on by improper movements in the shoulders.

My Experience with Shoulder Pain

Although I suffered for 8 months with unexplained shoulder and arm pain that prevented me from lifting my arms above my shoulders, I do not have a great deal of experience in healing shoulder pain because mine was healed instantly during a Reiki session. Frequently, people hold a lot of tension in their shoulders — the weight of the world can rest there when we are worried, stressed, or overburdened. If that stress-induced tension is part of the cause of your shoulder injury, then Reiki and meditation can be surprisingly helpful.

I witnessed my father experience a reduction in bursitis pain after some sessions with a Physical Therapist, but it returned when he did not continue the exercises. My mother has also dealt with a torn rotator cuff injury that healed with Physical Therapy.

Preventions, Treatments, and Coping Strategies for Shoulder Pain

Shoulder injuries are so common, many of us try to live with them, but it is best to attend to them before they create habitual inappropriate movement patterns.

Treat Shoulder Pain

1. **Do not move out of the appropriate range of motion**. Even though with hypermobile joints, you *can* do something, it doesn't mean that you *should*. Be especially careful when reaching behind yourself (like when you reach for your seatbelt) or when twisting your body while holding or pulling something. *Keep your shoulders safe by limiting your movements to an easy, comfortable range of motion.*
2. **Sleep on your back with pillow support**. *You cannot be aware of your shoulders becoming threatened or injured while you sleep, so try to sleep in a position and with support that will keep them safe.*
3. **Apply ice.** If the shoulder or muscles around it are inflamed due to an injury, ice will reduce the swelling and numb the pain. *Ice can be a useful treatment immediately after an injury, but it can slow healing and even cause damage if it is used for too long.*[628]
4. **Get massage**. It is possible but difficult to massage your own shoulder. You will also need to massage your back, neck, chest, and arm. If you are unable to do it sufficiently yourself, see a professional Massage Therapist. See Section VI: Seek Professional Help. *Massage will relax the muscles that freeze up around the shoulder to protect it from moving too far.*
5. **Get Physical Therapy**. Make sure that the therapist evaluates the movement of your shoulder blade; scapular dyskinesis (improper movement and positioning of the shoulder blade) is common among people who are hypermobile and can be a generative factor in shoulder injuries — scapular dyskinesis is often very subtle and easy for a therapist to miss upon first examination. See Section VI: Seek Professional Help. *A Physical Therapist has many tools with which to soothe pain and build muscle to rehabilitate your shoulders.*
6. **Get Myofascial Release Massage**. Your Physical Therapist or Massage Therapist may be able to do this for you. Often, it is easy to do this kind of massage on yourself, but the areas of the shoulder and back that you will need to treat are too difficult to reach without risking injuring your other shoulder. See Chapter 52: Myofascial Release Massage. *When your shoulder tissues are injured, the fascia locks up around the joint, limiting mobility and causing pain until you release the fascia with gentle massage.*
7. **Apply heat.** Use a heating pad for up to 30 minutes at a time; excessive use can harm the skin. *Heat will help relax the muscles and speed healing by increasing blood flow and clearance of waste products.*[629]
8. **Get Reiki.** Sometimes numerous Reiki treatments are needed to effectively cure a Joint Injury, but other times it is instantaneous. See Section VI: Seek Professional Help. *Reiki is very effective at relaxing tight muscles.*

TREAT SHOULDER PAIN

1. Do not move out of the appropriate range of motion.
2. Sleep on your back with pillow support.
3. Apply ice.
4. Get massage.
5. Get Physical Therapy.
6. Get Myofascial Release Massage.
7. Apply heat.
8. Get Reiki.

Ask your doctor before trying anything new.

34

Sinus Congestion

EVERY HUMAN BEING PROBABLY DEALS with Sinus Congestion at some point in time, but given all of the conditions we with hEDS/HSD are coping with, some of us experience it more often than most people.[630] Aside from the typical viral infections that all humans can expect to contract from time to time, Sinus Congestion is always a symptom of something else having gone wrong in the body — an MCAS flare or Migraine trigger, for example — but even when you cannot eliminate the primary cause of the congestion, you can take steps to reduce the discomfort without making things worse.

My Experience with Sinus Congestion

I have known multiple people who suffered from chronic sinus infections that only went away if they spent large amounts of time outside. Perhaps an air filter inside the home would have helped, but fresh air is certainly good for us.

I have also known many people who have gotten good results using neti pots (with which you pour warm salt water into your nostrils to clean the nasal passages), but I have never been able to make myself try it.

For my family, *Pulsatilla* homeopathic remedy and lymph drainage massage usually take care of any congestion we get.

Preventions, Treatments, and Coping Strategies for Sinus Congestion

Natural remedies for Sinus Congestion abound; here are a few that have worked for me.

Reduce Sinus Congestion

1. **Do Lymph Drainage Massage of the face and neck.** See Chapter 51: Lymph Drainage Massage. *This is a very effective technique that can sometimes stave off a cold that is developing and that can eliminate an ear infection.*
2. **Use Homeopathic Remedies *Pulsatilla* and *Phosphorus*.** *Pulsatilla* is good for congestion in the head, and *Phosphorus* for congestion in the lungs. See Chapter

50: Homeopathic Remedies. *Homeopathic remedies can easily be carried with you, they are safe to take, and they often affect an improvement within minutes.*

3. **Spend as much time outside as possible.** *Fresh air can clear the sinuses very effectively.*
4. **Use peppermint or other herbal teas.** *Because they are hot and steamy, herbal teas are especially good for flushing congestion out, and they are enjoyable, especially with some health-giving honey or real maple syrup in them.*[631]
5. **Use pseudoephedrine or ephedra.** As found in the oral form of Sudafed that requires you to show your driver's license to purchase, it is the best pharmaceutical decongestant I know of. There are not many medicines I would recommend, over-the-counter or prescription, but this one has been extremely helpful at times. However, it is a vasoconstrictor and, in large or frequent doses, can increase risk of stroke.[632] Sudafed is designed to mimic the natural plant, ephedra.[633] The tea of this plant's leaves is an even better decongestant. Unfortunately, because it was misused in weight-loss pills and caused heart problems and sometimes death in people who took too much, it is currently illegal to sell in the US. However, you can purchase seeds for the plant and grow it yourself — I didn't have much luck with the seeds, though; it is a desert plant and I live in a very humid environment. *Often just one dose of pseudoephedrine or ephedra tea is all you need to allow your body to get ahead of the congestion.*
6. **Breathe steam**, carefully so that you do not get burned.[634] *Steam or heat liquify the mucous so that it can flow out of the sinus passages more easily.*
7. **Use cotton handkerchiefs** to blow your nose rather than disposable tissues. As long as you are using a nontoxic laundry detergent, the handkerchiefs will be safer than the tissues that can contain harmful chemicals. (Just throw them in the laundry with your towels and you won't notice them as additional laundry.) They won't make your nose as raw, either. *Cotton handkerchiefs are yet another case of natural products being the most luxurious available.*
8. **Use a Neti Pot.** The warm saline solution can rinse irritants and excess mucous out of the nasal passages. *Many people report relief from Sinus Congestion after using a Neti Pot; it can also remove airborne particles from the nostrils that would otherwise incite an Allergy/MCAS/MCS reaction.*

REDUCE SINUS CONGESTION

1. Do Lymph Drainage Massage of the face and neck.
2. Use Homeopathic Remedies *Pulsatilla* and *Phosphorus*.
3. Spend as much time outside as possible.
4. Use peppermint or other herbal teas.
5. Use pseudoephedrine or ephedra.
6. Breathe steam.
7. Use cotton handkerchiefs.
8. Use a Neti Pot.

Ask your doctor before trying anything new.

LINKS FOR PRODUCTS MENTIONED IN THIS CHAPTER

Pulsatilla https://amzn.to/3vv0832
Phosphorus https://amzn.to/47xYESO
Peppermint Tea https://amzn.to/44sybWX
Handkerchiefs https://amzn.to/44chpuZ
Neti Pot https://amzn.to/4aLpskj

35

Thoracic Outlet Syndrome

THE THORACIC OUTLETS ARE THE SPACES in the upper chest near the shoulders where nerves and blood vessels channel from the neck into the arms and sides of the torso. The clavicles and upper ribs are intended to shield this space, but sometimes these bones or the soft tissues around them compress the area.[635] The resulting condition is called Thoracic Outlet Syndrome (TOS) and is characterized by loss of blood flow and nerve damage.

TOS-related loss of blood flow can cause pain, tingling, numbness, weakness, and coldness in the arms, hands, and sides of the torso. Nerve compression and damage in the thoracic outlet can also exacerbate these symptoms. Additionally, compression of the thoracic outlet can create a sort of dam where fluids cannot drain from above, which leads to swelling above the outlet, in the shoulders and neck. This swelling can be visible and uncomfortable. Additional symptoms can include vestibular dysfunction (problems with balance and spatial awareness), occipital headaches, Migraine, visual impairment, tinnitus (sounds heard when no external corresponding sound is present), fatigue, brain fog, speech problems, anxiety, and in severe cases, fainting, narcolepsy (neurologically impaired sleep cycles), and seizures.[636] TOS may also increase the risk of stroke.

TOS can be caused by anatomical anomalies, injuries, temporary skeletal malalignments, and tight muscles. For many people with TOS – probably between 25-60% — Physical Therapy can resolve the condition. There are also minimally invasive procedures, such as botulinum injections, that can temporarily relax the muscles that are constricting the nerves or veins.[637]

Some people who have TOS have an extra rib or two. Some even have an extra vertebra that gets in the way. In these cases, and sometimes even in the absence of extra bones, treatment is surgical removal of the offending bones.

Although surgery and the recovery from it is painful and often more problematic for people with hEDS (who may not respond well to anesthesia nor heal well), many people who go through the removal of extra bones in the thoracic outlet area find relief. Their pluck is endearing to me because they so often express pride in owning these removed bones. There is an entire social media group dedicated to sharing ideas for making jewelry and crafts out of removed ribs.

My Experience with TOS

For me, TOS caused my hands to fall asleep, becoming numb, tingly, and swollen while I was sleeping. Sometimes this was very painful and woke me up; it would take time for the swelling to abate from my hands, but otherwise, I rarely felt TOS symptoms during the day. It did cause visible swelling and discoloration where my shoulders met my neck, though it was not very uncomfortable. It also caused pain in my sides along the rib cage.

I had this condition temporarily though effectively treated by a Chiropractor and an Osteopath. My Doctor of Osteopathy light-heartedly laughed with me — while I stood in his examining room, he tried to take my pulse in my wrists and said, "Nope! No pulse! You're dead!" Following his Osteopathic treatment, he took my pulse again and pronounced that he had brought me back to life.

I am fortunate that I did not have symptoms severe enough to need more than gentle adjustments from these two professionals. However, the condition persisted until I became really dedicated to improving my posture.

By improving my posture, fascia and muscle tone, and muscular strength, I cured myself of this condition, with the help of my husband's massages. Chapter 56: Posture will be very helpful for eliminating the syndrome, as well as these recommendations:

Preventions, Treatments, and Coping Strategies for TOS

Treat Thoracic Outlet Syndrome

1. **Correct your back and shoulder posture.** Do not slump, but also do not pull your shoulders back too far. Feel that you are lifting your sternum up and being pulled by a string in the top of your head. Some people even get relief by lifting their shoulders; while this can open the thoracic outlet and relax muscles, it is not a long-term solution (unless in response to a habit of pulling the shoulders too low). *To make room for the thoracic outlet, you must lift your body up and keep your shoulders wide apart.*
2. **Get an adjustment from a Chiropractor or Osteopath.** *If any joints in the shoulders or back are out of alignment, they could be causing the compression of the thoracic outlet.*
3. **Stretch out your chest.** Sit on a large yoga ball and roll down until you can lean back over it. There are also stretches in the video linked in Number 9 below. *After letting your chest sink in, the ligaments and muscles may be shortened and need to be stretched.*
4. **Stretch the pectoralis muscles.** Stand in a doorway. Place a bent arm on the wall beside you with your thumb pointing up. Step forward and hold the position for a few seconds. *This stretch is unlikely to threaten the shoulder joint, but always be careful with stretching.*
5. **Do a Kneeling Thoracic Stretch.** Get on your knees in front of a cushioned sofa or chair. Place your elbows on the seat. Bend forward so that your head goes down between your arms, and your hands come back, possibly touching your back, though that is not necessary. *This stretch should be done cautiously, but it will stretch the thoracic area of the back in a way that might feel really good and is unlikely to hyperextend it.*

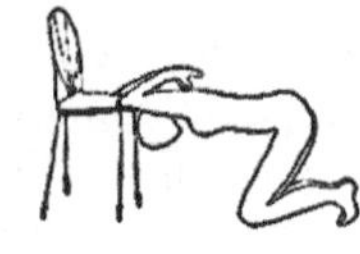

Figure 61: Kneeling Thoracic Stretch

6. **Strengthen your back by lifting weights** with your arms and doing rows, pullups, and pull overs. *The muscles in your back must have the strength to hold your chest and shoulders up and back, off of the thoracic outlet all throughout the day and even while you sleep.*
7. **Do Shoulder External Rotation exercises:** Tie a resistance band to a doorknob or hook on the wall somewhere between waist and shoulder height. Put a small pillow into the armpit under your working arm and squeeze it with your upper arm to hold it against your side, keeping your elbow in. Stand with the other arm closest to the resistance band. With your hand holding the resistance band in front of your stomach, move your hand out to your side. Repeat as many times as you can. During the repetitions, you can try different hand positions and different speeds. *These muscles are often very weak; building them up may be challenging, but it is worth it.*
8. **Breathe deeply into your belly and keep the ribs mobile** as you breathe. (See Chapter 30: Rib Cage Pain for more details.) Maintaining proper movement of all of the elements of the chest will help keep space for the thoracic outlet. *Also, deep belly breaths relax your body, which will relax the muscles that are too tight around the thoracic outlet.*
9. **Do self-massage.** Follow the self-massage instructions on the YouTube video by Train and Massage entitled "#1 Treatment for Thoracic Outlet Syndrome (It's NOT Stretching or Exercises!)" *In many cases, Thoracic Outlet Syndrome is caused purely by tight muscles, so massage can release the tightness and restore proper posture and space for the thoracic outlet.* https://www.YouTube.com/watch?v=-3OHGMte1lg&t=509s
10. **Do Myofascial Release Massage** and gentle massage of your chest, underarms, and sides. *If you have been in a compressed position for very long, the fascia will have tightened into the wrong position and you need to release it so that your bones and muscles can do what they are meant to do.*

TREAT THORACIC OUTLET SYNDROME

1. Correct your back and shoulder posture.
2. Get an adjustment from a Chiropractor or Osteopath.
3. Stretch out your chest.
4. Stretch the pectoralis muscles.
5. Do a Kneeling Thoracic Stretch.
6. Strengthen your back by lifting weights.
7. Do Shoulder External Rotation exercises.
8. Breathe deeply into your belly and keep the ribs mobile.
9. Do self-massage.
10. Do Myofascial Release Massage

Ask your doctor before trying anything new.

36
TMJ

Temporomandibular Disorder (TMJ) is a condition of pain in the Temporomandibular Joint, which is the joint of the jaw. TMJ causes pain in and around the jaw and loss of movement of the joint. It can interfere with eating and talking, and additionally may cause headaches, ear pain, dizziness, and more.[638] Thus, TMJ can diminish the psychosocial contentment of people with the disorder.[639] Unsurprisingly, the laxity of joints in hEDS greatly increases the risk of TMJ and can also make treatment more complicated.[640]

My Experience with TMJ

Many years ago, I had an episode of TMJ that lasted many months and was so severe I could not open my mouth very much and, for a number of weeks, had to take in all of my nutrients through a straw. The only medical treatment offered for my condition was surgery. At the time, two friends of mine went through the surgery for their TMJ pain, which included breaking the jaw and re-setting it. Although they were both happy with their results, I had no desire to go through that risk, pain, and change in the shape of my face. Fortunately, without any guidance from professionals, I was able to use my intuition and heal the condition completely, using mostly meditation and self-massage. I have also heard of patients being relieved of TMJ with hypnosis.

Preventions, Treatments, and Coping Strategies for TMJ

TMJ is a Joint Injury much like those discussed in Chapter 9: Joint Instability & Pain, so many treatments overlap. Still, the face is different from the rest of the body and so there are some specific treatments for TMJ.

Heal Symptoms of TMJ

1. **Meditate to relax the muscles of the face.** Sit or lie quietly with your eyes closed in a comfortable position. Focus on the areas in and around the jaw joint that hurt, and send them love. Send them feelings of safety and calm. Let any stress, tension, and emotion drip out of the muscles. Then, encourage the muscles to relax, melt into softness, be at ease. *Your mind can control your muscles; it can convince them to relax and allow the joint to relax into the proper position.*
2. **Eat soft foods.** Give the tissues a rest. *As long as pain persists, try not to aggravate the joint or increase the pain, which can exacerbate the problem.*
3. **Don't move the jaw in ways that hurt.** Do not chew gum. *Try to keep the muscles relaxed; in case of a partial dislocation or misalignment of the jaw bones, do not risk further Joint Injury.*
4. **Improve posture.** Forward head posture and rounded shoulder posture reduces the endurance capacity of deep neck flexor muscles, which can be a cause of TMJ.[641] See Chapter 56: Posture. *Proper posture will relieve the pressure on the jaw.*
5. **Use heat and/or ice.** When the jaw is particularly inflamed, ice can reduce swelling and pain. Use both temperature treatments in moderation so as not to damage the skin. Heat can help relax the muscles that have stiffened around the damaged joint. *Heat and ice are safe, inexpensive, and effective treatments.*

> Heal Symptoms of TMJ
>
> 1. Meditate to relax the muscles of the face.
> 2. Eat soft foods.
> 3. Don't move the jaw in ways that hurt.
> 4. Improve posture.
> 5. Use heat and/or ice.
> 6. Seek help from a professional therapist.
> 7. Get Craniosacral Therapy, Osteopathy, or Chiropractic care.
> 8. Massage.
> 9. Do Myofascial Release Massage.
> 10. Exercise and listen to music.
> 11. Treat Trigeminal Neuralgia, if present.
>
> Ask your doctor before trying anything new.

6. **Seek help from a professional therapist**. There are Physical Therapists, Speech Therapists, and Occupational Therapists who have treated TMJ. See Section VI: Seek Professional Help. *If you have adopted improper movement habits in the jaw, professionals can help, and they can offer soothing treatments.*
7. **Get Craniosacral Therapy, Osteopathy, or Chiropractic care**. These professionals can align the bones correctly. See Section VI: Seek Professional Help. *Outside help for realigning the jaw bones will be the easiest treatment to receive.*
8. **Massage**. Self-massage works well for the TMJ joint, but many professional Massage Therapists will know how to help as well. Gently massage the muscles of the jaw, neck, face, and head. Also, spend some time gently pulling on the ears — pull on different parts of the ear and in different directions to release tension. *Coerce the muscles to relax back into a normal state.*
9. **Do Myofascial Release Massage.** A therapist can help with this, or you can do it yourself. See Chapter 52: Myofascial Release Massage. *This is important for allowing the jaw to move back into the appropriate position; a lot of the pain you are feeling is probably in the fascia.*
10. **Exercise and listen to music**. One study has shown that those with TMJ got significant reduction in pain after 12 weeks of adding exercise and music to their lifestyle.[642] The exercise was not for the jaw – it was walking, running, working out at the gym, or whatever physical activity the subject chose, for 30 minutes at least

5 times per week. They listened to music for at least 15 minutes at least 5 times per week. *Participating in physical activity and listening to music both have analgesic (pain reducing) qualities.*

11. **Treat Trigeminal Neuralgia, if present**. Sometimes, damage to the cranial nerve that innervates the face can cause tension that appears like grimacing but that can actually activate the muscles improperly and pull on the jaw joints. See Chapter 28: Peripheral Neuropathy. *Get to the source of the problem.*

37

Other Comorbidities — Fibromyalgia, ME/CFS, Eating Disorders, Anxiety, ADHD, Insomnia, Hypersomnia, Sleep Apnea, Depression, Fear, Panic Disorders, Agoraphobia, Suicidal Thoughts & Attempts, Mood Disorders, Bipolar Disorder, Tic Disorder, Borderline Personality Disorder, Obsessive-Compulsive Disorder, Multiple Sclerosis, Rheumatoid Arthritis, Ankylosing Spondylitis, & Autism

THERE ARE FAR TOO MANY SECONDARY CONDITIONS and comorbidities for me to include all of them in this book, but there are some that have been left out for another reason — many people find that these conditions improve when they heal the other conditions that are listed in this book. I suppose that you could call these "tertiary conditions," and they include Fibromyalgia, ME/CFS, Eating Disorders, Anxiety, ADHD, Insomnia, Hypersomnia, Sleep Apnea, Depression, Fear, Panic Disorders, Agoraphobia, Suicidal Thoughts & Attempts, Mood Disorders, Bipolar Disorder, Tic

Disorder, Borderline Personality Disorder, Obsessive-Compulsive Disorder, Rheumatoid Arthritis, Ankylosing Spondylitis, and Autism.

Of course, for many people with these diagnoses, the conditions are genetic, primary conditions and will not be affected by the treatments and techniques in this book. They are beyond the scope of a hypermobility-focused book.

In other cases, though, it has been found that some of these diagnoses are inaccurate. Frequently, these misdiagnoses occur in what has been called the "odyssey" of seeking an hEDS diagnosis, when no one has yet figured out what is really wrong. On average, 42% of the diagnoses given to people with hEDS were inaccurate and were actually, simply, hEDS.[643] One study found that 95% of the patients who were diagnosed with neurological disorders and then later with hEDS did not actually have neurological disorders. The other most commonly misapplied diagnoses were Multiple Sclerosis (76%), Fibromyalgia (67%), and Bipolar Disorder (62%).

For yet other cases, the diagnoses are accurate but are indirectly caused by hEDS. These tertiary conditions may be improved by addressing hypermobility factors, and so I want to bring special awareness to some of these.

Fibromyalgia and ME/CFS

Fibromyalgia is a musculoskeletal disorder that causes long-lasting, widespread pain throughout the soft tissues of the body.[644] "Fibro" means fibers and indicates tendons, ligaments and connective tissues; "my" means muscles; and "algia" means pain. It is usually accompanied by fatigue, brain fog, and dysautonomia such as POTS. More than 56% of people with hEDS also have Fibromyalgia; those who have both conditions have much more severe and numerable symptoms than those who have just one condition or the other.[645]

Fibromyalgia has a lot of overlap in symptoms not only with hEDS but also with another condition called Myalgic Encephalomyelitis (ME) or Chronic Fatigue Syndrome (CFS). [646] Due to the confusion of having two names for a single syndrome, it has been suggested that the condition be called Systemic Exertion Intolerance Disease (SEID), but ME/CFS is the term that is usually used to describe it.[647] In essence, ME/CFS is fibromyalgia following exertion such as exercise or mental effort.

Fibromyalgia and ME/CFS may have a number of different initial triggers, including genetic inheritance or predisposition, injuries from playing sports or car accidents, severe viral or bacterial illnesses, and emotional trauma like sexual assault or military combat service.

It turns out that most people with Fibromyalgia and ME/CFS have lax joints and hypermobility. In fact, the higher the score on the Beighton Criteria, the more severe the symptoms of Fibromyalgia and ME/CFS. (For information about the Beighton Criteria, see Chapter 4: Diagnosing hEDS, HSD, & Pediatric Joint Hypermobility Disorder.) It could be that in some cases, Fibromyalgia and ME/CFS are a manifestation of hEDS/HSD.

A blood test is currently in the late stages of development that may simplify the diagnostic process, but at this time, Fibromyalgia is a clinical diagnosis and is actually considered a diagnosis of exclusion (tests are done to exclude the possibility that the symptoms are caused by a different condition).[648] For some people, Fibromyalgia may be a legitimate condition on its own, but it is often given as a diagnosis when the cause of pain throughout the body is unknown.

I have seen numerous reports of people discovering that what they had been suffering with was in fact Joint Injury and referred pain. Others have found that their pain was associated with Neuropathy, Migraine, Allergies/MCAS/MCS, or others of the common hEDS Secondary Conditions. It may be that your Fibromyalgia is not caused by any of these things, but if you have an awareness that it could improve with some of the treatments for the other conditions, you may be alert to any changes and more likely to correlate them correctly and make the best decisions for your health.

Similarly, ME/CFS could be a legitimate condition on its own, but it could be that the Insomnia brought on by joint pain has created the fatigue.[649] Pain even without Insomnia is exhausting, I can tell you (and I bet you already know). The other numerous symptoms of the secondary conditions and comorbidities of hEDS also can create a feeling of fatigue. It makes sense to treat the physical conditions of Joint Injuries and other aspects of connective tissue disorder, and then see if there is still fatigue left to be treated.

Eating Disorders

Eating Disorders, such as Anorexia, Bulimia, and ARFID (Avoidant/Restrictive Food Intake Disorder), are frequently diagnosed in people with hEDS — sometimes accurately but oftentimes not.[650] When pretty, young women suddenly lose dangerous amounts of weight and the doctors don't know why, sometimes the doctors jump to unfair conclusions and blame the women. I have seen it happen, and it is gut-wrenchingly devastating. Please be aware of this diagnostic problem.

In addition to naturally remarkably slender builds, among some with hEDS, there are a number of reasons it may look like a patient has an eating disorder. There are also a number of ways that hEDS can create eating disorders because eating can be unpleasant.

Many people with hEDS have difficulty swallowing because the collagen in the esophagus (the tube from the mouth to the stomach) doesn't keep it open well enough or squeezing in its wavelike motion to move food down. Trouble transferring food from the mouth to the throat is called oropharyngeal dysphagia, and it can cause pain in the throat, as well as gagging. It may feel like you've swallowed food wrong, or it may actually go down the wrong pipe. (You might experience oropharyngeal dysphagia less if you keep your head facing forward while you are swallowing.) Additionally, food can get stuck in the esophagus further down, behind the sternum. This is called esophageal dysphagia, and it can be very unpleasant.

People with hEDS often have texture-sensitivity. This is why so many of us cut tags out of our clothing, refuse to wear tight socks, and are picky about the fabrics we wear. Texture-sensitivity can happen in our mouths as well and make certain kinds of foods unpleasant and unappetizing.

For those with Allergies/MCAS/MCS, the smell of food often causes nausea and other symptoms, rather than a desire to eat. Allergies/MCAS/MCS often lead to anaphylactic reactions when we eat certain foods. For those with gastrointestinal problems, eating can cause really severe discomfort with nausea, bloating, indigestion, stomach pain, diarrhea, constipation, and other symptoms. Plus, having hEDS means that sometimes we feel full too soon.

Some of the symptoms that I have mentioned may be part of a legitimate eating disorder that can be treated medically, and it is important to do so for your survival. Technically, eating disorders are mental conditions with a psychological basis and behavioral disruption. However, if the eating disorder is caused by one of the physical symptoms of hEDS, then treatment will be different. I pray that healing the symptoms of the primary and secondary conditions in this book will be sufficient to establish normal and enjoyable patterns of eating for you.

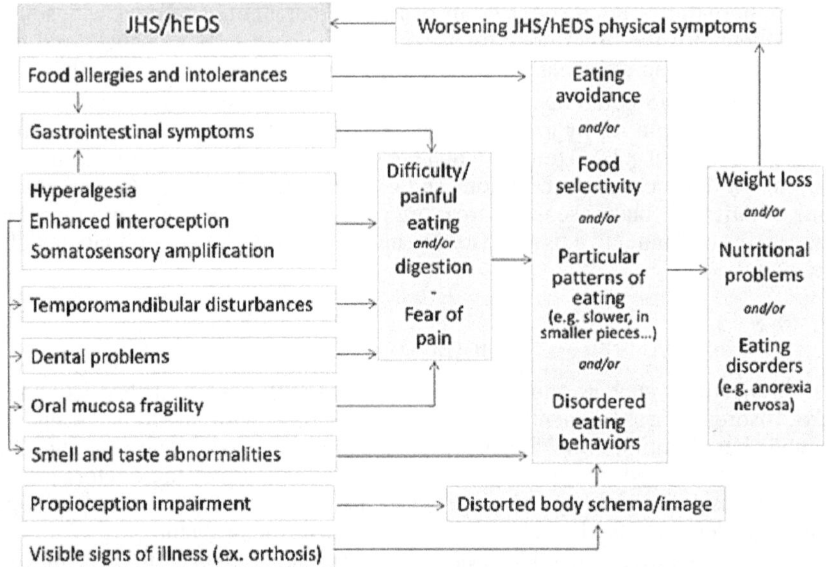

Figure 63. Reprinted with permission from Bulbena A, Baeza-Velasco C, Bulbena-Cabre A, Pailhez G, Critchley H, Chopra P, Mallorqui-Bague N, Frank C, Porges S. (2017).[651] *Note that JHS in the figure above stands for Joint Hypermobility Syndrome, an iteration of Hypermobility Spectrum Disorder.*

Anxiety Disorder

Anxiety is very common among hEDS/HSD patients. In fact, it is diagnosed in 70% (as opposed to 20% in the general population). Even dogs who are hypermobile exhibit emotional excitability, indicating that anxiety in response to hypermobility may be a positive evolutionary trait, protecting us from harming ourselves.[652]

Pathological Anxiety is a condition in which the detection of a fear- or worry-inducing stimulus occurs at lower levels than normal, the somatic (symptoms in the physical body) and emotional responses to the stimulus are out of proportion to the seriousness of the stimulus, and the avoidant or self-protective behaviors are excessive or inappropriate. [653]

Most of the common symptoms of Anxiety (heart palpitations, digestive upset, dizziness, etc.) are common symptoms of hEDS/HSD and their secondary conditions. Also, people with Anxiety are more likely than the general public to have a number of conditions that are common among hEDS/HSD (irritable bowel conditions, Fibromyalgia, thyroid dysfunction, TMJ, mitral valve prolapse (a heart condition), asthma, chronic pain, Migraine, interstitial cystitis (bladder pain), vulvodynia (female genital pain), etc.). Also, patients diagnosed with Anxiety Disorder tend to have long, slender limbs, and nearly 70% have joint hypermobility.

However, the question remains as to whether this Anxiety a) exists on its own and is comorbid with hEDS/HSD, b) is a symptom of hEDS/HSD, or c) is a secondary condition resulting from experiences like pain, dysautonomia, and sensitivities.

I have heard from numerous people who had been diagnosed with Anxiety and suffering with it for years before they received a POTS diagnosis. Soon, they started to realize that all of their Anxiety symptoms were actually POTS symptoms. Once the POTS was under control, there was very little Anxiety left, if any. Allergy/MCAS/MCS reactions can cause Anxiety as part of their regular symptom cluster as well. I and some of my clients at my holistic healing center discovered that if we wore polyester clothing, we would develop Anxiety or Social Anxiety that we didn't feel if we wore cotton clothing. Migraine and any kind of pain can also create Anxiety that does not have a psychological basis.

It is good to know the true cause of your problem, not only because you can then treat it appropriately, but also because you can respond to it appropriately. People with Anxiety must use mental effort to determine the validity of a feeling of anxiety, and understanding the possible causes of the feeling is crucial for making a good decision.

ADHD

A recent report on children with ADHD stated that 99% of them were hypermobile.[654] Adults with ADHD are also likely to have joint hypermobility. The need to move frequently to relieve the fatigue in muscles that are supporting lax joints could explain how hypermobility could cause ADHD, at least in part. The symptoms of many of the secondary conditions and comorbidities could be to blame — the pain, dizziness, fatigue, proprioceptive impairment, etc. could create emotional dysregulation, hyperactivity, inattention, and impulsivity.[655, 656] The changes that hEDS/HSD create in the brain could have an impact on the presence of ADHD, too.

Insomnia, Hypersomnia, and Sleep Apnea

Fatigue, sleep disturbance, daytime sleepiness, Hypersomnia, and Obstructive Sleep Apnea (OSA) are all prevalent among people with hEDS. In fact, it has been found that 42% of children with hEDS have OSA. This condition, in children and adults, could potentially be caused by the laxity of the tissues in the face, larynx, and pharynx.

For myself and others I know, Insomnia is a reliable component of Migraine, Allergy/MCAS/MCS, gastrointestinal problems, and all forms of pain. Yet, when we are not suffering with those other conditions, we sleep well. Treating for Insomnia with certain medications can be taxing on your liver, so it is best to understand the underlying cause, as it may change the treatment plan.

Other Psychiatric Disorders

Depression, Fear, Panic Disorders, Agoraphobia, Suicidal Thoughts and Attempts, Mood Disorders, Bipolar Disorder, Tic Disorder, Borderline Personality Disorder, and Obsessive-Compulsive Disorder are much more common among people with hEDS/HSD than the general population. [657, 658]

People with hEDS/HSD are 4.3 times more likely than the general population to be diagnosed with a Psychiatric Disorder. This is probably because the symptoms of hEDS/HSD create emotional distress and crises in identity and self-efficacy. People with hEDS/HSD must develop coping methods and psychological adaptations for their experience; frequently, these behaviors and adaptations appear to be or manifest as Psychiatric Disorders.

It is important for the Psychiatric Disorders to be treated with a knowledge of the underlying cause, and it is even more important for the underlying cause to be treated. It is also important for doctors to be aware of the prevalence of Psychiatric Disorders in association with hypermobility so that they will evaluate their hypermobile patients for Psychiatric Disorders and the whole patient can be treated to improve quality of life.

One of the most important findings in research about Psychiatric Disorders and hEDS/HSD is that suicide attempts are correlated with delay in diagnosis (as well as with Borderline Personality Disorder). Early diagnosis of hEDS is protective against suicide. This is especially poignant considering that psychological manifestations, apparent or real, in hypermobility are one of the primary causes of delayed diagnosis — doctors sometimes blame the reported symptoms on the psychological condition and do not look for a biological explanation. (As mentioned at the beginning of this chapter, this may happen in up to 95% of cases.) It is extremely important that the medical community become better informed about hypermobility disorders.

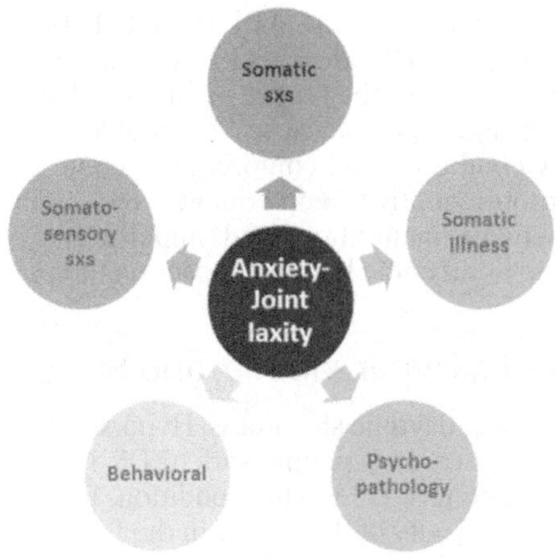

- Behavioral Dimensions are patterns of defensive mechanisms that are often identifiable at the extreme of a continuous axis (i.e., fight/flight, restriction (avoidance)/dependency
- Somatic symptoms include dysautonomia, asthenic somatotype, "blue sclera" "easy bruising," eczemas, dyskinesia, dislocations, prolapses, and hypertrophic scars
- Somatic illnesses: irritable bowel syndrome, dysfunctional esophagus, chemical sensitivities, dizziness, fatigue, fibromyalgia, dynias, hypothyroidism, asthma, migraines, temporomandibular dysfunction, and food intolerances.
- Somato-sensory symptoms include increased olfactory sensitivity, eye-contact difficulty, selective photophobia, dyspnea, dysphagia, choking, palpitations, joint pain and enhances sensitivity to weather and chemicals
- Psychopathology: increased interoception, exteroception, decreased proprioception, anticipatory anxiety, high loss sensitivity, and high positive confrontation.

Reprinted with permission from Bulbena-Cabré, A., Baeza-Velasco, C., Rosado-Figuerola, S., & Bulbena, A. (2021, November 9).[659]

Multiple Sclerosis

Multiple Sclerosis (MS) is a condition in which a body's immune cells damage components of the nervous system, leaving scar tissue called sclerosis, which doctors can see by using Magnetic Resonance Imaging (MRI).[660] Because different parts of the nervous system can be affected, MS can create a wide variety of symptoms, such as vision problems, muscle weakness, tingling, clumsiness, dizziness, and bladder control problems. As the disease progresses, it may also cause depression, cognitive problems, and mood changes.

MS is sometimes progressive but frequently goes through long periods of remission and sometimes full recovery. People with MS have a normal life expectancy.

There are a number of different factors that are thought to be potential causes of MS. It is not an inherited condition, but susceptibility to it may be inherited. The Epstein-Barr virus (which causes mononucleosis) is commonly found in people with MS, but only 5% of the general population has never had this virus, and MS is present in only 35.9 per 100,000 people worldwide (that is 0.000359%). Vitamin D deficiency and smoking are also highly correlated with MS.

Although only a tiny percentage of people have MS, one study showed that people with hEDS are at least 10 times as likely as the general population to get it.[661] As explained in the beginning of this chapter, people with hEDS are much more likely to be *mis*diagnosed with MS as well.

One of the possible connections between hEDS and MS is that mast cells (infamous because MCAS is present in 89% of people with hEDS) are also implicated in MS. Additionally hEDS has numerous impacts on the nervous system, which may have an as-yet undetermined effect on the pathology of MS.

Rheumatological Conditions: Rheumatoid Arthritis and Ankylosing Spondylitis

Rheumatoid Arthritis (RA) and Ankylosing Spondylitis (AS) are both autoimmune conditions in which the immune system becomes intolerant to a certain protein that is in the synovium of the joints.[662] The synovium is the slippery tissue and fluid that lines joints where bones meet.[663] The immune system begins to attack the synovium; this action of the immune system causes inflammation in the joint, which results in swollen, warm, red, painful joints.[664]

Many of the symptoms of RA and AS overlap with those of hEDS, but there are some differences. Both of these rheumatological conditions can be diagnosed based on a combination of factors as determined by a symptom and history report made by the patient, clinical observations made by the doctor, imaging test results that demonstrate the damage in the joints, and in the case of RA, lab tests that might reveal specific markers in the blood related to RA.[665]

In RA, the affected joints are usually in the hands and feet, progressing to the wrists, ankles, knees, elbows, shoulders, and hips. RA can also cause inflammation, damage, pain, and other forms of discomfort in the eyes, mouth, skin, lungs, blood vessels, blood, and heart. These symptoms frequently lead to a sedentary lifestyle that can result in weight gain that increases the risk of diabetes and heart disease.

AS primarily affects the lower spine and the sacroiliac joint (the joint where the spine meets the pelvis). Eventually, swelling, redness, warmth, and pain can occur in some other joints as well. AS can also cause symptoms in the rib cage, eyes, digestive tract, heart, and lungs.[666]

It is unknown what causes RA and AS — possibilities include viral or bacterial infections, traumatic events, a trigger in the environment, or some other external factor.[667] There is also a strong genetic factor.[668] However, someone with a family member with AS has only a 20% chance of having it also. Approximately 30% of the general population has the gene that indicates RA, but only 0.41% of people actually develop RA. Obviously, there is an epigenetic (environmental rather than genetic) factor to rheumatological conditions.

Interestingly, there is a correlation with hEDS.[669] Although most people with hEDS/HSD do not have RA or AS, there is a prevalence of it much higher than in the general population. According to a 2017 study, RA is present in as little as 0.41% of the general population but 6.8% of people with hEDS; AS is present in only 6.1% of the general population but 24% of people with hEDS.

Thus, it is important that RA/AS be considered as a differential diagnosis for those with hypermobility. Although there is overlap among the treatments for the various conditions, their treatments are different.

It is unknown why there is a correlation between hEDS/HSD and RA/AS, but it could be that the inflammation caused by hEDS/HSD increases the risk of RA or AS. Additionally, symptoms of hEDS/HSD and RA/AS can exacerbate each other, or at least, decrease quality of life as they occur simultaneously and create extreme discomfort. Thus, it would be my hope that treating hEDS/HSD in those who have it could reduce the number of people who develop RA/AS, and for those who have RA/AS that treating hEDS/HSD could improve their overall symptoms and quality of life.

Autism

Studies looking at both Autism and hEDS or hypermobility are very rare, but it has been seen that they co-exist much more often than would be expected by chance.[670] It has been found that more than 20% of mothers with hEDS have children with autism.[671] Autism and hEDS have a lot of overlapping symptoms, as well: Anxiety, chronic fatigue, dysautonomia, proprioceptive impairment, hyper- and hypo-skin sensitivity, light and sound sensitivity, autonomic dysregulation, gastrointestinal problems, Chiari malformations, Peripheral Neuropathy, immune system dysregulation, etc.

With the high correlation of hEDS with Autism, it stands to reason that hypermobility could be one of the causative factors of Autism for some people; joint hypermobility may be a subtype of Autism.[672] In fact, I have known people who had a reduction in Autism symptoms when they successfully treated their Allergies/MCAS/MCS, gluten intolerance, other gastrointestinal problems, and Sympathetic Nervous System hyperactivation in ways similar to those described in this book.

Although the brain of a person with Autism may be different, [673] it may be that at least some of the unpleasant symptoms that accompany the condition can best be treated with hEDS in mind.

Natural Treatments for All Conditions

Recently, I was outlining for a friend the basics of my recommendations for naturally healing symptoms of hEDS/HSD. He stopped me and said, “Shannon, what you're really telling me is to live a healthy lifestyle?”

Yes, a healthy lifestyle will support any of the health conditions in this book and probably any others. The keys to success are knowing how to live a truly healthy lifestyle and paying attention to your own body's unique needs within that lifestyle.

Many of the techniques listed in the next section, Healing Treatments, can be part of a happy and healthy lifestyle.

Section V

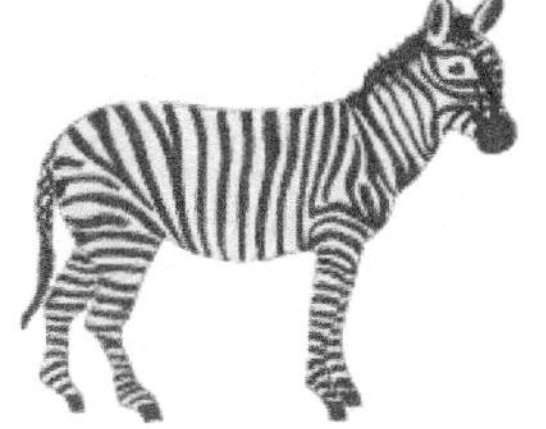

Healing Treatments

38

Self-Treatment Techniques for Healing Symptoms of hEDS/HSD, Secondary Conditions, & Comorbidities

OUR BODIES ARE MIRACULOUS, HEALING FORMS. Our ancestors have been developing healing abilities for millennia before us and passing down that information so that we can heal ourselves now.

Our minds are resourceful and inventive. As the world changes and we learn new things, we develop new, amazing healing techniques so that we can meet whatever challenges the changing world presents.

Whether or not you have the assistance of a doctor or other medical professional, you can benefit from using alternative and complementary therapies to heal yourself. I pray that you increase in knowledge, confidence, self-agency,[674] and ability by trying the techniques listed below, and that you are able to completely heal yourself.

39

Abhyanga Oil Massage

THIS IS A TRADITION FROM INDIA THAT HELPS to remove toxic chemicals from the body.[675] It is relaxing and leaves the skin soft and beautiful.[676] It may also help alleviate muscular hypertonicity.

My Experience with Abhyanga Oil Massage

Abhyanga Oil Massage has been very healing for me at times when I was reacting most strongly to chemicals. It is enjoyable to me, and it requires that I spend a little extra time on myself.

Step-By-Step Instructions for Abhyanga Oil Massage

As you follow these instructions, luxuriate in the pleasure of it and let your body be healed by the oil and your self-loving touch.

Abhyanga Oil Massage Steps

1. Rub olive oil onto all of the body. Use only a good quality organic olive oil. Stand over a towel so that you will not drip on the floor and make it slippery. Rub each body part for about a minute until the entire body is massaged and oiled.
2. Get into a very warm shower.
3. Use a washcloth to gently scrub away the oil. Do not use soap; a trace of the oil will be left behind on your skin. Be careful because the shower may become slippery; using some kind of non-slip surface in your shower is a good idea.
4. Use soap to clean your hairiest parts (head, underarms, and private areas). Make sure to use only an all-natural, fragrance-free soap.
5. After the shower, dry off as usual. You probably won't need any moisturizer.
6. The washcloth may become very oily and may not be safe to wash and dry in your laundry machines; it is recommended that you continue to use it until it is overused and then throw it away, but I always just wash the washcloth in hot water with Borax to supplement the laundry soap.

40

Affirmations

ONE OF MY FAVORITE WAYS OF IMPROVING health and healing injuries is by using the mantras Louise Hay developed for her book, *You Can Heal Your Life*. I do not believe that our emotions always cause diseases nor that all diseases are caused by emotions, but I do believe that our bodies record everything we experience, and this can lead to problems that are related to our experiences. In order to clear the emotional blocks that might be impacting our health and to leverage our emotional power to transform our illnesses into wellness, we can use Affirmations.

Affirmations or declarations can help convince us of our adequacy and ability to meet challenges successfully. Additionally, when a person's belief in herself is affirmed, she is likely to make better health decisions, both because she is more likely to make decisions based on factual information rather than defensive or fear-based reactions, and because she is more likely to have success making the lifestyle changes that can make a difference.[677] Positive Affirmations can also reduce the feeling of stress, including biomarkers like cortisol, as well as the negative effects of stress, such as Insomnia, inability to adapt to situations, obesity, and even an increase in threatening or harmful events. Not only that, but there may be a supernatural effect taking place, so that if you speak it, it will be so.

In her book, Hay first lists "Probable Mental Patterns that create disease" for each of a long list of diseases or body parts, and then she lists "New Thought Patterns" or Affirmations that create health to go with each disease or body part.

This is a very easy healing method, and it is free! Although her book is worth reading, you can also find her list if you search Spiritual Meanings Underlying Diseases for free online in many places; here is one of them:

https://lovehonourandrespect.org/emotional-health/louise-hay-Affirmations-for-illnesses/

Not only can you easily find Hay's Affirmations, but as she wrote, you can invent your own Affirmations whenever you need them. She explained further that all diseases are related to either fear or anger, and the New Thought Pattern you really need is to love yourself. Many of her Affirmations are about trusting.

One change that may be beneficial to make to Hay's Affirmations is to translate them into third person and say your name to yourself.[678] So, when using her Affirmation for Joint Pain, instead of saying to myself, "My life is Divinely guided, and I am always going in the right direction," I say, *"Shannon, your life is Divinely guided, and you are always going in the right direction."*

Another source of Affirmations that I have especially enjoyed is Silent Unity. You can submit a prayer request online or by phone, and if you request a reply, they will send you an email with an Affirmation for your current need. These are always uplifting and encouraging to me, and I have felt the power of their prayers.

https://www.unity.org/request-prayer

While writing this book, I submitted a prayer request to Silent Unity that all of the people who read this book will receive healing. Silent Unity replied with a beautifully enheartening email, which included this Affirmation, which I invite you now to use as your own personal Affirmation as you enact the changes inspired by this book (note that it is sometimes helpful to say a new affirmation three times; this is to confirm that you agree with this affirmation on all levels — mental, physical, and spiritual):

> *The healing love of God flows through you now, restoring energy and vitality*
>
> *The healing love of God flows through you now, restoring energy and vitality*
>
> *The healing love of God flows through you now, restoring energy and vitality.*

My Experience with Affirmations

About 25 years ago, a wise woman I was friends with gasped, widened her eyes, and with reverence said to me, "Oh, everything that you look upon will become more beautiful because you have looked upon it."

What a valuable gift that proved to be for me, and to everyone around me. I held that phrase to my heart as an Affirmation, and I made it become true, though it usually felt like a magical congruence of energy rather than my own effort. When I looked upon a dance student, I gave her confidence and knowledge, and she became a more beautiful dancer with a more beautiful personality. When I looked upon a healing client, she became healthier and more empowered, filled with beauty and self-agency[679] to make the world a better place. When I looked upon the yard in front of my house, I planted flowers. When I walked in the forest, I picked up trash. When I looked upon a friend and felt love for her, she became more beautiful in my eyes and, I believe, in her own.

Especially when I am feeling down, Affirmations can empower me and help me believe in the good in myself and the world. When they are health-focused, optimistic attitudes make a difference in my body's ability to be well and heal more quickly than I believe I would heal otherwise.

As I have been writing this book for you, I have practiced this technique: "Shannon, your thorough research, candid openness, attention to detail, and concern for your readers is evident on every page. You are doing a brilliant job of writing a valuable book that is going to help millions of people live better."

Step-By-Step Instructions for Affirmations

Affirmations can be used in many ways, including in meditation and prayer. The following ideas do not need to be done in order; simply choose whichever of these options is most powerful and convenient in your life right now. Ask your doctor before trying anything new.

Use Affirmations for Healing

1. Find an Affirmation in Louise Hay's *You Can Heal Your Life*, from a prayer request to Silent Unity, from a spiritual book, or make one up yourself. Affirmations are most effective when you say your own name and use third-person voice (say to yourself "you" rather than "I").
2. Repeat the affirmative thought in your head whenever it comes to mind.
3. Write the Affirmation on paper or a Post-It note and stick it up on walls and mirrors around the house.
4. Set alarms on your phone to remind you of your Affirmation on a regular schedule.
5. Ask a friend to remind you of this Affirmation whenever you talk to each other.
6. Truly believe the Affirmation. You do not have to start out believing it; repeating the Affirmation for many days is one way of convincing yourself that it could be true.
7. Feel the emotions of the truth or fruition of the Affirmation.
8. If you cannot come to believe that the Affirmation is true, analyze the situation. What is holding you back from believing it? What created the problem? What could possibly change to make this Affirmation a possibility? As you work through these kinds of questions, you awaken intuition or memories that lead to concrete answers regarding which healing techniques to use. Otherwise, rephrase the Affirmation beginning with, "You are beginning to believe that..." or switch to using a different Affirmation — one that is a step toward making the original Affirmation a possibility.

LINKS FOR PRODUCTS MENTIONED IN THIS CHAPTER

You Can Heal Your Life https://amzn.to/41YAoby

41

The Basic Exercise

STANLEY ROSENBERG HAS WRITTEN A FASCINATING book called *Accessing the Healing Power of the Vagus Nerve*. In it, he introduced The Basic Exercise, but there are also other healing techniques described in it. I highly recommend that you read it for a better understanding of the Vagus Nerve, which is the longest and most complex nerve system in the body.

The Basic Exercise is designed to switch your nervous system from the stress response to the rest-and-digest state, as well as to increase proper mobility of the neck. It can be especially helpful to do this exercise if you have had a stressful social encounter, if you are having neck or head pain, or if you feel anxious.

Here is a video that explains how to do it: "The Basic Exercise by Stanley Rosenberg" by yoopod on YouTube https://www.YouTube.com/watch?v=rbowIy6kONY&t=19s .

I have adjusted the exercise slightly, as follows.

My Experience with The Basic Exercise

When I first started doing The Basic Exercise, it made quite a surprisingly large difference. I did it multiple times every hour. I did it every night before going to sleep and every morning before getting out of bed. It could instantly reduce my neck pain and restore my ability to breathe deeply.

As time has gone on, I have needed to do The Basic Exercise less and less. Apparently, my body has learned to exist in the rest-and-digest state more of the time, and my neck has gotten used to being in a proper alignment. I do still find that The Basic Exercise helps me after any kind of stressful experience, especially social activities.

Step-By-Step Instructions for the Basic Exercise

This exercise is basic because it is as simple as an exercise can be, but it can still be powerful. Ask your doctor before trying anything new.

The Basic Exercise Steps

1. Lie down.
2. Lace your fingers together and place them behind your head.
3. Close your eyes.
4. With your eyes closed and keeping your nose straight toward the ceiling, move your eyes all the way to the right. Hold them there for a count of 60.
5. Slowly, very slowly, move your eyes to the left. Hold them there for a count of 60.
6. Slowly, very slowly, move your eyes to the front. Open your eyes.

When you have become very comfortable with doing this exercise, you will be able to achieve the desired result while sitting or standing and without putting your hands behind your head. You may also feel a release or relaxation before reaching the count of 60, at which time you can move to the next step. You may also want to try moving your eyes to various positions as if looking up.

LINKS FOR PRODUCTS MENTIONED IN THIS CHAPTER

Accessing the Healing Power of the Vagus Nerve https://amzn.to/3T3rfdE

42

Cusack Protocol

This is a supplement protocol developed by Deborah Cusack, a woman who has hEDS and whose four children also have it; they were all suffering severely, needing medications, surgeries, and braces. She went to great lengths to determine the best supplements to help her family cope with hEDS. It was so successful that she felt she should share it with the world, which she has done, along with encouragement and help from other people who have been helped by the protocol.

The Cusack Protocol has not yet been studied for its efficacy or safety. It is not known if the supplements, though generally deemed safe, have contraindications, work safely in conjunction with each other, or have effects beyond the placebo effect. It has been found that aloe, one of the most important supplements in the protocol, has a beneficial effect on the fibroblast cells that create collagen in order to repair connective tissues.[680, 681]

Self-reports on social media indicate that many people get positive results from it, though it does not seem to help everyone who tries it. Faithful implementation of the protocol could have an influence on the effectiveness of it, but with self-reports rather than a scientific study, the methods and fidelity of implementation that have been used are unknown. The supplements on the protocol are polysaccharides (George's Aloe Vera Juice, Host Defense Maitake Capsules, or PharmAloe), pyrroloquinoline quinone (PQQ), *L-rhamnosus GG*, L-arginine with L-lysine, D-ribose, lions mane mushroom, diatomaceous earth (DE), glucosamine chondroitin, astragalus, and hyaluronic acid.

Deborah Cusack has a small website and a YouTube channel about the protocol:

https://ouredsjourney.weebly.com/resources.html

https://www.youtube.com/@deborahcusack8782

Extensive information about following the Cusack Protocol is available in a private Facebook group's guides and files. There are many details to consider, such as the brands to choose, the timing of supplements, and whether to take them with or without food, so it is best for you to consult the original recommendations on the Facebook group. https://www.facebook.com/groups/497844976982140

My Experience with the Cusack Protocol

Soon after discovering that I had hEDS, I began the first step of the Cusack Protocol, the Culturelle probiotic. I almost immediately noticed that I got less bloating and indigestion, though it did not go away completely, as it is triggered by my MCAS triggers and CCI.

Once I knew that I could tolerate the probiotic, I started taking PQQ. I did not notice any changes with the PQQ. In fact, once I had used the entire bottle, I stopped taking it, and again, I noticed no changes. It could be that it helped me in ways I didn't notice, or it could be that my body did not need the PQQ. I have heard through the Facebook group that it can take a long time for PQQ's benefits to become apparent, so I believe it will be worthwhile for me to try it again in the future.

After a week or so on the PQQ, I started drinking George's Aloe Juice. A few days after starting it, I lay down on my side and noticed that my hip wasn't immediately slipping right out of position. It seemed that my joints were magically firming up. I attribute a lot of the Joint Injury healing that I managed in the following months to be due in part to the George's Aloe. Any joints that I have been able to get back into position have tightened up.

The biggest difference I have noticed due to the George's Aloe is in my skin. My skin looks smooth and beautiful all over my body, hands, and face. It feels plump and youthful. It feels good to the touch. I look much younger and feel better. I had previously gotten some of these skin improvement results from using the Near Infrared and Red Light Therapy box, but the George's Aloe has made an even bigger improvement.

I also found that my POTS symptoms diminished. I have not noticed a change regarding my chemical sensitivities that I would relate to the Cusack Protocol, but there are other supplements on the protocol that I have not yet tried that are purported to help with sensitivities.

My son and mother have also had good results from the Culturelle probiotic and George's Aloe.

I have not felt a need to try the other supplements on the Cusack Protocol, but I am grateful to know that they are there in case I experience the symptoms they can treat.

Step-By-Step Instructions for the Cusack Protocol

Give yourself several months with each supplement because it can take a long time for results to be recognizable. Some people report continuing to improve for up to a year and beyond. Ask your doctor before trying anything new.

Follow the Cusack Protocol

1. Study the instructions on the Ehlers Danlos Syndrome and the Cusack Protocol facebook page: https://www.facebook.com/groups/497844976982140 . There are so many details to consider when following the protocol, you must read all of the Guides before you get started.
2. Always start one supplement at a time, at a reduced dosage so that you can determine if you have had a reaction or improvement with it.
3. Increase dosages slowly until you reach the full dosage, and continue to take the supplement.

4. Keep notes of the supplements you try and how your symptoms change so that you can make appropriate adjustments and personalize the protocol. Also, be patient; many of the supplements will not result in recognizable differences right away, and even once improvements are noted, you may continue to gain improvements for a year or more, according to testimonials in the facebook group.

LINKS FOR PRODUCTS MENTIONED IN THIS CHAPTER

George's Aloe Vera Liquid https://amzn.to/3Uzvz6h

Host Defense Maitake Mushroom https://amzn.to/3WldYQT

PharmAloe Capsules https://pharmaloe.com/products/aloe-vera-capsules?variant=31048939798607

Pyrroloquinoline Quinone https://amzn.to/4aXP1iU

L.Rhamnosus https://amzn.to/3HkFUeX

L-Arginine https://amzn.to/3UH63fG

D-Ribose https://amzn.to/4dx0WWP

Lions Mane Mushroom https://amzn.to/3UEQuFh

Diatomaceous Earth https://amzn.to/3JZTIgt

Glucosamine Chondroitin https://amzn.to/44nh4G2

Hyaluronic Acid.

https://amzn.to/4dfsGyN

43
Deodorant

IF YOU ARE SENSITIVE TO CHEMICALS or if your body has a difficult time detoxing, you may do best going without deodorant. I know it may sound crazy. It might be a big surprise, but human bodies do not always need deodorant. It is possible to go without deodorant and still smell good.

Some of the benefits of going without deodorant are obvious: saving money and hassle, but also, going without deodorant is good for you. The glands under the arms are designed to release fluids containing many chemicals, including heavy metals and other toxins. Sweating is one of the ways our body detoxes. Deodorants and antiperspirants can block pores, reducing sweating and also reducing the body's ability to detox.[682]

Additionally, the glands in the armpits are designed to absorb chemicals — partly, they reabsorb their own sweat to manage the amount of fluid under the arms, but they also absorb chemicals from deodorants and antiperspirants.[683] Some of the chemicals in these products, such as fragrance and aluminum (both of which are mast cell activators), are very dangerous to your health.[684]

There are a number of natural deodorants on the market, and there are a lot of homemade options like apple cider vinegar that are far safer than the mainstream deodorants and antiperspirants. These are good choices in circumstances when it is really necessary to reduce your odor. However, they still change your skin's natural bacterial biome and prevent you from detoxing as effectively as possible. In my holistic clinic, I noticed that clients whose sweat ducts appeared to be blocked by the product they were using under their arms developed swollen lymph nodes under their arms. This can be uncomfortable, unsightly, and concerning for health.

Really, the key to not being stinky is to live a nontoxic lifestyle — no harmful chemicals, no chronic stresses, and no (or little) junk food — and stay clean. A natural soap and clean water are all you really need to smell good.

In most cases, you do not need to bathe daily, but you likely will need to bathe anytime you have experienced something that could make you stinky. Viruses and anger can make you stinky, and no amount of washing will cure that until the viral infection or anger have passed — our smells really tell us about what is going on in our bodies. Still, if you are wearing clothing that covers your armpits and bathe frequently, it is unlikely that other people will notice your smell during these times.

The best deodorant for your health is none, but the transition from using deodorant to not using deodorant can be embarrassingly smelly if you don't do it right. This is because all those poisons and waste products that have been building up in your body are stinky. You need to detox your armpits.

My Experience with Living Deodorant-Free

I have gone without deodorant for over 6 years, even when I was working as a performer in a professional dance company. My husband, who loves to work out at the gym, stopped wearing it after he met me. I have known musicians who never wore deodorant, even when performing with a band in front of thousands of people.

I feel better without deodorant on, and I find that my shirts actually stay cleaner most of the time and even last longer before getting discolored or thread-bare under the arms. I love how easy it is not to have to pack deodorant for trips. I especially love saving money and never having to worry about having a bad reaction to deodorant.

Step-By-Step Instructions for Transitioning to No Deodorant

These steps will be of help even if you are choosing to transition to a more natural deodorant option rather than none. Ask your doctor before trying anything new.

Use an Underarm Clay Mask for Detoxing and Eliminating Body Odor[685]

1. Wash your underarms thoroughly with a natural soap and water.
2. Mix together water and bentonite clay. It is not always easy to get the right consistency that is spreadable and will cling to the skin. I like to mix up a small jar of it several days in advance so I can adjust the ratio of water and clay (which varies, probably depending on humidity in the air) and let it become homogeneous over time. In the jar, it will become silky smooth. See Appendix A: Recipes.
3. Spread the bentonite clay paste onto the skin under your arms.
4. Allow the clay mask to dry completely.
5. Use a warm wet washcloth to wash the clay off.
6. Repeat this any time you notice body odor on yourself. At first, you will possibly need to do this mask daily, but eventually you will need it less and less. Within a few weeks, you will probably not need a mask anymore. Within a few months, you might kind of forget that you ever wore deodorant or were ever smelly. Once you have detoxed, you will not smell stinky unless something unusual happens: you eat too much junk food, you get exposed to toxic chemicals, you have an MCS/MCAS reaction, you get sick with a viral or bacterial illness, you get really upset/angry/sad/stressed out. Most of the time, it will be sufficient to wash with soap and water, but you can always do another bentonite clay mask when needed.

LINKS FOR PRODUCTS MENTIONED IN THIS CHAPTER

Bentonite Clay https://amzn.to/4aetcut

Jars https://amzn.to/49oQlua

Soap http://azsungoldsoaps.com/mobile/order/liquid/products_shampoo.html

44

Detox

THERE ARE MANY METHODS OF DETOXING the body, and the first step in detoxing is to switch to only non-toxic products. For some of you lucky people, this may be the only step you need. It's easier than you think, and it is really important, not only for your own body but also for the entire planet. Toxic toiletries and household products are poisoning the Earth's air, water, and creatures. Taking the step to make yourself healthier will make everyone healthier.

In fact, 50% of the petroleum pollution in the air comes from household products.[686] One of the worst offenders is "fragrance." You will see fragrance on the ingredient labels of most perfumes, body sprays, colognes, laundry products, scented candles, wax warmers, soaps, shampoos, lotions, deodorants, cleaning products, air fresheners, trash can liners, facial tissues, and other products.

There are more than 3,500 chemicals that can be called "fragrance," and the companies that sell these products are not required to disclose which chemicals these are.[687] Up to 95% of them are derived from petroleum, the crude oil fossil fuel that we put in our vehicles. We know that vehicle exhaust air pollution is damaging human and ecosystem health, but most people are surprised to find that the chemicals in household products are implicated in air pollution just as much as vehicle exhaust.

Chemicals that can be listed as fragrance are usually harmful to your health. Many are neurotoxins, which means they poison the nervous system and can cause nausea, weakness, memory problems, vision problems, sexual dysfunction, Parkinson's-like symptoms, Alzheimer's-like symptoms, and other health conditions.[688, 689]

Many are endocrine disrupters, which means that they disrupt the hormone balance in the body and can cause reproductive problems, sexual behavior dysfunctions, developmental problems, diabetes, fatty liver disease, abnormal social behavior, neurological deficits, heart disease, obesity, many kinds of hormone-sensitive cancers, and more. These chemicals can even cause diseases that manifest long after exposure or even in the next generation.[690]

Many are carcinogenic, which means that they cause cancer.[691] It is also suspected that fragrance can play a role in the development of autism.[692] Most frightening is the fact that fragrances can be mutagenic, which means that they can permanently change your DNA.[693]

Many hEDS people and also many in the general public report symptoms such as headaches, brought on by fragrance exposure, but even if you don't notice the effects, it would be kind to everyone you come in contact with if you limited or eliminated the use of fragrance. More than a third of the population reports adverse effects from exposure to fragrance. These effects can include things like respiratory problems, congestion, Migraine attacks, asthma, brain fog, digestive problems, skin problems, musculoskeletal problems, and more.[694]

To make it simple, start by looking at the cleaning products you have in your kitchen and bathroom cupboards — if the ingredients list contains the word "fragrance," throw it out and replace it with a non-toxic option.

I know what you're thinking: "But I spent my hard-earned money on this!" I have counseled countless clients and friends through the transition to a healthy, non-toxic lifestyle, and each one of them, at some point, has said something along these lines: "I'll just use up this bottle and buy something better next time." I can fully understand this sentiment, but I encourage you not to wait until next month to get healthy.

Consider what your response would be if someone said to you, "I will pay you $5 to poison yourself a little bit." You would say, "I don't want to be poisoned! I don't need $5 that badly."

Therefore, go ahead and throw out that fragranced lotion without using it up, even if it was a gift from a loved one. Feel the relief of not smearing poison all over yourself every day. Feel proud of taking a stand for your health even though it means changing things up.

Also, you will want to avoid many of the popular beauty treatments, which are toxic, such as tattoos, hair dye, fingernail polish, Botox, fillers, and implants. Clean, pure health is beautiful. Once you are detoxed, you will not need the assistance of these treatments to look beautiful.

The hardest part of getting rid of toxic products is finding healthy versions to replace them. Look carefully at products labeled "unscented;" many of them contain Volatile Organic Compounds (VOCs) plus fragrance that covers up the smells. VOCs are molecules that can float in the air and be smelled — fragrances are VOCs.

Although some natural products do not contain fragrance, they still may contain essential oils. While essential oils are not composed of as many toxic chemicals as fragranced products are, and they have some beneficial uses for healing when used cautiously and sparingly, they also can be harmful, especially to sensitive or allergic individuals. Instead, always choose fragrance free. Save essential oils for the occasional but important acute healing needs.

You will also want to avoid using any toxic chemicals in your home, such as pesticides, fungicides, and herbicides. Although they are not as harmful to us as they are to the pests, molds, and plants they are designed to kill, they can cause problems for sensitive people or those with impaired detoxification systems.

Be careful about choosing any building or remodeling products; many building supplies contain dangerous chemicals. A good resource for guidance in these matters is https://www.mychemicalfreehouse.net/ , but "green building" is becoming much more popular and known throughout the country. Do your due diligence, though, because this is another area where "green washing" is rampant. Green washing is the act of deceptively calling something "green" or "non-toxic" when it is not.

Avoid standing where you can smell the exhaust of vehicles. Stand far away from vehicles that are getting gas. Do not use scented waxes or conditioners on or in your vehicle.

When you buy a new product, furniture, or appliance, give it some time to "off gas" outside before bringing it into your home. Many products release toxic gases when they are new, but once they have released the gases, they become safer to use. Wash all of your new clothes before wearing them. You may need to avoid second-hand stores, as the items there may have become so saturated with the persistent fragrances that other people have used that you either may never get the smell out or may get sick trying.

After you have avoided toxins for a while, your condition will probably improve, and you may not react so strongly when you are exposed to them. However, it is best to avoid them always, whenever possible, so that your body can be as healthy as possible. Besides, the products you will have replaced them with are more luxurious and better for the environment.

Once your lifestyle is detoxed, if you do not start feeling better, you may need to detox your body. There are many options for doing this — fasting, herbs, zeolites, body work, etc. One supplement that is considered safe and helps to support the liver, which is responsible for much of our detoxing, is milk thistle extract. Very few people will need a great deal of assistance in getting their bodies to detox once the toxic load they are exposed to every day has significantly decreased. However, you may need to treat for MTHFR to support your body's detox system. See Chapter 24: MTHFR.

My Experience with Detoxing

It has taken my family years to finally discover and throw out all of the products and items we had that were fragranced, but we have noticed our sense of smell coming back. We hadn't known it was missing before, but now the flowers, the rain, the sun-soaked earth all smell surprisingly good.

In my holistic healing center, approximately 90% of the clients who came in with physical or emotional complaints experienced significant improvement when they detoxed their lifestyles.

Step-By-Step Instructions to Detox

Get rid of the toxic products in your home and replace them with nontoxic versions. In addition to this, you may want to take measures to ensure the air in your home and vehicle are clean — guidance on this is in Chapter 11: Allergy, MCAS, & MCS. Ask your doctor before trying anything new.

Nontoxic Home and Personal Products

1. Soap: Arizona Sungold Soap's Hi Suds Shampoo is an all-natural, fragrance-free castile soap that can be used as a hand soap, body wash, shampoo, dishwashing soap, floor cleaner, and for every use that soap could be needed for. (Note that when it is used as a shampoo, you may want to use a little Borax along with it sometimes. Borax is the mineral boron, an essential mineral that some people are deficient in and that can balance hormones, reduce arthritis, protect against damage from toxins, improve cognitive performance, and treat cancer.[695] Boron can be absorbed through the skin in small amounts when it is dissolved in water, but it is not recommended to take it orally as a supplement without the oversight of a doctor because high doses can be dangerous.[696] No Borax is needed when this soap is used

for all other purposes, like hand washing and dishwashing. (Also note that it is not a good idea to mix castile soap with vinegar.)

2. Moisturizers: Simplest is almost always best. Look for the lowest number of ingredients in any product you purchase. I have three recommendations for full-body moisturizers. In the winter, I use organic olive oil. It feels very luxurious, but you must give it a little time to dry before you put on clothes or walk across the floor (leaving oil footprints). So, use it sparingly, and slow down and enjoy the sensation of rich, health-giving oil soaking into your skin; break your addiction to the disease-promoting rush and hurry of modern life. In the summer, I prefer Seven Minerals Aloe Vera Gel. (Again, allow it to dry before your skin touches anything; the high vitamin C content of the gel is very good for you but can cause brown stains on some items when it is exposed to sunlight before it is dry.) For my face, I use the Oil Cleansing Method (See Chapter 54: Oil Cleansing Method) for both cleaning and moisturizing. For this method, I use an organic olive oil mixed with_castor oil. For lips and hands and as a primer for my face before putting on makeup, I use Mountain Rose Herbs Refined Shea Butter. Scoop out a little bit of the solid shea butter, use your fingers to rub it into the palm of your other hand, and it melts into a smooth, thick coating.
3. Multipurpose Cleaning and Disinfecting Spray: For most cleaning needs, I use vinegar. When a little extra scrubbing power is desired, I use Orange Peel Vinegar (See Appendix A: Recipes).
4. Dishwasher Detergent: Biokleen Free & Clear Dishwashing Detergent Powder.
5. Bath or Kitchen Scrubbing: Borax and baking soda give scouring friction when used dry with a moist washcloth or scouring pad. Borax disinfects surfaces, and baking soda is very gentle. Baking soda also works well as a nontoxic silver polish.
6. Pots and Pans: Stainless steel, cast iron, and ceramic coated pans are usually good. Avoid anything with Teflon or aluminum.
7. Food Storage Containers: Avoid using plastic. Glass or stainless-steel containers with plastic or metal lids are acceptable.
8. Natural Scouring Pad: Sisal pads are made of a plant material instead of foam made from petroleum waste.
9. Laundry Detergent: Biokleen Free and Clear Laundry Detergent and Biokleen Oxygen Bleach.
10. Dryer Sheets or Fabric Softener: Do not use those poisonous things. Instead choose wool dryer balls. However, if you are washing only all-natural fabrics, you will not need dryer balls; only synthetic fibers tend to get static electricity build-up. Still, you may want the dryer balls for washing pillows and down-filled items.
11. Trash Bags: Most people haven't noticed it yet, but most of the trash bags for sale in our local grocery stores are fragranced, and those that aren't fragranced are contaminated with fragrance from other items. Fortunately, Hippo Saks Tall Kitchen Bags with Handles are made from plants, not petroleum, so they are better for the environment. Plus, they are fragrance-free, and the handle design is really nice.
12. Paper Cups: When a reusable drinking vessel isn't the best option, plain, uncoated paper cups are dye-free and plastic-free.
13. Duster: A feather duster is all natural, effective, and lasts a long time. You can use it to brush dust onto the floor before you vacuum or sweep.
14. Shower Curtain: Use a cotton shower curtain (or two of them layered) instead of a poisonous vinyl one.
15. Clothes: Wear all-natural fibers because your skin can absorb chemicals from your clothes, especially when you are hot.[697] Avoid polyester, nylon, and other synthetic

fibers. Although bamboo and rayon are considered natural fibers, they are usually processed with so many chemicals that they are not a good choice. Natural fiber clothing is usually cotton, silk, wool, cashmere, or linen.

16. Makeup: Due to my personal sensitivities, the only makeup I can recommend is Mineral Fusion's pressed powders.
17. Hairspray: AZ's Own Hairspray is made of prickly pear plant extract. It works well, though it needs to be reapplied frequently.
18. Feminine Products: Avoid bleached and chemical-containing menstrual products. Cotton pads and period underwear are preferrable. There are also natural tampons available, but I prefer Sea Pearls Premium Ultra Soft Sea Sponges. See Chapter 15: Female Reproductive Concerns.
19. Insect Repellant: Many of these are very toxic. Depending on your susceptibility, you may be able to use a milder product that I, my family, and even the guests at my country wedding used, rose geranium hydrosol.
20. Sleeping Supplies: Most mattresses are made almost exclusively with toxic materials that off-gas for years. During the 8 hours that you are sleeping, at a time when your body wants to go into healing mode, you are bombarded with these chemicals. I can recommend My Green Mattress for chemically sensitive people, along with a Whisper Organics Mattress Protector. Make sure that your sheets and blankets are all natural materials, too.
21. Drinking water: In many parts of the country and the world, tap water is not filtered to a state that is safe for people who are sensitive. It can still contain toxic chemicals and pharmaceuticals, not to mention the fluoride and chlorine that is purposefully added. A Reverse Osmosis filter with a remineralizer is my recommendation. You will want to take your filtered water with you wherever you go, so carry it in a bottle that is nontoxic, preferably glass or stainless steel.
22. Tea and coffee makers: Most tea bags are bleached and contain harmful chemicals. Most coffeemakers incorporate plastic that gets heated and leaches into the water. Stainless steel tea strainers and stainless-steel-and-glass French press-style coffeemakers are easy to use and make your drinks taste purely delicious.
23. Once your lifestyle is detoxed, it is time to clean out your body. To some extent, once the toxic load that comes in every day is reduced, your body will start detoxing itself automatically. Sometimes it needs some help, though. Many different methods exist for detoxing the body, some of which are safe and some of which are not. You will need to do some research to see what method will be best for you; some people get good results by working with a naturopathic doctor to do this. Some of the methods you might consider include fasting, taking herbs, using a steam or Infrared Sauna, using TRS, chelating with the Andy Cutler protocol, doing Abhyanga Oil Massage (See Chapter 39: Abhyanga Oil Massage), and moving lymph (See Chapter 51: Lymph Drainage Massage). While you are detoxing, I generally recommend supporting the liver with milk thistle extract. Other herbs or treatments may be appropriate for supporting other body parts that are active in detoxing, such as the kidneys and skin.

LINKS FOR PRODUCTS MENTIONED IN THIS CHAPTER

Milk thistle extract https://amzn.to/48LdF4S

Soap http://www.azsungoldsoaps.com/products_liquidsoap_level_H.html

Aloe Vera Gel https://amzn.to/3ciygCB

Refined Shea Butter https://amzn.to/4aTnwa1

Funnel with Strainer https://amzn.to/3SmxgTE

Spray Bottle https://amzn.to/3y6U251

Dishwasher Detergent https://amzn.to/3VhUYlG

Scouring Pad https://amzn.to/3x2Ncgt

Laundry Detergent https://amzn.to/3vTx40u

Oxygen Bleach https://amzn.to/2TGgrqS

Wool Dryer Balls https://amzn.to/4azJxL9

Trash Bags https://amzn.to/3gagrXF

Paper Cups https://amzn.to/3pjqqOu

Makeup https://amzn.to/3A6jGIM

Hairspray http://azsungoldsoaps.com/mobile/order/samples/products_hairspray.html

Sea Sponges https://amzn.to/3h0eY7O

Rose Geranium Hydrosol https://amzn.to/3x0Flp3

My Green Mattress https://www.shareasale.com/r.cfm?b=997038&u=2860296&m=71414

Mattress Protector https://amzn.to/3hjnOg9

Reverse Osmosis Filter https://amzn.to/43m3qSZ

Water Bottle https://amzn.to/3TDiW9N

Tea Strainer Basket https://amzn.to/3TC7wTE

French Press Coffeemaker https://amzn.to/3VkWVOd

45 Earthing

EARTHING OR GROUNDING IS THE ACT OF BEING in contact with the Earth, which allows you to absorb some of the Earth's free electrons, which is highly beneficial for your health.[698] Many benefits come from Earthing, such as speedy wound healing, activation of the Parasympathetic Nervous System and deactivation of the Sympathetic Nervous System, improved blood oxygenation, improvement in Heart Rate Variability, improved ratios of electrolytes and minerals in the blood, balanced hormones, enhanced stability of neurons, and reduced swelling, inflammation, pain, and anxiety.[699, 700, 701, 702] A measurable health difference can be found after just 20 minutes of contact with the Earth. Some scientists have found evidence that the lack of grounding in our modern lifestyle may be responsible for the development of chronic diseases.[703]

Contact with the Earth is free and easy some of the time — just take off your shoes and walk around on the grass or sand. Sitting or lying on the earth brings about even better results, as long as you are either naked or wearing cotton clothing; you can also lie on a cotton sheet. The more time you spend in contact with the Earth, the better.

But we all know that you don't always have time to linger on the ground, and sometimes the ground isn't friendly, if there is broken glass, sharp burs, pinecones, cacti, biting or stinging insects, mud, etc. And when the weather is cold — or really hot — being bare and touching the ground doesn't make sense. In those cases, you will want to use an Earthing product, which transmits the Earth's electrons to your body. Earthing products can be easily plugged into a regular electrical outlet, or you can get an Earthing pole that plugs the wire for the product directly into the dirt outside your home.

My Experience with Earthing

I got my first earthing sheet when my son was a baby. I still had pregnancy edema, which had caused swelling in my extremities — closing all those snaps on the baby clothes with my swollen fingers was agonizing! The first night I slept on the earthing sheet, the swelling went away and my fingers felt OK when I snapped the snaps.

I often wonder if some of the treatments I try are successful due to the placebo effect — after all, even pharmaceutical medications are sometimes effective only due to the placebo effect. In this case, my tiny baby proved to me that the earthing was good for him.

I had always lain my baby down for the night with his head on a sheet but his body on a cotton waterproof pad because he often had diaper leaks during the night. He had always slept still and soundly this way. The first night and every night that I put him down with his head on an earthing sheet, he would wiggle his way in his sleep until his entire body was on the earthing sheet.

Even our dogs and cats always prefer to sleep on the earthing sheet.

In my holistic healing clinic, the earthing electrodes were always appreciated during healing sessions. Many clients reported that the pain they had come in with disappeared completely after an hour with earthing electrodes on the spot of the pain.

I continue to use earthing electrodes whenever I have pain. I especially like to put them on my neck after exposure to an Allergy/MCAS/MCS or Migraine trigger. I sleep with them on my neck when I'm not feeling well, and I am often surprised by how much better I feel in the morning. They are also helpful on Joint Injuries and can relieve swelling and pressure.

Step-By-Step Instructions for Earthing

When you are healthy, you may not notice very much of a difference when you Earth, but when you have ailments, you may want to Earth daily. Ask your doctor before trying anything new.

Make Electrical Contact with the Earth for Health

1. Make physical contact with the Earth. It is best if your skin touches the Earth, but a thin layer of cotton fabric may be acceptable, especially if there is some moisture in it from the earth or your skin.
2. Use products from the Earthing store or another brand so that you can Earth every day, regardless of weather.
3. Put Earthing Therapy Patches directly on whatever body part is in pain.
4. Use an Earthing tester by holding the metal with your fingers while pressing the button to see if you are connected to the Earth's electric field. Also periodically check your products to make sure they are still working.

LINKS FOR PRODUCTS MENTIONED IN THIS CHAPTER

Earthing Products https://amzn.to/49TV8Dr

Earthing Tester https://amzn.to/43YH0aZ

Earthing Therapy Patches https://amzn.to/4aFvdjY

46

Emotional Regulation

HAVING A CHRONIC ILLNESS CAN BE REALLY depressing. Suffering with pain — many different kinds of pain, some of them excruciating — can make you furious. Being clumsy and scatterbrained from Ataxia and brain fog can be frustrating and embarrassing. Digestive problems that can strike at any minute can make you afraid to do simple daily things like eating and going places. Having limited mobility from Joint Injuries can make you feel defeated and hopeless — how can things ever get better if you can't even do anything for yourself? Searching for answers to your health problems and finding no doctors who can help can make you feel lost or crazy or angry. And when all of these things happen at once and you end up accidentally lashing out at a loved one for some tiny infraction like not having put their dishes in the dishwasher, you really feel miserable because you hate yourself.

Not only that, but the kinds of conditions that people with hEDS often live with sometimes cause hormonal imbalances, and these messed-up chemicals can create mood swings that make it hard to see things clearly.

A lot of days, the outlook is bleak. It feels like everyone is against you, even your own body. Everything is bad, and there is no way it will ever get better.

If these thoughts are going through your head, stop and take a look at them. Right now, you will not be able to convince yourself they are not true, so don't even try. Instead, look at them and recognize that they are caused by the disease. Just hold on.

Hold on. Wait a minute. Get through today. It doesn't have to be pretty.

The fact of the matter is that our emotions are not us. A lot of the times, they aren't even real. They aren't necessarily caused by our experiences. Sometimes, they are just a bunch of hormones doing something that doesn't relate to our actual life or who we are.

Look at the emotions, be aware of these underlying feelings that will color everything you see and do today, and understand that they are just chemicals.

Do whatever you can to keep hold of yourself. Do whatever you can to treat people the way you want to treat them, to move through your day the way you want to be — despite what you feel. Just don't make any big decisions while you're feeling this way. When you feel the world is against you is not the day to decide to get a different job or buy a new car or end a longstanding relationship or tear down the wall between your kitchen and living room or throw out your dirty sofa. All of the big decisions can wait until your mood has normalized. Things will look different then.

It won't take long living with this awareness until you can really experience that your emotions are not always real and that your behavior does not have to be dictated by your emotions. Your emotions, your thoughts, your intuitions, your physical sensations, they are all separate, and more importantly, when something is out of whack in your body, they can tell you lies.

You may not be able to skip around smiling when you're really feeling depressed, but when you recognize that at least some of the depression is just chemicals, you will feel enough relief to be able to hold onto yourself and be who you are and act how you want to act, at least for part of the day.

One of the books that gave me a really good sense of how to manage emotional regulation is *No-Drama Discipline: The Whole-Brain Way to Calm the Chaos and Nurture Your Child's Developing Mind* by Daniel J. Siegel and Tina Payne Bryson. This book is not actually about what we are going through; it is mostly about relationships. The recommendations in *No-Drama Discipline* are based on new information about how the brain works that has become available with recent technological developments for imaging the brain.

I apply the teachings of *No-Drama Discipline* not only to parenting my son but also to how I react in the relationships I have with other family members and friends. It has excellent information about emotional regulation and how it works. You may not have been taught it by a parent as this book is aiming for people to do, but you can learn it as an adult and you will surely become happier, with healthier relationships, including the relationship with yourself.

Eventually, for most of us, we will move out of the flare-up, the critical state of hormonal dysregulation will fade away, and our brain chemicals will become normalized again. The Ataxia and brain fog will diminish, at least for a little while. Given enough time, we will find ways to reduce the pain and manage our lives even with limited mobility. Jesus will bless us or the stars will align, and we will find a doctor, a friend, or a book to help us improve some.

That is when we will know that our emotions weren't real. The world wasn't against us. We hadn't lost ourselves forever.

So, you have to take your moments of joy when you can get them. Find delight in the little things. Snatch up every opportunity that comes to you (and that won't harm you) on a day when you're not stuck in bed. Even on days when it is hard to believe that goodness exists, it helps to remember that an optimistic and grateful attitude is good for our health.[704, 705] Whether based in truth or not, these "good" feelings encourage and enable our bodies to heal.

Just keep in mind that, as the Bible says, "This too shall pass." The good and the bad — everything will change. Nothing lasts forever. Most of us have flares and remissions of some of our symptoms, whether we try to or not. We will go through unpredictable patterns of getting better and worse and then even worse and then better again and then, when we're lucky, even better.

Let's pray that we continue most of the time and for a very long time on that upward slope of getting even better and even better, but always sit in the peace and comfort of knowing that this too shall pass.

My Experience with Emotional Regulation

I was once told by an astrologist that my star chart shows me to be very much a water sign, but that I am not the wishy-washy or slippery type of water. My version of water sign is like the water at the deepest depths of the greatest ocean — although it is fluid and can feel the touch of great storms or gentle winds on the surface, it is stable and massive.

This seems to me a good metaphor for my emotional life, especially since I read *No-Drama Discipline*. I feel emotions and experience the constant changes of daily life, but it does not impact who I am or what my inherent outlook is.

I feel this has served me well. Once I could look at my emotions as being separate from me, and more than that, as being chemicals that are somewhat meaningless, I understood life and myself much better. This emotional regulation can get me through difficulties in life and illnesses in my body. I will come out of these challenges slightly different, but I will still be myself.

My sister asked, if the unhappy emotions aren't real, how do we know that the happy emotions are real? Well, they aren't who we are, and they may not be related to our circumstances — but I believe that God's Creation is miraculous in and of itself. It is a beautiful, joyous miracle that we are alive. There is much of beauty and joy around us that we can turn our focus to.

Step-By-Step Instructions for Emotional Regulation

Emotional regulation is not always common sensical. Sometimes it is contrary to what you feel like you should do. It takes concerted effort. However, when you later look back on the decisions you made in the effort to regulate your emotions, you will most likely recognize that you did the right thing. Ask your doctor before trying anything new.

Maintain Emotional Regulation

1. Read *No-Drama Discipline* by Daniel Siegel and Tina Bryson.
2. When you are feeling down or angry, take a moment to look at the emotions and see if they are just the messed-up chemicals in your body making you feel things that aren't real.
3. Find joy everywhere you can, whenever you can, but keep in mind that this too shall pass.
4. Be yourself and keep hold of yourself. Act like the person you want to be, even when it's hard.

LINKS FOR PRODUCTS MENTIONED IN THIS CHAPTER

No Drama Discipline https://amzn.to/3S0SvsG

47

Enjoy Life

THERE ARE PEOPLE EVERYWHERE WHO ARE curmudgeonly and enjoy being unhappy, but most people will experience much better health if they can enjoy their lives.[706, 707] There are scientifically shown healing effects from smiling, laughing, cuddling, and doing other fun things.[708, 709, 710, 711] Although you might be working hard to cope with your condition or improve your health, and although you might feel too miserable to do much besides lie in bed, it is still important to find ways to enjoy your life.

The kind of entertainment you choose matters. Seeing a smiling face actually makes people physically stronger, while seeing a sad face makes them physically weaker.[712] So, find books and movies that are wholesome and uplifting. Avoid violence, depravity, and depressing media. Take a break from following the news when your mood is getting anxious or depressed. Hang out with people who do not gossip or try to get revenge on people. Surround yourself with things that build up life and encourage joy.

When you're not feeling good, read a book, listen to a podcast, smell a flower, fantasize about your happy place, let a fan blow on your face, hold someone's hand. Simply pay attention to what feels good. Pay attention to what you appreciate. Pay attention to what you like.

When you're up to it, have a cup of tea with a friend. Watch a movie with your sibling. Go for a walk around the block. Pet a dog or cat. Think of what you most liked to do when you were a child and find a way to do just a little version of that.

When you're feeling really good, go to parties. Take a walk around the downtown of your city or out in the woods. Go to church or the library. Go on an easy trip and spend a few days enjoying the view of an ocean or mountain or desert.

When you're feeling like yourself, do your favorite hobbies. Make crafts. Play music. Bike ride. Kayak. Rock climb. Zip line. Snorkel. Horse ride. Run. Skate. Cook. Climb trees. Take an art class. Make pottery. Build furniture. Paint.

And end every day with gratitude for the pleasures you experienced that day, no matter how large or small.

My Experience with Enjoying Life

My greatest enjoyment in life is spending time with my family, so we play a lot of board games and go on a lot of hikes in the woods. They are always willing to climb into bed with me on days when I'm not feeling well, and they're always willing to go on adventures with me when I'm feeling like myself. I am very blessed.

Step-By-Step Instructions for Enjoying Life

1. Pay attention to what feels good.
2. Give yourself permission to have fun even if you've been lazy, spent money on healing treatments, or acted grumpier than you should have.
3. Feel gratitude for everything you enjoy.

48

Forest Bathing or Immersion in Nature

I showed up at my Physical Therapist's office one day to find that every wall suddenly had a large framed photograph of trees on it. My PT told me that a compelling scientific study had just been published that showed that just looking at a tree made a person healthier according to a number of different measures.[713] I hadn't known that just looking at photos of trees made a difference, but I had known my entire life that the forest will always make me feel better.

Forest Bathing is the translation of a Japanese term for spending time immersed in nature for relaxation, enjoyment, and health.[714, 715, 716] Some scientists have begun talking about people suffering from Nature Deprivation Disorder.[717] The strongest symptoms they mention are usually regarding mental health and behavior, but the symptoms of the disorder can reach into all of the systems of the body. For those of us with chronic illness and pain, we can be especially deprived of contact with nature, but it is worth it to try to find a way to Forest Bathe.

I have known a number of people who, once they started spending large amounts of time outside in nature, had sudden remissions of whatever symptoms had been troubling them. They didn't even have to do any work or go on any diets or make any other changes besides being outside. Fresh air; sunshine; the sounds of birds, wind, and water; the smells of the leaves, the earth, and flowers; and the beauty of the landscape are really good for us.[718, 719]

One of the benefits of spending time outside is improved eyesight.[720, 721, 722, 723, 724] One study showed that prison inmates, who are required to spend 2 hours per day outside, end up developing better eyesight than school children, who often get 20 minutes or less outside on a daily basis.[725] As William Bates explained in *The Bates Method for Better Eyesight Without Glasses*, looking into a far distance relaxes the eye muscles, allowing the eye to return to health and improved vision. You can really only see far distances when you are outside.

Earthing is also possible when outside, not only if you have your skin physically in contact with the earth. The electric field beneath a tree is different from that in the open air, and it can enact healing benefits for you, albeit milder than when you are in touch with the earth.[726] Go ahead and hug some trees!

Additionally, plants and especially trees produce chemicals that we inhale, such as oxygen and phytoncides, which are antimicrobial and produce myriad benefits for our health.[727]

The studies show that frequent visits into natural settings are more effective than short annual vacations, so get out whenever you have the time and energy.[728] Ask your friends where their favorite parks are. Look at your state's State Park website. Ask a local farmer if there are any safe trails on his property. Enjoy the bench outside the library or other public building. Plant trees in your own yard.

Natural areas with trees have consistently shown stronger results in improving health than natural areas without trees, but I understand that some people feel nervous in the forest — the light is dimmer there, it is cooler, there are strange sounds, and the trees and bushes could be hiding a threat. For those people, the meadows and plains might give healing, with their waving grasses and big skies. Some people love the desert or the lake, or the snowcapped mountain.

The ocean is certainly a healing natural place. The salt water can be full of nutrients, and it is an excellent conductor of the earth's electrical energy. The rhythmic sound of the waves is soothing, and the salty air can be good for the lungs. For millennia, doctors and healers have been prescribing time at the seaside for their patients for good reason.[729]

Benefits of being in nature are shown whether you are participating in a sport, working out, walking, or sitting. It is recommended to find a few moments, at least, to stop whatever you are doing to notice the elements of nature that surround you. It is especially enjoyable to see how they vary from location to location and season to season.

My Experience with Forest Bathing

When I go into nature, I usually find out that I have a lot of things on my mind. I can't help but spend some of the time when I'm walking on a forest path thinking about homeschool lesson plans, the conversation I had with my friend last week, that horrible thing that happened two years ago, the gift I want to knit for my husband, and writing this book.

Eventually, though, while I'm walking, I start to notice the leaf shaped just like a heart, the sweet trill of the bird high above me, the moss carpeting the shady spot beside the trail. Suddenly, everything I look at and hear is beautiful. And then, the breeze in my hair gives me such a sense of relief that I stop dead in my tracks and sigh deeply. The sun hits my face, and the tension drops out of my shoulders.

Now, I am no longer in my head. I am really in the woods. Here I am, amidst the trees, my new friends. I can walk on the path, absorbing the beauty of the forest, and feel the health streaming through me. My hips move more fluidly as I walk, my lungs fill and empty more easily, my limbs are filled with energy, my heart is filled with peace. This is life.

Step-By-Step Instructions for Forest Bathing

The most important thing to do in order to have a successful Forest Bathing experience is to wear clothes and shoes appropriate to the place and weather conditions. As they say, there is no bad weather, just bad clothing. If you are uncomfortable while you are in nature, it is most likely because you didn't dress appropriately. Ask your doctor before trying anything new.

Proper Preparation for Nature Immersion

1. Go barefoot when you can. Otherwise, wear barefoot/minimalist boots, shoes, or sandals so that you can feel the vagaries of the path you walk on. Make sure you wear footwear that keeps your feet dry, especially if it is cold, unless you are wading in streams, in which case water shoes might be appropriate.
2. In warm weather, make sure to take plenty of water to drink, preferably with electrolytes.
3. For sunny weather, a hat with a wide brim is a must. Find shade frequently to prevent sunburn. A lightweight, long-sleeve, cotton shirt will help protect your arms from excessive sun exposure.
4. For cold weather, layers and coverings for every body part are necessary. I like to wear cashmere on every body part except my face — cashmere socks, cashmere pants and sweater (over cotton or silk long underwear), cashmere-lined leather gloves, cashmere hat (under the hood of my coat), long down-filled coat, and a scarf. My favorite winter boots are Mukluks. On my face, I apply refined shea butter to protect it from the cold wind.
5. Layers of clothing are always best, no matter the weather, as long as you can tie them around your waist or shoulders if you need to remove them.
6. Use only natural scents on your body. The only creatures attracted to synthetic scents are bears and stinging insects; all other creatures will flee from synthetic fragrances and you won't get to view the wildlife. Make sure that your laundry detergent, toiletries, and insect repellants are all scent-free.
7. When you are in a state of chronic illness, do not be too ambitious. Stay within range of cell phone service. Bring a loved one who will care for you or ask a loved one to have their phone on in case you need to call for help. Start with short trips and rest frequently. You can always walk the same trail twice if it turns out that you have energy to spare.
8. In populated parks, take only pictures and leave only footprints. But, if you can find a safe location that is not very populated, you can have an even better experience by interacting with nature. Throw pebbles into the stream, hug trees, pick berries, pet soft leaves, run your fingers through waves of grass, crinkle up dried leaves, sit on a cushion of moss, strike a stick against a rock, dig down into the mud, tear open a seedpod to see what is inside, build a rudimentary shelter out of sticks and leaves, create mandalas on the ground with different colors of leaves, balance rocks on top of each other, see who's hiding under the ledge at the edge of the creek, collect snail shells and pinecones, watch the butterflies alight when you walk through their field, pick a bouquet of flowers. Interacting with nature is better for you than just observing it, and it is also better for nature because nature is tough enough to take it, and the bond you make with the place, the appreciation you gain for it, will most likely translate into you wanting to protect the wild places rather than devastatingly harvest their resources.[730, 731]
9. Depending on the location of your sojourn in nature, you may need to do a "tick check" immediately upon leaving the park or arriving at home. Take off all of your clothes and look at all of your body – especially in creases and hairy areas. If chiggers are a concern in your area, use your hands to wipe down your legs every 15 minutes while on your walk. Chiggers, which are virtually invisible and too tiny to feel, might be on you without biting until hours later, so take a bath or shower as soon as you get home.

LINKS FOR PRODUCTS MENTIONED IN THIS CHAPTER

Bates Method https://amzn.to/48VlXac

Mukluks https://amzn.to/3W7zFnu

49

Haka & Other Methods of Shaking for Trauma Release

IF YOU HAVE EVER WITNESSED A CAT ESCAPE a chasing dog, you probably saw it walk away shaking its limbs one at a time. Many times, after an athlete achieves an exceptionally challenging goal, he or she will shake parts of their body in celebration. I'm sure after someone sustained a minor injury, you've heard a coach say, "Shake it off!"

Shaking after an intense event is a normal reaction for our bodies, but our society has mostly trained this behavior out of us. Now, when we experience stress, perhaps we tremble, but we rarely give ourselves a good shake. This leaves the tension trapped in our muscles, and Dr. David Berceli has developed a way to release it, called TRE (Trauma Release Exercises). His method has been taught to practitioners around the country, and his website lists numerous published research papers and other information about shaking for trauma release. https://traumaprevention.com/

I have friends who have gotten excellent results by visiting a teacher of TRE, and also others who have read about other shaking methods of trauma release and then cured themselves of various ailments. I, however, had a bad experience when I tried it on my own. I actually got severe amounts of uncontrollable shaking that lasted for days and completely disrupted my life. It was scary and uncomfortable; I do not recommend trying it on your own.

Instead, when faced with severe stress, I got similar but safer healing and preventative results by inventing my own Haka dances. Haka is a traditional war dance of the Māori people of New Zealand. They performed it to call on the War God to bring them victory, to give themselves courage, and to frighten their enemies before a battle. They still conduct Haka prior to sports matches, and there are many videos, even some of actor Jason Momoa doing Haka, on YouTube.

https://hakatours.com/blog/haka-meaning/

One of the features of Haka that is especially beneficial is thumping the thymus with the fist or open palm. The thymus is located in the upper chest and controls the immune system. By thumping or tapping it, you help regulate it; you get it ready for whatever immune-system need is coming.[732, 733]

My Experience with Shaking

When faced with nerve-wracking situations, nothing gives me more confidence than doing a private Haka dance in my home.

Step-By-Step Instructions for Using Haka for Trauma Release

To prevent trauma lodging in and harming the body, create your own Haka. It is helpful to conduct this dance prior to stress, if you know it is coming, and after a stressful situation. You can do it in the privacy of your bedroom or in front of friends who will cheer and support you. You can follow a video of a Haka, or you can choreograph or improvise your own. Ask your doctor before trying anything new.

Haka Dance for Releasing Stress and Trauma

1. Maintain a strong stance with the feet wide apart for most of the dance. Kneeling on one knee can be implemented as well.
2. Stomp your feet rhythmically. The pattern can change and pause throughout the dance.
3. Slap your hands against body parts. Slap your thighs, your arms, your chest. Cup your hand so that the sound is loud but you do not hurt yourself. The slaps should be rhythmic and repetitive and change position occasionally.
4. Make one hand into a fist and hit it into your other hand or against your chest (where the thymus is).[734, 735] Beat this fist rhythmically and repetitively.
5. Shake body parts fiercely. Your hands should tremble greatly as your arms extend. Different parts of the body or even the whole body should shake at different times.
6. Move your arms into various positions of strength. The legs can be moved into positions of strength as well. Move quickly and hit the position sharply with a tightening of the muscles. Show how fiercely you can hit or kick your opponents from any direction.
7. Stick out your tongue very far and make fearsome faces. Bulge your eyes and tilt your head in menacing ways. Bare your teeth. Frighten your enemies with your expressions.
8. Vocalize. Yell, grunt, or chant in English or Māori or nonsense words. Your vocalization does not have to continue the whole time you are dancing, but it should be rhythmic and repetitive at least some of the time.
9. End by holding for several seconds a particularly strong and fearsome pose, facial expression, and yell.

50

Homeopathic Remedies

HOMEOPATHIC REMEDIES ARE SO SAFE THAT if a child eats an entire bottle of 80 pills and the parent calls the Poison Control Center, they will be told not to worry. The child may act as if they have eaten a large piece of candy, but the sugar rush is all there is to worry about.[736] Not only are homeopathic remedies very safe, they are very inexpensive and can be very effective.[737]

It is possible for homeopathic remedies to cause adverse symptoms, but it is very rare. It happens when someone takes a remedy that is not indicated for the symptoms they are experiencing and "proves" the remedy. Proving the remedy means creating the symptoms the remedy is intended to heal. In most cases, the remedies are made from plants, usually poisonous plants — whatever symptoms the plant would cause are the symptoms the remedy will heal. When a remedy is proved, the symptoms can be stopped by sniffing or ingesting the antidotes: coffee or peppermint. For this reason, you should not ingest coffee or peppermint when using homeopathic remedies — they can also negate the remedies' healing effects.

Fortunately, proving a remedy is a very rare occurrence. The remedies are a type of energy healing and contain only sugar; they are so diluted that scientists cannot measure the components that they are made from. It is safe to give even newborn babies homeopathic remedies.

The remedies serve as a communication with the body so that the body can heal itself. When the correct remedy is found for the situation, it can be very effective because the body is doing the healing rather than having something done to it.

My Experience with Homeopathic Remedies

I began using Homeopathic Remedies at my midwife's suggestion when my baby was little. When he had a fever from a virus, I gave him a little easily-dissolved sugar pill homeopathic remedy from Hyland's, and within 15 minutes, his fever had gone away. My family and I have continued to have similar experiences with homeopathic remedies ever since. I believe that they have helped my body learn how to cope with my triggers and stay calm instead of reacting with Allergy/MCAS/MCS symptoms.

Step-By-Step Instructions for Using Homeopathic Remedies

Often, the most difficult part of taking homeopathic remedies is deciding which one to take. Do an online search for your symptoms and the words "homeopathic remedy," and then read through the options — consider as many of the indications as you can.

There are many homeopaths online, especially in social media groups, who will give advice about how to take remedies, which remedies to take, how to do "water plussing" or "paper plussing" to make your remedies go further, and how to store your remedies. I have a lovely wooden tool box from Harbor Freight that I keep my remedies in at home, and I have an attractive cotton, copper-lined fabric pouch to hold the remedies I carry with me. (Homeopathics can be negatively affected by EMFs, so you want to store them where they are protected from electricity, WIFI, etc., which is why my travel case is lined with copper.) Ask your doctor before trying anything new.

Homeopathic Remedy Use

1. Do not ingest or smell coffee or peppermint.
2. Once you have decided which remedy to try, take one pill by letting it melt under your tongue.
3. After waiting 15 minutes, assess how your symptoms have changed.
   a. If you are worse, sniff some coffee or peppermint, which act as antidotes to homeopathic remedies. Then, try a different remedy.
   b. If you are unchanged, then you have chosen the wrong remedy and should try a different one.
   c. If you are better, then you have chosen the correct remedy.
4. As more time passes, if you stop getting better, take one more pill by letting it melt under your tongue. (Often, I find that taking one pill every 15 minutes for an hour is very helpful.)
5. If you continue to get better, no more pills are needed.
6. If you notice different symptoms appearing, then find another remedy to take; you can take as many remedies at once or in succession as you need.

Homeopathic Remedies I've Used for Specific Symptoms

Every homeopathic remedy has numerous uses. It is quite a complex system. However, I have certain remedies that I have successfully used for certain purposes for years. Here are my most frequent remedies. Note that most of the remedies I have recommended are Boiron brand; I really like these — they are effective and have a lid that dispenses one at a time when you twist it. However, if you are giving remedies to babies or elderly who will have a hard time keeping the pill under the tongue until it dissolves, give Hylands brand, which dissolves almost immediately.

Note that I use homeopathic remedies to treat acute symptoms as they occur. Some homeopathic doctors believe this is not an appropriate way to use remedies. Despite the excellent results I have gotten, I recognize that I am very uneducated regarding homeopathics and that it may be much more effective to use them in a way that a homeopathic doctor would prescribe. Many of these doctors use constitutional remedies; I believe this facet of homeopathics could be highly effective, but although there are homeopathic doctors in all of the big cities and some of the smaller ones, I have not had the pleasure of seeing one.

1. Allergic reaction initial stage and anxiety: *Ignatia amara*
2. Bee or wasp sting: *Apis mellifica*
3. Body aches and exhaustion: *Chamomilla*

4. Colds: *ColdCalm*
5. Cough and chest congestion: *Phosphorous*
6. Deep-seated fear: *Stramonium*
7. Diarrhea: *Diaralia*
8. Difficulty breathing, fatigue, exposure to poisonous chemicals, food poisoning: *Arsenicum album*
9. Exposure to petroleum products like synthetic fragrances and gasoline, skin rashes: *Petroleum*
10. Fatigue: *Silicea*
11. Flu, Motion Sickness: *Oscillococcinum*
12. Hopelessness, overwhelm, menstrual cramps, mood swings, sense of being overworked at home: *Sepia*
13. Inflamed mucous membranes, sore throat, Sinus Congestion, fever: *Belladonna*
14. Indigestion: *Carbo vegetabilis*
15. Itchy bug bites, prevention of bug bites: *Ledum palustre*
16. Motion sickness: *Tabacum*
17. Muscle tension and anxiety: *Magnesium phosphorica*
18. Nausea, Motion Sickness, Insomnia caused by worry: *Nux vomica*
19. Nerve pain: *Hypericum perforatum*
20. Overexertion, physical or emotional trauma, bumps, bruises, scratches, emotional shock, hurt feelings, sore muscles from working out, pain: *Arnica montana*
21. Poison ivy rash, itchy rashes: *Poison ivy and oak*
22. Prevention of flu or cold if taken immediately at onset of symptoms: *Aconitum napellus*
23. Sinus pressure, sneezing, colds: *Pulsatilla*
24. Social stress, nervousness about talking in front of a crowd, bloating, gas: *Lycopodium clavatum*
25. Sores in mouth, sore throat: *Mercurius solubus*
26. Stiff neck, tension headache, stage fright, fever, muscle tension: *Gelsemium sempervirons*
27. Sunburn, blisters, urinary tract infection: *Cantharis*
28. Swelling in face, sneezing, coughing, allergen exposure: *Histaminum hydrochloricum*
29. Vomiting, nausea: *Ipecacuanha*
30. Personalized symptoms: You can create your own homeopathic remedies, which is especially useful if you are allergic to something in your environment. You put a small amount of that item (a cat hair, for example) into a glass jar filled with filtered water, put the lid on, and then concuss it (hit it) 100 times. Search online for more detailed instructions.

LINKS FOR PRODUCTS MENTIONED IN THIS CHAPTER

Tool Box
https://www.harborfreight.com/eight-drawer-wood-tool-chest-94538.html

Homeopathics Carry Case
https://www.etsy.com/listing/1192344121/pouch-for-15426090-homeopathy-tubes-reve?click_key=e622d87c7ac4308fa3cb8919bd9a5342fb407529%3A1192344121&click_sum=134aa88c&ref=related-1&frs=1&sts=1)

Boiron Store https://amzn.to/44jAziO

Hylands Store https://amzn.to/49XKrzO

51

Lymph Drainage Massage

LYMPH CHANNELS OR VESSELS ARE TUBES that run through the layers of the skin, circulating bodily fluids and nutrients and flushing waste products, toxins, and pathogens away from the body's cells. Because the outer layer of the lymph channels is made of collagen,[738] people with connective tissue disorders often have weak lymph channels. Even in someone who does not have a connective tissue disorder, lymph channels temporarily collapse very easily; the pressure of a massage will push them closed. However, they generally re-establish themselves quickly, too, although this is probably less true for people with hEDS.

Lymph Drainage Massage is very gentle so that it does not collapse the lymph channels. Instead, it activates them. Once you get lymph flowing in one area, it will begin flowing in other areas too, because the channels are connected throughout the body. Lymph Drainage Massage is also very relaxing because it is so gentle. If you have it done by a professional, you just might fall asleep on the massage table.

Massage Therapists who specialize in this can get amazing results.[739] It is also worthwhile for you to do Lymph Drainage Massage on yourself. In order to do this, you very softly pet your skin in a slow, rhythmic fashion. Your strokes will be just a few inches long and will overlap themselves. Always try to stroke toward the heart, armpit, or groin. Lymph channels are one-way roads, so you won't be able to cause a problem by going in the wrong direction, but you also won't be moving the lymph.

My Experience with Lymph Drainage Massage

The first time I received a professional Lymph Drainage Massage, I lost two clothing sizes while I was lying on the massage table. I got dressed after the session and my pants fell down! Those clothing sizes did not come back, either.

One of the ways in which my family has proven the effectiveness of Lymph Drainage Massage time and again is by using the technique on the face, neck, and chest when one of us has a sore throat or earache. We can often halt the development of an oncoming cold or cure an aching ear. In order to get this result, we usually do the massage for about 30 minutes and repeat it throughout the day as needed.

Step-By-Step Instructions for Lymph Drainage Massage

Lymph Drainage Massage is my favorite way of moving lymph fluids, but there are a number of other ways to get lymph moving: dry brushing, rebounding (jumping), riding shaking vehicles, Abhyanga Oil Massage, gua sha scraping, exercising, and more. Look into these ideas, because some may work better for you. Ask your doctor before trying anything new.

Lymph Drainage Self-Massage

1. With the flat part of the fingers and or palm of the hand, pet the skin toward the armpit, groin, or heart.
2. Use the gentlest of pressure to brush the skin.
3. Make each stroke short — a few inches — and then overlap it with the next pet, moving by degrees along the body.
4. Pet slowly and rhythmically toward the armpit, heart, or groin.
5. Once you have pet rhythmically along an area of the body, go back to the beginning and do it again several times.
6. For sore throats, colds, and congestion in the head, pet the face and around the ears, down the throat, and along the chest to the arm pits for about 30 minutes at a time. Repeat as needed.
7. You can also gently pull on the ears in various directions to release congestion.
8. If you are not having success getting lymph flowing, you can use your fingertips to gently press or pump repeatedly and rhythmically into the soft spots below the ears, at the base of the neck, and/or in the armpits. This should help the lymph begin to move.
9. Doing a Lymph Drainage Massage on one part of the body will help to get lymph flowing in all parts of the body, but it is still nice to do the massage on the entire body if you have the time and ability.
10. Drink an extra glass of water to give the lymph system plenty of fluid to work with and to replace any fluids that are flushed out.
11. If you are not getting the results you hoped for, hire a professional who will teach you how to do lymph drainage massage properly on yourself.

52

Myofascial Release Massage

ONE OF THE MOST UBIQUITOUS TISSUES in our bodies is fascia. Made mostly of collagen, fascia is a net-like structure that connects, separates, and provides structure for all of the parts of the body. It covers, gives shape to, and interpenetrates the skin, blood vessels, bones, organs, lymph channels, and nerves. It is the scaffold of the body, and all of the fluids that flow between cells (known as interstitial fluids) are carried in the fascia.[740]

Much of the pain that people with hEDS experience comes from the fascia.[741] In some cases, the fascia is also responsible for at least some of the pain that is diagnosed as fibromyalgia. Often, when joints are threatened or injured, the fascia will tighten and thicken in an attempt to stabilize the joint. Where fascia is thick or adhered, it will probably cause pain.

Whereas most people who do not have hypermobility experience pain emanating from muscles when they are injured, in people with hypermobility, their pain usually emanates from the fascia. Their fascia also tends to be thicker and tighter than that of those in the general population. Massage Therapists report that it does not have as much "slide" as it normally should. (Because a layer of fascia lies between the muscles and skin, gentle pressure with the fingers on the skin can cause healthy fascia tissue to slide over the muscles.)

Additionally, the fascia can entrap and compress nerves, creating Peripheral Neuropathy. This is what happens in Carpal Tunnel Syndrome, for example, and releasing the fascia around the involved ligament can provide relief.[742]

Another nice benefit of myofascial release is that it can reduce wrinkles and creases in your face (or elsewhere). Gentle myofascial release of your face can make you look younger.

There are a number of different ways to release the fascia when it is thickened, tightened, or adhered. Some of the ways that are mentioned online are so extreme they are dangerous. The most famous of these dangerous techniques is using the Fascia Blaster tool; it has been helpful for many people but harmful for many other people. Other techniques for releasing fascia include forcefully stretching the skin, simultaneous compression and "flossing" or working the underlying muscle, and foam rolling . Fascia release will sometimes result from these techniques, but it may not last very long, and damage to the fascia or other tissues is possible. The release experience may be painful as well.

Subtler techniques are usually more effective for hEDS patients, and they last longer although they may require more patience during treatment. These include regular massage, gentle movement release (such as instructed in Jeannie di Bon's YouTube videos for Rib Subluxation), using a small jade roller, and Myofascial Release Massage.

My favorite form of myofascial release is massage by a professional. Some Massage Therapists are good at this and some are not, so if you don't get the results you want, try someone else. Some PTs are also able to offer Myofascial Release Massage. When a practitioner is doing this kind of massage, they will put their hand(s) on you and then barely move. You will think they are doing nothing. For what feels like a long time. You may wonder why you are paying them for this. Even when the release happens and the practitioner moves or exclaims — "Ah, there we go!" — you may not feel it happen...and yet, you will notice it when you begin to move around. You may stand up from the massage table with the pain reduced and movement freed to the extent that you feel like a new person. Myofascial Release Massage can make the most remarkable difference of any of the treatments listed in this book.

My Experience with Myofascial Release Massage.

I treat myself with this massage any time I have pain, and at this point, it almost always relieves the pain completely. When I was in the midst of my healing journey, I frequently work up during the night, but self-Myofascial Release Massage relaxed me back to sleep and helped me feel better in the morning.

One time, I released fascia before I was strong enough — in my neck, and I ended up with headache and numerous neuropathy symptoms for weeks afterward. Because of that experience, I knew to be cautious, and from then on, I only had beneficial results.

Myofascial Release Massage was imperative for me especially whenever I made a posture correction — after building strength for the new position, the fascia release allowed my body to hold the position comfortably and removed any remaining pain. Occasionally, the fascia release was required early in the process in order for me to be able to move into the improved position, but generally, it was better to work on strengthening the position first.

Although I have frequently released fascia through self-massage, I appreciate having someone work on my back where I cannot reach well enough to do it myself. This is a healing technique that is helpful again and again.

Step-By-Step Instructions for Self-Myofascial Release Massage

Much more cost-effective and readily available than professional Myofascial Release Massage is self-massage. Proceed with caution, as with all self-treatments. If an area of fascia is stabilizing a joint and the muscles around that joint are not strong enough to support it without the help of the fascia, you may injure the joint following a myofascial release. I would guess that this happens only rarely because following a release, the fascia will resume its job of holding the structure of the body but in a more appropriate position. Still, I advise muscle strengthening for some days in advance of (and after) releasing fascia. Ask your doctor before trying anything new.

Myofascial Release Self-Massage

1. Make sure that the muscles in the area of release are strong enough to stabilize your joints. Take time to do strength-building exercises before going further.
2. You may want to take a warm bath before doing the Myofascial Release Self-Massage to help relax and prepare the tissues.
3. Very gently rub the affected area. Work in small areas to start with. This should feel good and simply warm up and relax you.
4. To begin the myofascial release, place the pads of your fingers against the skin. Use the friction between fingers and skin to slide the skin gently over the muscle. Do gentle micro movements on one tiny spot in different directions. I usually think of the points of the compass and rub with mild to moderate pressure about an inch or less north and south and then east and west. Do this for just a few seconds. (This work can achieve some fascia release if you continue with it, but the following steps can have faster results.)
5. To gauge the condition of the fascia, in exactly the same spot you just rubbed, place the pads of your fingers on the skin but do not press down. Keeping the touch light, press the skin to slide it over the muscle; move the skin to the east about ¼ inch. Release it and repeat it in each of the cardinal directions. If the skin slides easily in a direction, you do not need to treat it in that direction.
6. For any direction in which the skin does not slide easily, move it again ⅛ of an inch in that direction and hold it there for a few seconds. If you feel it beginning to slide slightly, slowly push further. Continue to hold it, but do not push very far. Be gentle. When you feel a release or become tired of holding the position, release the pressure.
7. Repeat this treatment in each direction that does not slide easily on that spot.
8. For large areas, you can use the palm of your hand instead of your finger pads to slide the skin, but be very gentle. It is easy to apply too much pressure when using the whole hand.
9. Very gently rub the affected area again, and then move to another area. You can repeat the procedure on the same area, but give it a rest first. Repetition may not be necessary.
10. After doing the massage, do slow, gentle movements of the body to stretch the area through its normal range of motion. Repeat these slow range of motion movements at least daily.
11. After releasing the fascia in an area, continue to do exercises and postural adjustments so that it will not retighten into the wrong position but will support the posture and movements that are best for you.
12. Alternate repeated sessions of regular tissue massage and Myofascial Release Massage on subsequent days.

53

Near Infrared & Red Light Therapy

NEAR INFRARED (NIR) AND RED LIGHT THERAPY is recognized to speed the healing of injuries, relieve fatigue, improve blood circulation, protect the nervous system from degrading, treat cancer and chronic diseases, prevent vision problems, improve the appearance of the skin, and much, much more.[743, 744, 745] It is also thought to increase female fertility and prevent Alzheimer's Disease. It can even induce production of collagen[746] — although people with hEDS may still produce an inferior form of collagen, a deficit of collagen is a more pronounced problem when the collagen is faulty.

NIR Therapy not only heals you and makes you look better, it feels wonderful, especially in the wintertime since it is warming. It is easy to do and relaxing. It is also possible to get a Full Spectrum Infrared Sauna, which includes both near and far infrared, which is even more beneficial.

My Experience with NIR Light Therapy

My family and I use NIR Light Therapy whenever we have an injured joint, and sometimes it will heal it immediately. I also use it to firm my skin and remove dark spots and other imperfections, and I use it as the lamp for the sunning exercise from the Bates Method on cloudy or cold days. (See Chapter 14: Eye Strain.) And, I use it to fight off a virus more quickly. It gives me energy and just makes me feel good.

The device I use is the Hooga. It is affordable and effective, and it is a size that is easy to handle. I have had it for over 4 years, and it is still operating well, despite it being treated more roughly than it should be. Although the size is easy to manipulate, a larger size would allow for quicker treatment of more of the body; Hooga makes larger sizes, but they are more expensive, of course.

Step-By-Step Instructions for Near Infrared and Red Light Therapy

Treatment with NIR and Red Light Therapy is relaxing and enjoyable. Ask your doctor before trying anything new.

Near Infrared and Red Light Therapy at Home

1. Remove clothing from the area you want to treat.
2. Turn on the light box and warm it up by holding it a few inches from your skin in the area you want to treat. Once it is warm, you can continue to treat the same area or move on to another one.
3. Place the glass of the box against your skin.
4. Leave it there until you begin to feel uncomfortably warm inside that area of your body. This usually takes up to 10 minutes. (The glass should stay fairly cool for much longer.) It should never become painful.
5. Move it to another body part or end the session.
6. Do this once or twice daily, as little as once a week, or as frequently as you desire.

LINKS FOR PRODUCTS MENTIONED IN THIS CHAPTER

NIR Light Therapy https://amzn.to/48ritwy

54
Oil Cleansing Method

THIS IS AN ALL-NATURAL METHOD OF CLEANING your face. It works well because the skin on your face produces oils, which hold onto the dirt and clog your pores, but oil is dissolved by oil. Also, the cleansing oils have antibacterial, anti-inflammatory, and antioxidant qualities and can repair the skin barrier, heal wounds, and prevent skin aging.[747]

Even though people with acne often complain of oily skin and can't imagine applying oil, because this method dissolves the oil that is in the pores, it can actually reduce or eliminate acne.

There are a number of different carrier oils that you can choose for this method, such as organic olive oil, jojoba oil, sunflower seed oil, coconut oil, argan oil, oat oil, and rosehip oil. Many of these oils are expensive and more appropriate for spot treatment rather than daily cleansing purposes unless you have a specific need that they address. Make sure that you use high quality oils; I have seen people break out with a lot of acne when they tried using a cheap, generic brand of oil.

My Experience with Oil Cleansing

When I first started using this method, the blemishes on my skin went away, the dark spots slowly faded, and even some sebaceous cysts disappeared. The most stunning change was that people started telling me that I looked well rested (even though I wasn't). I believe that part of that effect may have come from releasing the fascia through massage (see Chapter 52: Myofascial Release Massage) as part of the cleansing method.

Step-By-Step Instructions for Oil Cleansing

I really love the antibacterial, anti-inflammatory, and antioxidant qualities of organic olive oil, which is also easy to find and fairly inexpensive. Jojoba oil is highly respected for use on the skin, and it is purported to improve the skin barrier, which could reduce the "leakiness" of your hypermobile skin. Jojoba is thinner, lighter, and more thoroughly absorbed than olive oil, but in my experience, it can grow mold, which I have never seen happen with olive oil.

Oil Cleansing Method for the Face

Every once in a blue moon, I accidentally drip oil on my chest when I am putting it on my face, so you might want to cleanse your face while wearing pajamas, lounge clothes, or nothing, instead of your nice blouse or dress. Ask your doctor before trying anything new.

1. Blend together 3 parts carrier oil (such as olive oil) and 1 part castor oil in a 3-ounce bottle. You must use good quality, organic oils. Poor quality oils will only clog your pores and cause breakouts. Olive oil is moisturizing and castor oil is drying, so adjust the ratio according to your skin's needs. I often use a higher ratio of olive oil in the winter than summer. I mix the oils in a small travel toiletry bottle so it is always ready for me.
2. If your skin needs some extra exfoliating, put about ⅛ teaspoon of food grade diatomaceous earth into the palm of your hand. Be careful not to create clouds of dust of the DE because it is not good to breathe it in; it will damage your lungs.
3. Pour about one teaspoon of oil into the palm of your hand; if you are using DE, blend the oil and DE together with the fingertips of your other hand. Using your fingertips, massage the oil into the skin of your face (and neck and hands, if you wish). Massage gently for about one minute. Make sure to keep all of your face muscles very relaxed while you massage.
4. Make good use of the oil by rubbing the excess after the massage into the backs of your hands.
5. Get a cotton washcloth wet with very warm water. Spread it over your face and hold it there to steam your skin for about one minute.
6. Use the washcloth and more warm water to gently scrub the oil off your face until it feels clean. There will still be a little bit of oil on your face; it will not be completely dry.
7. While washing your face, be sure not to jut your head forward or hinge your neck. You may have a habit of doing this, but you need to protect your cervical spine. See Chapter 25: Neck Pain & CCI and Chapter 56: Posture.
8. If your skin is too dry at any time, use a tiny bit of the oil mixture as a moisturizer. In the beginning, you are likely to need to do this, but once your skin has adjusted, you will possibly never need to moisturize your face again, except maybe on the driest days of the winter.
9. When you wash your washcloths that were used for oil, they can go in with the other towel laundry, just add a little Borax to boost your regular laundry soap. If the washcloth stays oily, do not put it in the dryer; you will not likely have this problem until you have used the washcloth for this purpose for a long time.
10. If you are experiencing acne or black heads, use a Face Mask made of equal parts water and bentonite clay; add jojoba oil for extra moisturizing and to help keep the skin barrier strong.[748] See Appendix A: Recipes.
11. If you are going to apply make-up, use organic refined shea butter as a moisturizer after doing the Oil Cleansing. Melt a tiny amount in your hand with the friction of your fingers of your other hand. Massage it into your skin and allow it to dry completely. This will give a good base for makeup.

LINKS FOR PRODUCTS MENTIONED IN THIS CHAPTER

Castor Oil https://amzn.to/3UF3iKD
Refined Shea Butter https://amzn.to/4aTnwa1

55

Positive Prayer

I HAVE WITNESSED PRAYER HELP PEOPLE of a variety of religions, as well as those who are spiritual but do not relate to a specific religion. Scientists have shown that patients who are prayed for — even if they don't know that they're being prayed for or don't practice a religion — fare better than their counterparts who are not prayed for.[749] Somehow, prayer works.

Prayers made by other people for us, especially by prayer groups, seem to be especially powerful. Still, prayer does not always work, and we can't understand why. Why did prayer not save the life of my young friend? Why did it take so long for me to meet my now-husband? If we want to have faith in prayer working, we have to find a way to accept that it works when it is meant to, in God's timing.

One of the most powerful actions we can take is to pray for others. Saying Positive Prayers on behalf of loved ones, friends, strangers, or the world can benefit not only those you are praying for but also yourself. Joining a prayer group can be especially rewarding. There are many that meet virtually these days, in addition to those at churches and other organizations in every town.

Positive prayers not only work, but they can get you through tough times. When you are in a flare and feel miserable, spend your time praying for other people or world peace. It might help. It might get you through.

Probably, all kinds of prayer work. Anything you say silently in your head, aloud to your empty room, to your friends or family around the dinner table, or in a prayer group can count as a prayer, and it can work. The most successful prayers that I have witnessed, though, have been positive prayers.

My Experience with Positive Prayer

Prayers have been answered for me in astounding ways. My mother prayed for my husband to come into my life, and though it took a long time for our stars to align for us to meet, when he came to me, he was exactly what she had prayed for.

At a time when I had faced some hardships and was so poor that I could not buy food but was too proud to ask family for help, a Hopi prayer circle prayed for me, and immediately I had food even though I kept my need a secret from everyone else — the volunteer and as-of-yet unrecognized mulberry tree in my yard fruited for the first time; one of my holistic center volunteers started working at the nearby bakery and began bringing me the day's leftover baked goods when she came to volunteer after work each day; a friend felt an urge and started bringing me leftovers from her family's meals since I was a single mother of a young baby; the community garden director started dropping off the garden's extra vegetables at my doorstep because he just didn't know what to do with them; a local farmer asked if he could give me a free CSA share if I would host a weekly CSA pickup at my business; previously unknown, kind men asked me out on dates and paid for my meals; the restaurant next door to my business asked if they could give me money and free meals in exchange for setting up tables on my sidewalk during busy dinnertimes; a food truck owner asked if he could set up in front of my center on weekends and give me money and burgers. When the Hopi community prayed for me, I went from being hungry to having to give food away to friends because I had more than I could eat!

Most importantly, when I prayed to Jesus to heal me, he led me to find out about hEDS/HSD, and within months, I was significantly healed.

Although the Hopi tradition has greatly influenced my method of Positive Prayer, most of the time when I pray, I am talking to the Holy Mother Mary or Jesus Christ. Mary has been by my side, along with some of my ancestors, intimately helping me with all of the details of my life. But my knowledge and healing of hEDS came in response to a prayer to Jesus. He is the most famous of all healers. Most of his miracles were healing. I encourage you to turn to Him when you need healing.

Jesus, thank you beyond all thanks for loving me. Thank you for healing me of all of the conditions related to hEDS that have troubled me. Thank you for healing every little ailment in my body, my mind, my emotions, and my spirit. Thank you for returning me to full and glorious health and happiness.

And thank you, Jesus, for giving me the ability and opportunity to provide all of this healing information to other people in the world with hypermobility. Thank you for guiding my words to be exactly what will most help them, and thank you for rewarding me for my long, diligent work. Most of all, thank you for healing all of the people who read this book. Amen.

Step-By-Step Instructions for Positive Prayer

Many cultures have their own version of positive prayers. I especially like Ho'Oponopono, a Hawaiian tradition of prayer. This tradition focuses on love and gratitude but has the distinct attitude that we are responsible for everything, not just our own actions. Anything we see, hear, feel, or experience exists, at least in part, because of us, or else we would not be experiencing it. We cannot be an uninvolved observer, but we can heal others by healing ourselves.

Ho'Oponopono follows this pattern:

Ho'Oponopono Prayer

I love you.
I'm sorry.
Please forgive me.
Thank you.

Each of these phrases, if you expand upon them as you speak to the divine, can mean many different things. As you repeat the prayer while trying to heal yourself of whatever problems you see in others and become closer to God, you will discover many different meanings, and if you keep praying, you will discover even more.

You can learn more about Ho'Oponopono Prayer in the book *Zero Limits: The Secret Hawaiian System for Wealth, Health, Peace, and More* by Joe Vitale and Ihaleakala Hew Len.

My favorite method of Positive Prayer is developed from the Hopi tradition. I have outlined my personal way of posing these prayers, below. Ask your doctor before trying anything new.

Positive Prayers

1. Begin in an attitude of gratitude and awe. Notice and express how wonderful is whatever is wonderful to you right now, even if it is something from your memories, or even if it is in your hopes for the future. This is the most important step, to praise God for His creation, and you can stay on this step forever.
2. Recognize your connection to God and all things. Concentrate on the qualities of God — goodness, love, joy, and peace.[750] Whatever spiritual feeling and lesson has been relevant to you recently is appropriate to focus on for a few minutes.
3. Speak with reverence, gratitude, and love to the Spirit being who is most relevant and meaningful to you. I encourage you to reach out to Jesus, as he is a powerful healer.
4. Imagine in specific detail that whatever it is you desire to see come to be, has come to be. That moment right after it has happened — what is that moment like? Picture that moment. Visualize the setting, the people, and what they say. In your mind, live the realization that your prayer has come to be. Feel what you would feel, and even feel what the other people involved would feel. As if it has already occurred, feel gratitude for it having happened.
5. Sit in peace with the knowledge that what you have prayed for is already so.

56
Posture

WHEN I AM INTERACTING IN HEDS, MCAS, CCI, TOS, and other groups on social media, the most common question I get asked is, "How did you correct your posture?"

First of all, it is important to accept that your body will always change and circumstances will always change. We might be in pursuit of "Perfect Posture," but there is no absolute when it comes to the body. Further, there is no wrong position for your body to be in as it moves throughout the day or your exercise routine, but there are certainly positions that can lead to problems if you become habituated to them. And, there are positions that generate health when you use them as your home base in between all of the other movements you do.

Posture applies to every body part from the top of the head to the tip of the toes. Improving your posture will be a lengthy endeavor. I advise that you focus on one body part at a time, usually for about three months, and then move on to another body part. You may repeat body parts whenever necessary. It makes sense to focus on whichever part of the body is feeling the most pain so that you can relieve yourself of the pain.

If you are worried about how your shoulders slump forward, it may seem silly to work on your knees, for example, but I assure you that they are all connected. For example, according to one of my Physical Therapists, there is a nearly 100% correlation between people who cannot move their pinky toes independently and people who have pelvic dysfunction.

Because people with hEDS/HSD don't have strong ligaments holding our posture for us, and our muscles might be weak, we need to do Strength Training to build the capacity of the muscles that hold us in position. If our muscles are just strong enough to hold our posture, we will always struggle. We have to get our muscles so strong that they can do more than hold our posture — they need to be so strong that holding our posture is the easiest thing they do.

My Experience with Posture

One of the best things I have done for my health is to improve my posture. I have had so much success with it that I have even gotten almost two inches taller! Other people I have helped with posture have gained inches in height also.

One of the most important things I learned when fixing my posture is not to get discouraged and to keep working on different sections of the body. I worked and worked on my abdominal and rib cage positioning, but I could never accomplish deep, full belly breaths until I fixed my forward head posture, and then suddenly I could breathe with ease. [751] I worked and worked on curing my Bunions with proper foot posture, but they never got all the way better until I stopped hyperextending my knees.

I believe that correcting my posture has reduced my number of extant Joint Injuries, improved my digestion, reduced my headaches and Migraine attacks, and reduced symptoms of neuralgia and neuropathy.

It has also given me confidence because I look more attractive. I can move more easily when hiking or playing sports. Even chairs and sofas feel more comfortable when I have good posture. People are friendlier to me, too.

I often feel like it's not fair that hypermobile people have to work so hard to have good posture, but it is what it is. It is worth it to work on posture, and Strength Training is worth it, too, because that is what gives my body the ability to hold good posture for long periods of time.

Also aim to reduce any inflammation caused by the other conditions discussed in this book, as that inflammation will make it more challenging for your muscles to do the work you are asking them to do; but don't wait for the inflammation to go away. You have to start work on your posture today; it could be that your posture is directly or indirectly responsible for the inflammation.

Step-By-Step Instructions for Posture

A general guideline that applies to most body parts is to aim for a neutral posture. In a neutral posture, you will not be at the far end of your range of motion for that body part. You will be able to move from this position in every direction; up, down, front, back, and side to side. In some cases, you may need to do exercises or other releases to restore range of motion in order for this ability to move in every direction to be possible. Your goal is not to be stiff and straight; posture is meant to be flexible and allow a variety of movements for all body parts, though it will make you seem to be standing straighter and may actually make you taller. Ask your doctor before trying anything new.

Feet

Foot posture is often overlooked by people who are treating someone for improper posture, especially if they are focused on head posture or slumping shoulders. Yet, foot posture makes a big difference to how you can hold the rest of your body. The feet are the foundation of your body, and they are intricately made to do some amazing work — standing, walking, running, jumping, and dancing. Your feet must work correctly in all of the movements you do in order for the rest of your body to be able to do what it is meant to do.

1. If you are having symptoms of Bunions, Plantar Fasciitis, or Flat Feet, do the treatments recommended in Chapter 16: Foot Pain.
2. Make sure that your arches are kept raised. This requires you to use the muscles on the inside of the ankle and foot to lift the arches from the ground. Do *tendus* and *relevés* to strengthen the arches if needed, always keeping the ankles straight. (See Chapter 16: Foot Pain for descriptions of these movements.) Also, do side-to-side movements of the foot (but not too far to the side) to strengthen the ankles, since it is their strength that will hold the arches up.
3. Spend time walking barefoot to keep the feet strong. Walking barefoot on a smooth floor is a great start, but walking barefoot on uneven ground will be especially helpful in strengthening as well as maintaining the mobility of each little joint.

4. Massage. Loosen tight muscles and fascia with gentle massage.
5. Take foot baths with magnesium flakes to relax muscles and fascia.
6. Pay attention to where the weight of your body is. Your leg should come straight up out of your heel. If your weight is too much on your toes, your leg will come up at an angle. Most of your weight should be on your heel, with a small amount spread across your toes.
7. Keep your toes splayed (and make sure your shoes are wide enough to allow this).

Knees

In my experience, my hyperextended knees were never painful, and they didn't hyperextend nearly as far as some of my friends' and students' knees, so I thought they were not problematic, but once I started adjusting them, I found that they had been causing pain in my lower back, hips, thighs, calves, and feet.

If you have tightness and knots in your calf muscles, specifically the soleus that runs from the back of the knee to the heel, it is possibly caused by hyperextended knees. If your knees go back too far, they can perpetually shorten the soleus and cause it to spasm. This can lead to Plantar Fasciitis and foot pain and also potentially exacerbate POTS symptoms.

I had painful, knotted calves my entire life, and no treatment that I did myself or received from any of a number of professionals was ever able to make a bit of difference in the soleus. But then after just two days of not hyperextending my knees, my soleus relaxed and the pain was miraculously gone. It was one of the easiest treatments I've ever accomplished for myself. By the third day, the pain in my back was gone, too.

Treating knee posture is quite easy.

1. Do not rest into your knees at their hyperextended extreme. Do not lock your knees back.
2. Stay in the muscle; do not rest into the bones and ligaments. Bend your knees just enough for them to be straight instead of hyperextended. Keep them here by activating the quadriceps muscles.
3. Gently stretch and massage the soleus, hamstring, and quadriceps so that they can return to optimal condition and make it easy to keep the knees in appropriate posture. Apply comfrey oil as needed to reduce pain and to return tendons to optimum strength.
4. Strengthen the quadriceps with the knee exercise described in Chapter 19: Knee Pain.
5. If you are correcting a hyperextended knee posture, you likely need to correct the tilt of your pelvis. You will need to lengthen some pelvic muscles and strengthen others. Massage will help, but most effective will be the anterior pelvic tilt correction exercise described in the next section, Hips.

Hips

In general, I would recommend starting posture work with the pelvis because this area can become more twisted and malfunctioning than most of the body. It is a complex area that really needs the help of a pelvic specialist Physical Therapist. The pelvis can become so hypertonic that any exercises you try will only be counterproductive. However, I can give these pointers.

1. Do not keep the gluteus maximus tightened while standing. Its work is meant to be done while you are doing things like climbing stairs or hills. If you are squeezing

your rear end while standing still, you probably have your pelvis pushed forward too far.

2. Tighten the pelvic floor muscles when you need more stability, but do not squeeze them all the time. These are the muscles that are involved in doing Kegel exercises; they help stop the flow of urine, but also support the entire pelvis. I recommend that you see a PT to find out if you are doing Kegel exercises (including the relaxation phase) correctly.
3. Keep the pelvis neutral, not tilted forward or backward. Look for the front of your thigh and the base of your torso to rise along the same line. The pubic area (where the hair grows) should be plumb vertical. If you have an anterior pelvic tilt, which is common especially with hyperextended knees, do a bridge exercise to strengthen the muscles to hold the pelvis neutral: lie on a bed or yoga mat with your knees bent and soles of the feet flat on the surface. Tilt your pelvis up as if beginning a bridge, but lift the pelvis only until you feel the pull in your back and hold the position for 30 seconds. Release and then repeat as much as you feel you need. Do not go past the position of the pull, even though this is probably only a small raise. Keep pressure in your heels, not toes, as you hold the position. Once you have strengthened yourself with this exercise for a month or so, have someone do Myofascial Release Massage on your lower back, and it will become even easier to maintain the good, neutral pelvis position.

Abdomen

Tightness in the abdomen can cause you to curl up into a partial fetal position. Tightness in the abdomen is often caused by stress, fear, and anxiety; it is the body's well-intended and valiant effort to protect the soft, tender areas and organs that are so important to survival. The abdomen is the container of the digestive system and the reproductive system, two very busy and productive components of the body. Improving the posture of the abdomen can improve digestion, relieve constipation, diminish menstrual cramps, restore fertility, and more.

1. Visit a Physical Therapist if you think that your abdominal muscles may not be doing their work. I was told by a PT that most of the people she sees do not have proper engagement of their obliques.
2. When standing still, keep your stomach muscles soft enough that your belly can move in and out as you breathe. Tighten the muscles only when you are lifting, jumping, scrubbing, or doing other movements that require extra stability in the abdomen.
3. Massage the stomach to loosen hypertonic muscles and tight fascia. Deep tissue massage works along the outer areas of the stomach — beneath the rib cage and above the hip bones. To release the muscles in the inner areas of the stomach, lie on your back and press your fingers slowly into the tissue. Keep breathing. Let your fingers move deeper in as the tissues relax. Raise your fingers slowly, and then move up or down along a line between the pelvis and rib cage. Repeat this until you have done the entire line, then go to another line. As the tissues relax, you will be able to feel your heart beat pulse in your fingertips as the blood flow is returned to the area.

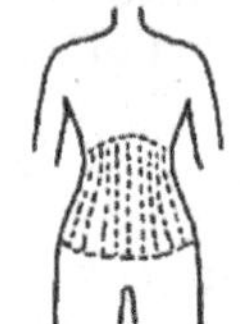

Figure 66: Abdominal Massage

4. Exercise the abdomen not by doing crunches, which can be hard on your vertebrae, but by lifting the legs. This can be done while hanging from a bar or while lying on your back. After contracting the abdominal muscles by raising the legs, always return to a full extension by lowering the legs and taking a deep belly breath.

Back

The back is what most people think of when they think of posture, though in my experience, it has less to contribute than other parts of the body. Still, it is obviously very important to posture and also extremely important because it houses the spinal cord, which is ultimately responsible for everything that happens in the body.

1. Do a Kneeling Thoracic Stretch. Get on your knees in front of a cushioned sofa or chair. Place your elbows on the seat. Bend forward so that your head goes down between your arms, and your hands come back, possibly touching your back, though that is not necessary.

Figure 67. Kneeling Thoracic

2. Strengthen the back by doing rows and pull overs with resistance. For rows, you can sit on the floor with straight legs in front of you; hold onto both ends of a resistance band (one hand on each end) that is wrapped across the soles of your feet. Pull the band back so that your elbows go slightly behind you, then release and repeat. For pull overs, mount a resistance band securely above you (perhaps in a door frame), with straight arms over your head, grasp each end of the resistance band and pull your straight arms down to your thighs.
3. Visit a Myofascial Release Massage Therapist and ask them to treat your back so that it can move into new positions as you strengthen it and make changes to the posture of other body parts.
4. If you have any abnormal curvature or pain, visit a PT and/or an Osteopath.
5. Swimming is very good for straightening and strengthening the back. See Chapter 31: Scoliosis.
6. Do the bird dog stretch to relieve lower back pain. On hands and knees, lift and extend opposite hand and foot and hold for 10 seconds. Then repeat on the other side.
7. When sitting or standing, keep the back plumb, not leaning forward or back.

Rib Cage

The rib cage is actually a series of joints in the front where the ribs connect to the sternum and in the back where they connect to the spine. Between the ribs, intercostal muscles and other connective tissues control the ribs' spacing and movements. All of these joints are intended to articulate in a variety of directions, depending on the movement of the body.

The intercostal muscles can be caused to retract inappropriately during MCAS/MCS/allergic reactions, especially in the case of mild-to-moderate anaphylaxis. Many people with hEDS get frozen rib cages, which limits the ability to improve posture.

You may need to return to this body part many times to regain flexibility so that the rib cage can adjust to other posture adjustments you have made.

1. Do deep breathing exercises, feeling the rib cage move alternately in the front, sides, or back, or in all directions at once. Keep the rib cage moving fluidly.
2. Visit a Myofascial Release Massage Therapist and ask them to focus on the fascia surrounding your rib cage. You can also do self-massage for the parts you can easily reach — do not dislocate your shoulder by trying to do too much on your own. See Chapter 52: Myofascial Release Massage.
3. Lift the front of the rib cage. For most people, the front of the rib cage collapses down and restricts the diaphragm. Consciously lift it up. You will probably be forced

to take a big breath of air when you lift your rib cage, as it makes extra room for your lungs to inflate. At first it may feel that you are leaning back when you do this, but as your muscles strengthen you will aim for a sensation of lifting the sternum up.

4. Use heat, in moderation, to relax these complex joints.
5. Do pull overs and rows to strengthen the back of the rib cage. See the previous section, Back, for a description of these exercises.
6. Do exercises to strengthen the serratus anterior. These muscles on the sides of the rib cage are frequently forgotten in Strength Training plans, but they are easy to include. One of the many exercises that target these muscles is the dumbbell pullover: lie on the floor or a bench (with your head at the end of the bench), hold one dumbbell above you so that your arms are stretched straight up toward the ceiling. Keeping the arms as straight (but not hyperextended) as you can, lower the dumbbell beyond your head. If you are on a bench, you will be able to lower the dumbbell lower than your head. Then return the dumbbell to the starting position, again with straight (not hyperextended) arms.

Chest

The most overlooked aspect of posture is the chest, but it is very important to give it some attention. Generally, when posture is bad, the muscles on the upper part of the torso, between the shoulders and where the sternum is, tend to get shortened and tight. Until you release the tension in the chest muscles and fascia, you will have a very difficult time getting your back and shoulders into position.

1. Gently massage the chest and shoulders to relax the fascia. See Chapter 52: Myofascial Release Massage.
2. Do deeper massage to relax the muscles.
3. Stretch in a doorway with one arm bent against the wall at shoulder height; step forward to enact the stretch.
4. Imagine that your sternum is being lifted by a string toward the sky.
5. Feel your love energy pulsing out of your sternum toward the people you see; it will attract them and make them want you around.

Shoulders

The shoulders are the most noticeable aspect of posture. If your shoulders are rounded, people will assume that you lack confidence or maybe you feel beaten down. If your shoulders are raised, people will perceive you to be on edge and nervous.

You can probably get some information about your shoulder posture when you look in the mirror. Face the mirror and stand as you normally do. If your shoulders are rounded, then the back of your hands may be facing the mirror. If you lift your chest and rotate your shoulders back as far as they should go, you will see the sides of your thumbs and pointer fingers in the mirror.

Think about how long your neck was when you were younger. When you look in the mirror, does it still look that long? If not, you may be raising your shoulders. Alternatively, you may have swelling in your neck due to TOS, or you may have a forward head posture; look at your body and see if you can tell what is going on.

1. Relax the shoulders into a nicely squared position. If you tend to keep them up by your ears, then drop them down. If you tend to pull them all the way down, then release them into a horizontal instead of drastically sloping position.

2. Keep your shoulders far apart. You can feel the tissues on the top of your shoulders stretch out to the side.
3. Do not squeeze the shoulders too far back. The way to pull your shoulders back is not to focus on the shoulders going back but to lift the chest so that the chest pushes the shoulders back. You probably need to lift your chest further than feels appropriate to get your shoulders into position; you'll get used to the position in time.
4. Do external rotation exercises with a resistance band. See Chapter 35: Thoracic Outlet Syndrome.
5. Let the arms hang loosely from the shoulders whenever they are not working. Tension in your arms will lead to tension in the shoulders.
6. Keep the fingers relaxed. Tension in your fingers will lead to tension in the arms and shoulders. Wiggle them every once in a while to make sure they are comfortable.

Neck

One of the most common problems with posture among both the hEDS/HSD population and the general public is forward head posture or military neck.[752] This can lead to a number of problems, including neck pain, headache, and neuropathy. It is also responsible for some unattractive qualities like dowager's hump, turkey neck, jowls, and oversized, hypertonic trapezius muscles.

The neck is a very delicate and complicated area. It is highly recommended to do these exercises under the supervision of a Physical Therapist or Personal Trainer. Remember to go very, very slowly. Do only a few reps of one or two exercises each day as you are building your strength. It is exceptionally easy to fatigue your neck, which introduces more instability and prohibits you from going about regular life.

1. Strengthen, straighten, and tone the neck using the exercises and techniques discussed in Chapter 25: Neck Pain & CCI.
2. Once you have built strength and improved alignment in the neck, add some additional, more advanced exercises. Be very careful. It is recommended to have the supervision of a Physical Therapist or other professional when learning new neck exercises. There is a high risk of injuring yourself and causing Occipital or Trigeminal Neuralgia or other serious problems when doing neck exercises. However, strengthening the neck is one of the most important things that you can do for your health and for some people could potentially eliminate MCAS, Cerebellar Ataxia, Dystonia, Digestive System Problems, Eye Strain, Migraine, Neck Pain, Peripheral Neuropathy, POTS, Shoulder Pain, Sinus Congestion, Thoracic Outlet Syndrome, and TMJ.
    a. Scalene strengthening: lie on your side, turn your chin toward your upper shoulder. Without moving anything except your head, nod your head so that your forehead moves toward your upper shoulder, then return it to its starting place. Repeat as many times as appropriate for your strength condition.
    b. Forward head posture correction: stand with the back of your head against a Red Ball you hold on the wall. Keeping your back straight and shoulders pulled back (but not too far), step your feet a few inches forward so that your body is leaning on a diagonal line. Hold this position for 30 seconds; increase the time as you get stronger.
    c. Red Ball Exercises Phase II: Do presses into the ball against the wall similarly to Phase I (see Chapter 25: Neck Pain & CCI), but instead of keeping the neck stable and moving the body, now you should move the neck while the body stays

still. Do this only to the back and sides, not the front; do not lift or lower the chin but keep it neutral. Be very cautious adding this neck exercise; it took a long time before I could do this one without creating pain and misalignment.

d. Reclined Nod: to strengthen the longus colli, in a reclined position, very slowly nod the head forward (chin traveling toward chest) and then return to the starting position and repeat.

e. Side Nod: to strengthen the sternocleidomastoids: lie down, turn the head to the side, raise the ear toward the chest and then lower the head back down to the bed, and repeat. Then, turn the head to the other side and do the exercise with the other ear nodding.

3. Seek professional guidance for next-level neck strengthening using weights and specialized tools.

Head

The head is mostly controlled by the neck, but it is helpful to take some time to pay attention to this uppermost body part. It is especially important to maintain good tongue posture (See Chapter 23: Mouth Health) because it increases your stability while standing.[753]

1. Hold your head at a neutral angle so that when you are looking straight forward, your eyes are centered in their sockets. You should not be looking up from under your eyelids or down over your nose.
2. Hold your tongue and jaw in the correct posture. Tongue should be broadly spread, suctioned across the roof of the mouth, and the teeth should be lightly touching with the lips together but relaxed.
3. Practice what I call a Resting Bliss Face. Smile, whether small or large, as much of the time as you can.
4. Try not to squint your eyes. Wear a wide-brimmed hat when the sun is bright. Take breaks from looking at screens.
5. Allow your jaw muscles to be relaxed.
6. Breathe through the nose, deeply and slowly.

Posture Practice

1. Focus on each body part, one at a time. Make a change, and then take a few days to a week to continue making it, correcting yourself each time you notice that you are not in the improved position. Take it easy with your workout routines, doing the exercises that are easiest for you — or give yourself a day or two off. Even though you aren't doing a lot of rigorous exercise, it takes a lot of energy and mental focus to hold your body in a new posture continuously. Your muscles need a chance to strengthen without being overly challenged. Lie down on your back when your muscles are too exhausted to continue in the new position.
2. Once you are feeling comfortable and strong in your new position, start going for walks. At first, choose smoothly paved, level paths — easy walking and short trips. Lengthen the walks until you feel quite comfortable walking in your new position. Then graduate to unpaved, uneven terrain, again starting with short trips and lengthening as you grow stronger. Also increase the steepness of the hills that you climb up and down.
3. When you can walk on a rough trail and keep your position without hurting or becoming overly fatigued, it is time to increase the challenge in your workout routine. Choose the exercises that are difficult for you, and do them slowly, focusing on your new posture position. Do not do as many reps as you used to do, but build

up slowly over the next week or so. Leave time in your workout routine to go for a walk or use a treadmill at the end of the session. This walk will give your mind an opportunity to focus again on the posture while your body has an opportunity to reclaim the new posture after having used other muscles.

4. Keep your new posture in mind during your daily tasks as well. For example, do not let your chest collapse or your head hinge back when you bend over or squat down to pick up something from the floor.
5. Usually, three months is the right amount of time to focus on one posture correction. After that amount of time, the correction is likely to feel pretty habitual and the muscles will have strengthened to be able to maintain the position without fatiguing.
6. When you move on to another body part, you will want to try to maintain the posture that you were just working on as well. There can be some complications here. You can assume that you haven't achieved perfect posture yet, and the correction you just made might be incompatible with the new correction you are trying to make. The only time this wouldn't be a problem would be if you got to where every single aspect of your posture was perfect except for the very last step — that last correction is going to be the easiest one of all.
7. If you are finding one of your corrections too challenging to make, skip that one and try a different one. If you can't find a correction that feels possible to make, see about fine-tuning the one you just finished with.
8. You will likely have to focus on each body part multiple times. You can only correct yourself so far at once. When you try to do too much at once, you may make yourself miserable. There were a number of times that a posture correction gave me a Migraine, sometimes lasting many days. Although I recommend making subtler changes that won't hurt while you're doing them, I also don't regret going quickly. The worst Migraine I got was after a correction of my head position, and although I was miserable for a week, after that, I stopped getting Migraines altogether. Also, my neck stopped hurting, my breathing improved, my eyes felt better, and my Rib Subluxations decreased even more.

Posture Review

Numerous times throughout the day, I say the following reminders to myself. Depending on the direction in which you corrected any body part, you may need to adjust the list for yourself. For example, if you always stood with your weight too far on your heels, then instead of, "Weight in heels," you may need to remind yourself, "Weight on toes,"

1. Toes spread.
2. Arches lifted.
3. Weight in heels.
4. Ankles straight.
5. Knees in the muscles.
6. Pelvis neutral.
7. Glutes relaxed.
8. Pelvic floor lifted.
9. Deep belly breaths.
10. Rib cage lifted.
11. Ribs moving out with breaths.
12. Sternum pulled toward the sky.
13. Back plumb straight.
14. Shoulders wide and relaxed.
15. Arms hanging.
16. Fingers loose.
17. Ears pulled back and up.
18. Chin neutral.
19. Tongue on roof of mouth.
20. Teeth lightly touching.
21. Jaw relaxed.
22. Lips happy.
23. Be mobile.

57

Range of Motion Exercises & Dynamic Stretching

PEOPLE WITH HEDS ARE ADVISED TO avoid hyperextending and ideally reduce the hypermobility of their joints, yet it is important to maintain a healthy range of motion. My favorite ways to do this are with Range of Motion Exercises and Dynamic Stretching.[754]

Range of Motion Exercises

Whereas long-held stretching can be a danger to hypermobile joints, moving slowly without stopping is safer. I recommend doing this every day, first thing in the morning, so that your body will be ready for whatever comes that day. This is also an efficient and effective way to warm up before doing any other kind of exercise routine. On days when you are feeling weak or sensitive, this can be the bulk of your workout.

For each joint in the body, one at a time, move through the joint's entire range of motion several times at least. For most joints, it will be best to move in a back-and-forth or side-to-side motion. When you get strong, it will become appropriate for some of the joints to be moved in circles. When the joint is weak, do not do circles; only use back-and-forth or side-to-side movements. Move slowly and do several repetitions.

The trickiest part of doing range-of-movement exercises is knowing how far to go. For a joint like the elbow or knee, it can be pretty easy to see what is straight — don't go beyond that. For other joints, you will have to pay closer attention. When you are within your range of motion, you will feel strong; when you move past your joint's optimal range, the movement will become mechanically disadvantaged and you will feel weaker; you might feel a pull on the tendons or ligaments. It can be very helpful to have a hypermobility specialist Physical Therapist advise you on your proper range of motion.

It's especially nice to listen to music while doing your Range of Motion exercises — let your movements be an easy dance. And, when you have gone through all of the motions, your body will be warmed up and your joints will be lubricated. This is the perfect time to do some fun dancing or Strength Training.

Dynamic Stretching

When you are weak, it is not advised to do stretching; your joints are too vulnerable. Wait to do any kind of stretching until you can do Range of Motion exercises easily, through the full range of motion that seems right to you.

When you are ready or being assisted by a hypermobility specialist Physical Therapist, you can try adding some careful stretching back into your routine if you feel it is necessary or helpful.

The kind of stretching that I would recommend is dynamic stretching, which means that the muscles are active while you are stretching. You do not get to the end point of your flexibility and then hang on the joint, stretching out the ligament. That is a very bad idea for hypermobile people.

What you aim to do is to get to near the end point of your comfortable and appropriate flexibility, then use your muscles of that body part to extend your stretch. If your muscle is under load (working) and feels strong and stable, your body will not freak out about the stretch.

If you have lost mobility in a joint, stretching cautiously can be one of the many tools you use to regain mobility through your full appropriate range of motion. Even in this case, you do not want to hang on the ligament. You can use pressure from your hand or a solid structure, moving slowly in and out of the stretch. Do not bounce with any force, but press, slow and steady.

Do not use your hand or gravity to force a stretch past a natural end point. Use the strength of the muscles that control the joint being stretched.

There is a form of dynamic stretching called Strain/Counterstrain, which can be used to release tension and regain mobility when you have healed a Joint Injury but are still experiencing stiffness. I strongly recommend that you do this with a therapist who is certified in it and understands hypermobility. You do not want to stretch too far.

With Strain-Counterstrain, you press against a force that is stretching you. Your muscles are working, and the force should never be so hard that you are trembling or feeling exhausted by it. When you have pushed long enough that the body begins to feel relaxed, then the stretch can be pushed just a tiny bit further. It should never hurt.

My Experience with Range of Motion Exercises and Dynamic Stretching

Range of Motion exercises have always been my favorite kind of movement. I have almost always started every day with some of them, as well as many of the dance classes I taught.

Many times, any kinks or pains that I have will disappear simply from doing a few minutes of Range of Motion exercises for all of the different joints of the body. It rarely works to focus only on the injured joint, but loosening up and lubricating all of the joints can make a difference for the specific ones that are troubled.

I received Strain/Counterstrain therapy from a Physical Therapist, and it was wonderful. She also taught me how to do it for myself using a jump rope for the force, but I found that her assistance was much preferred and safer.

My husband has been developing a protocol of dynamic stretching. The best thing about it is that I am no longer afraid of stretching. All fear is leaving my life, and so my Parasympathetic Nervous System is having a chance to heal me even further.

Step-By-Step Instructions for Range of Motion Exercises and Dynamic Stretching

When you are starting a Range of Motion and Dynamic Stretching routine, it will probably be helpful for you first to implement the body positioning described in Chapter 56: Posture; that chapter also explains some of the terms used in this exercise routine.

When you begin doing the exercise routine, start with very, very slow movements. You will also want to use these very slow movements any time you have had an injury or feel any misalignment. Sometimes, these slow movements can cue the body to return to the proper alignment and operation.[755, 756]

Depending on your condition, at first you may be able to do only a portion of this routine as your workout for the day, but eventually this will become a warm-up for other more strenuous workouts. When you are stronger, it is appropriate to do the Range of Motion and Dynamic Stretching routine at different speeds on different days. Or, perhaps you will go through the entire routine slowly and then repeat the entire routine at a faster speed. You can also change the order of the exercises on different days, and try adding in some new things for fun.

Let your muscles experience all of the dynamics they are capable of, and keep your mind interested. Have fun with it! Ask your doctor before trying anything new.

Sample Wake-Up Exercise Routine

For this routine, I usually repeat each movement 4 times on each side. Do the number of repetitions that feels right to you on any given day. If there are any motions that hurt even when kept small, skip them. Before beginning, use the restroom and drink a glass of water.

1. Stand (or sit or lie) with the best posture you can manage. I sometimes prefer to be in front of a full-length mirror so that I can see what my body is doing. (Other times, I like to be out in nature, really relaxing into the movements and feeling peace flow into every nook of my body.) Take some good deep breaths, allowing the rib cage to move out in every direction and enjoying your expanded position.
2. Lift the arms in front of you until they are comfortably overhead, remembering to move slowly. Make sure to keep good posture with relaxed shoulders and a long neck. Keep breathing. Lower the arms back down in front of you to your sides.
3. Lift the arms out to the side, bring them up until they are comfortably overhead, then lower them back down.
4. Raise the arms to the back as far as is easy and comfortable without bending forward or moving the shoulders out of position, then bring them forward to cross and very gently hug the front of the body.
5. Resuming your best posture, turn your head side to side, keeping your shoulders relaxed and neck long.
6. Nod your head up and down. Do not go too far up.
7. Tilt your head so that your right ear travels a little way toward your right shoulder, and then tilt your head to your left side.
8. Lift your shoulders gently and then lower them.
9. Raise your right arm over your head, keep the elbow in place and reach your hand down toward your upper back; it does not matter whether you touch your upper back or not. Arch to the side so that you make a long curve from your raised elbow to your hip. Keep your neck strong, and do not let your head rest on the neck. Try

to make your stationary side stay tall and make your working side get longer to create the curve. Then do it on the other side.

10. Hold your arms out to the side so that you make a T. Turn to the right until your right arm is pointing behind you at whatever angle is comfortable for you but not past your center in the back. As you twist at the waist, make sure that your feet stay strong on the floor with toes spread and knees in the muscles. Allow the opposite arm to bend so that your hand comes to the opposite shoulder. Repeat on the other side. Continue breathing.
11. Relax your arms down and bend your knees a little further. Gently shake your hips side to side.
12. Maintaining the bent knees, and upright back, rock your pelvis front and back.
13. Stand behind a chair or in front of a counter or bar; hold on gently with your hands just enough to help you keep your balance. Wiggle your toes and then make sure they are spread out on the floor.
14. Holding the chair, stand on one leg with the other leg slightly bent, only the toes of the foot touching the floor. Twist the leg in and out so that the knee points to right side and then the left to lubricate and activate the hip. Repeat with the other leg.
15. Holding the chair, do shallow knee bends, keeping your back straight and toes spread. Make sure your knees are going straight forward over your feet; do not lift your heels from the ground. When you straighten, do not hyperextend your knees.
16. Still holding the chair, do *relevés* or raises. With good posture, lift your heels and rise up on the balls of your feet, keeping your toes spread. Make sure to keep your ankles straight – you can weaken rather than strengthen your ankles if you let them fall to the side. If this is extremely difficult for you, put a tennis ball in between your ankles, and hold it there as you rise and lower; it will prevent you from being able to drop your ankles in or out. Lower back down even more slowly and touch the ground with your heels very gently.
17. Still holding the chair, lift your toes so that you are standing on your heels. If you are not strong enough to keep good posture (don't stick your rear end out), then do one foot at a time.
18. Turn to hold the chair with one hand, lift one leg slightly in front of you, and activate the ankle by holding the leg still while you move your toes up and down and then side to side. Then use the other leg.
19. Step away from the chair and make gentle circles with your hands to activate your wrists.
20. Hold your arms out to the side, keeping the upper arm mostly still, and circle the lower arm to activate the elbows.
21. Lift your knee toward your chest, keeping your body stable with a strong supporting leg and straight back; do not let your stomach become hollowed. Lower to standing position, and then repeat on the other side.
22. Lift your heel toward your rear to activate your hamstring, and then place your foot back down. Repeat on the other side.
23. Give yourself a gentle wiggle or shake all over and take a few deep breaths.
24. On strong days, you can add in some more active exercises:
    a. Standing behind a chair and holding onto the back of it, do deep knee bends (*grands pliés* in parallel). Keeping your back straight, bend all of the way down, allowing your heels to come off of the floor and your knees to go past your toes. Keeping your back straight, lower your heels as you stand back up. If you are having trouble balancing, place one foot slightly forward of the other foot and squeeze your knees together while you *plié*.

b. Do pushups against the wall for ease or on the floor if you're strong enough and won't get a POTS episode.
c. Hold onto the chair back with one hand and lift your leg, slowly, as high as you comfortably can to the front, then the side, then the back.
d. Do goddess bends (*grands pliés* in second turned out): spread your feet apart with your toes facing on an angle toward the side (but not necessarily all of the way to the side), and bend your knees until your thighs are horizontal to the ground. Keep your back straight; hold onto the back of the chair if necessary. Straighten up to standing but do not hyperextend your knees.
e. Jump little jumps in place or do jumping jacks. It is also fun to jump and punch the arms (not too hard) in different directions.
f. Take a large step forward into a lunge position, then push yourself back into a standing position. Repeat with the other leg lunging forward.
g. Lying on your back with your supporting leg bent and foot on the floor (easier) or stretched straight out (harder), bend the other leg toward your chest. Straighten the leg as far as comfortable to stretch the back of the leg, allowing it to move away from your torso as necessary; do not hyperextend the knee. Try to bring the leg closer to your torso, then slowly lower the straight leg to the ground. Switch legs.
h. Standing tall, reach the arms overhead, then fold the body and touch the ground. Go slowly to avoid overstretching or instigating a POTS episode.

58

Rebounding

REBOUNDING IS A FANCY WORD FOR JUMPING on a mini-trampoline. Jumping on a full-size trampoline or the floor counts, too. Bouncing or jumping are recommended to prevent osteoporosis, and they help get lymph fluids flowing. Rebounding will also build strength and stamina — and you might just have fun.

First of all, be safe. Jumping on a trampoline is dangerous. The moving surface means that you may hit the downward bounce unevenly, threatening your balance and challenging your joints. It may help to hold balance handles and not jump too high. Still, jump only if you are feeling strong and are not nursing any injuries.

You can jump in any pattern you desire. Sometimes I treat jumping like a HIIT (High Intensity Interval Training) workout, jumping as much as I can until I'm breathless and my heart rate is raised; then I rest until I feel ready to go again — be careful not to instigate a POTS episode if you try this. Another pattern to try is to jump for 20 seconds and rest for 10 seconds, repeating up to 8 times.

My Experience with Rebounding

Jumping is fun! It makes me feel like a kid again. Although it is recommended for getting lymph fluid flowing, I have not really noticed this. I do find that it is good for building my exercise stamina, and considering the results of my mother's bone density tests and all of the scientific research studies I've read on the matter, I trust that it is helping my bones stay strong. (See Chapter 26: Osteopenia & Osteoporosis.)

My parents bought my son a back-yard trampoline, so that is where I usually jump, in the good ol' outdoors. We also enjoy going to a local trampoline park, though I have to be cautious regarding fragrance exposures there, and I have to be careful not to overdo it and only go when I am feeling particularly strong.

Step-By-Step Instructions for Rebounding

Ask your doctor before trying anything new.

Rebound for Health

1. If you have a Joint Injury or weak joint that is likely to be injured during rebounding, heal this condition with the help of a Physical Therapist before beginning a rebounding routine.
2. Go to the bathroom before you begin jumping.
3. Do range of motion exercises first to warm up and lubricate your joints.
4. If you are inexperienced with rebounding or feeling weak at all, use a handlebar.
5. Keep your core strong, pulling up on the pelvic floor muscles while you jump. Relax your muscles whenever you rest.
6. Start by bouncing without letting your feet leave the trampoline surface. If this feels good, just do this for however long you like.
7. When you are ready for more challenge, start jumping. Keep your posture good, bend your knees when you land, remain conscious of your neck staying straight.
8. If straight jumping feels good, you can add some of the fun tricks you might have done as a child — dance moves, gymnastics or diving tricks, seat bounces, or children's games.
9. To build stamina, do HIIT jumping. High Intensity Interval Training means you jump as hard as you can for as long as it feels good. Do not go so long that you instigate a POTS or MCAS episode; just get yourself breathing a little bit harder than normal. Then rest until you feel like jumping again. Repeat as many times as you like.
10. For advanced jumping that may build bone even better, jump on the ground. Only do this when your joints are nice and strong. Choosing a spot with carpeting or a yoga mat may provide some protection without reducing the effectiveness of jumping on the floor. My mother's doctor insisted she needed to jump on the ground in order to improve her bone density, but I have not found any scientific studies to confirm this and in fact, many say that bouncing on a trampoline is sufficient. Still, jumping on the ground will increase your strength and potentially reduce your risk of injury in regular life, as long as you are careful enough not to injure yourself while jumping.
11. When you finish rebounding, do range of motion exercises again to stretch out any muscles that might have reacted by tensing up.

LINKS FOR PRODUCTS MENTIONED IN THIS CHAPTER

Mini Trampoline https://amzn.to/4b14wH2

59

Rest – Take a Break from Healing

IT WILL BE BEST IF THE RECOMMENDATIONS in this book become habits that you do easily, without thought or effort. But it will not happen instantly, and while you are learning new habits, it will take a lot of effort. You may have to correct yourself 5,000 times a day to keep your head posture correct. You may have to correct yourself every single time you go down the stairs for two weeks not to lean on the handrail.

While you are going through these transitions, making extra efforts and working hard to heal yourself, you will get tired. Not only is your body going to be working in new ways, but your brain is going to be burning more calories thinking about it and building the connections for it. You will sometimes feel worn out, tired, and even, if you keep going too long and overexert yourself, weary.

The feeling of weariness can be dangerous for me. It can lead to sadness and hopelessness. It can make me feel defeated. I've learned to try to avoid weariness, but if I land there anyway, I've learned to see it as a passing experience. If I rest, the weariness will pass. I will feel better.

Take a rest. Take a break. Do not do anything stupid that is going to set you back several steps in your healing journey...but if you do, don't beat yourself up about it. In fact, don't call it stupid. Maybe call it sub-optimal. It will probably happen to you at some time on this journey, and if you are reading books like this and doing the things you can do to heal yourself, you are obviously not stupid. You are, in fact, brilliant.

When you need a rest, it might not even be at a time when you're feeling really bad. Your body might be in good shape and it is your emotions that seem inexplicably taxed. Just tell your boss and your family that you aren't feeling well. Cancel your appointments and responsibilities if you can. Spend the day in bed. Or walk out into the woods and spend the day on a blanket or camp chair. Read a book. Or don't. Perhaps don't do anything but lie there in silence. Or spend all day talking on the phone to the friends you haven't talked to enough lately. Whatever it is that will take your mind off of your healing journey and recharge your batteries is what you should do.

You can take a break from your healing journey without taking a break from life, too. This might cause more of a risk of moving backwards in your journey, but a break like this is manageable and does not disrupt your life. Just go about your day as normal, but don't remind yourself not to close the drawer with your hip. Don't remind yourself to keep your posture correct. Don't do your exercises or healing treatments. Ask your doctor before taking a break from any medication or exercise he/she has prescribed for you.

Most of the time, one day is just the right amount of time for me to take a break, but sometimes I have needed two days, or only a morning. Take what time you need, even if it is a week, a month, or 5 minutes. When I'm stuck sitting at the longest traffic light in town, I have learned to sit in an enormous amount of gratitude for that little break. I even feel gratitude for the rest I get waiting for the tea pot to fill up with water from the Reverse Osmosis filter and for the time it takes for the water to boil. In those moments, I thank God and Jesus for that rest, and then I thank them for whatever wonderful things come to mind next.

Resting in a posture of gratitude and prayer is not really resting. When you have the energy to do it, it is wonderfully healing, but when you are really weary, even thoughts of gratitude and prayer are too much. You can rest in nothingness. Rest in the void out of which God created the world. All traditions around the world that I have learned about have believed that before God created this world, there was nothing, there was a great, dark void. Some people believe that a piece(s) of that void still exists and that you can sense it: the source of all creation. The beginning of all ingenuity. The place where unknown directions can begin. Rest in the void and be inspired; discover a new and brighter path forward. Come out of it refreshed, renewed, and ready to thrive. You are embarking on this healing journey, so I know that you have the courage to do it.

60

Rice Bucket Exercises

RICE BUCKET EXERCISES ARE A SAFE AND effective way to increase the strength of your hands and wrists, which will help you prevent hyperextending these delicate joints. Originally developed by the Shaolin monk warriors in China who were famous for empty-hand fighting, it has since been used by weightlifters, baseball players, rock climbers, and pianists. Physical Therapists rehabilitate their patients' hand and forearm injuries with rice bucket exercises as well.[757, 758]

A wonderful bonus to doing Rice Bucket exercises is that they help reduce inflammation and lubricate joints. Plus, your skin will be exfoliated and nourished by the rice.[759] My hands always feel better in every way after doing the Rice Bucket.

I have adapted a series of Rice Bucket exercises for hypermobile people, who must be cautious not to hyperextend finger or wrist joints while working to strengthen them. The hope is that if you do this, you will be able to write, chop vegetables, crochet, and do other tasks with your hands without pain. If you become strong enough, you may be able to resist accidental hyperextensions as well.

As always with hEDS exercising, stop immediately if it hurts and either rest or adapt the movement to something you can do painlessly. I recommend 30-second training sessions, but you should judge your own timing needs. If you do all of these exercises for 30 seconds the first time you do Rice Bucket exercises, you will probably fatigue your hands, so start with less and build up over weeks.

My Experience with Rice Bucket Exercises

I love doing Rice Bucket Exercises. I look forward to it every day because I know that it won't take long, it won't be hard, and afterward, my hands will feel comfortable, look pretty, and be soft to the touch.

It seems as if the rice pulls inflammation out of my hands and at the same time nourishes them with the vitamins and minerals in the rice. I definitely feel that the repeated movements of my fingers and wrists lubricate the joints.

During my healing journey, as I paid close attention to what caused various symptoms I experienced, I figured out that the Essential Tremor or Dystonia that I had after having been triggered for Allergies/MCAS/MCS sometimes got worse if I was doing something (like holding a dinner plate) with my fingers hyperextended and my wrist bending sideways. Sometimes, if I rounded my fingers and supported my wrist, the trembling stopped. Other times the trembling was just too strong to stop.

I wasn't previously strong enough to keep my fingers rounded when holding a dish, but in time, with the Rice Bucket exercises, the habit developed. Now when I notice that my finger joints are hyperextended, I am able to round them and continue holding the dish without pain or weakness. I even believe that my wimpy, skinny wrists have gained enough muscle that they are slightly thicker than they used to be. Note that I must keep my fingernails fairly short and my thumb nails even shorter so that they are out of the way when I hold a dish or push a button with rounded fingers.

I also have my son do Rice Bucket Exercises most days. He thinks it is fun for the sensory experience. I see that it has recognizably strengthened his hands. Before he started doing these exercises, my son hated to write. His handwriting of both print and cursive looked good, but he never wanted to practice it. He didn't complain about pain in his hand, but he did complain about overall fatigue when he was required to write. He is creative and prolific about making up stories and poems or detailing facts, but he never wanted to write them down. He is homeschooled, and it would sometimes be like pulling teeth for me to get him to write just one or two sentences.

About three weeks after he'd started the Rice Bucket Exercises, I gave him an assignment to write about a nonfiction book he had read. Nonfiction is not his greatest interest, and based on all of our previous experiences, I expected him to barely write two sentences. I was focused on my lesson planning for the next activity while he worked, and when he said, "I'm done!" I looked up from my work to see that he had written enough to cover an entire piece of paper front and back. I credit the Rice Bucket Exercises.

Step-By-Step Instructions for Rice Bucket Exercises

When starting off, do the exercises at the top of the rice, just barely dipping your fingers in for some resistance. As you get stronger, reach down further into the rice. It is like using heavier weights when you are deeper down into the rice bucket. Always make sure to stay within an appropriate range of motion. Ask your doctor before trying anything new.

Rice Bucket Exercises

1. Fill a 5-gallon bucket or pot with 10-15 pounds of rice (you can choose the least expensive rice at the store).
2. Remove your ring splints and wrist braces, except from especially weak and painful joints.
3. Grasp and Release: Open your fingers, reach into the rice and grasp some, lift it up, drop it. Repeat for about 30 seconds.
4. Front and Back Wrists: Grab handfuls of rice (this is to prevent your hand from being crushed in while you do the exercise; people without hypermobility would simply make fists to do this exercise). Holding the handfuls of rice, move your wrists front and back, digging down into the rice. When you reach a comfortable depth, continue to do the forward and back wrist movement for about 30 seconds. Do not move your wrists too far forward or back. When your hands are stronger, you can try doing this without rice filling your hands but with empty fists, trying not to let the pressure of the rice crush your hand in.

5. Side to Side Wrists: Grab handfuls of rice (as above), move your wrists side to side, digging down into the rice for 30 seconds. Do not move your wrists too far to the sides.
6. Wrist Circles: Grab handfuls of rice (as above), move your wrists in a circular motion, digging down into the rice for 30 seconds. Stay within an appropriate range of motion.
7. Stable Flicks: With one or two fingers of each hand, hold the finger in an almost-straight position, and flick the rice away from you, using movement of the wrist to make the flick happen and careful not to straighten your fingers so far that they hyperextend. You may need to start with a very rounded finger to build strength, and each week hold your finger a little straighter. Go slowly at first to learn what the limit feels like. Start at the top of the rice and then go deeper as you get stronger. Start with 15 seconds of flicking and then do 15 seconds with the next finger(s) until you have used them all.
8. Finger Flicks: With one or two fingers of each hand, keeping the wrist still, use the movement of the finger from very bent to almost straight to flick the rice. Start at the top of the rice and then go deeper as you get stronger. Do not hyperextend the fingers. Start with 15 seconds of flicking and then do 15 seconds with the next finger(s) until you have used them all.
9. Merry Go Round: Using one hand at a time, hold the fingers in an almost straight position, keep the wrist in the center of the bucket, and make circles with the wrist so that the fingers draw a circle in the rice around the outside of the bucket. Do not let the fingers hyperextend, and keep the wrist within the appropriate range of motion. Start at the top of the rice and then go deeper as you get stronger. Do 15 seconds or more with each hand.
10. Swimming: Cup your hands so that all of your fingers are round, then dig the fingertips into the rice, using a front-and-back, flipper-like motion and digging down deeper and deeper. When you have gone as deep as you want to go, pull your hands up and do it again, as many times as you desire. As you get stronger, make your cupped fingers straighter until they are all the way straight and wiggling like flippers, careful as always not to let them hyperextend.
11. Finger Grasps: Pinch rice between your pointer finger(s) and your thumb(s) and pick it up, then drop it. Keep your fingers and thumbs curved, and repeat for 30 seconds. Then, pinch rice using your middle finger(s) and thumb(s) and then ring and pinkies with thumbs as well. As you get stronger over weeks or months, reduce the curve of your fingers until you can do it with fingers straight and not hyperextended.
12. Shaolin Monk Prayer: With cupped hands, twist your wrists to scoop rice into the palms of the hands, lift it up, twist your wrists to let the rice fall, and bring your hands together into a prayer clap. Your fingers should be pressed together, completely straight; make sure that neither hand is being pressed so hard that the finger joints hyperextend. Your movements should begin slowly, but as you get stronger, the prayer clap at the end should get faster. Once you can do this well, do not touch your hands together when they do the prayer clap position — keep them a few inches apart so that instead of your hands stopping each other in the straight position, they are using their own strength to stop themselves in the straight position. Make this silent clap sudden, and hold it for a moment before repeating; it may take a long time before you can get all of your fingers to behave — my pinkie fingers gave me particular trouble. You may try using a brace or splint to support those particularly troublesome joints but be sure to exercise them bare as well.

61

Sports & Hobbies

SPORTS AND HOBBIES ARE FUN AND GOOD FOR YOU.[760, 761] As mentioned in Chapter 3: The Benefits of hEDS/HSD, hypermobility can be seen as an asset, not a liability, and this is potentially most obvious when participating in sports and hobbies. Your easy flexibility can give you a tactical advantage, agility, and grace, whether you are playing soccer, dancing, holding a paintbrush, or crocheting. That always feels good.

Sports and hobbies also bring us enjoyment as well as beneficial exercise for the mind and body. These activities are likely to be building the strength that you need in order to protect your joints and keep your mind young, but they can be so much fun that you don't even notice that you're doing something to build your health. Frequently, there is a social aspect that is health giving as well.

However, we need to be careful. Most obviously, we need to protect ourselves from injury. (See Chapter 9: Joint Instability & Pain.) Try not to get so caught up in the competition or the artistry that you don't notice when you are pushing your limits. Use the braces or tools that you need to keep yourself in a safe zone.

As far as I know, no scientists have rigorously studied the effects of various sports and hobbies on people with hEDS. For now, with very little to go on, I would guess that sports, including those that use a lot of flexibility like dancing, but not including those that are particularly rough and come with a high risk of injury like American football, are mostly good for you, as long as they are done with caution.

I have seen comments in social media groups from several professionally performing contortionists who regretted their careers — although they did not feel pain at the time that they were doing the contortions, the joints that they routinely hyperextended have since degraded into arthritis.

I don't want you to stop dancing — or doing whatever you love to do, but if you are in a state of chronic illness, I do recommend avoiding hyperextending no matter what. Be more cautious than you will be once you get back to a state of health. You have to give your body a chance to heal without activating the fight/flight response that comes up when a joint is being threatened. During the time that you are healing, kick your leg, but don't kick it so high.

And remember that mast cells can be activated by the stress of strenuous exercise. Don't go overboard; pay attention to your body and its limits.

While you are observing your limits, go ahead and have fun. One of the benefits of sports and hobbies is that they are so much fun you don't even realize that you are exercising your body and mind. Even just looking at a drawing of a happy face makes a person stronger in the moment, so enjoy yourself![762] Happiness is good for your health![763]

My Experience with Sports and Hobbies

I myself and numerous people I have known have suffered an injury and then been told by the doctor to stop moving. "Don't ever dance again," my doctor told me. Two men I knew were told, "Don't ever lift weights again." For a time, we obeyed the doctors, but our injuries did not improve and our happiness certainly decreased. So, each of us soon began to move again, to do exercises that would strengthen the injured area, and to carefully become involved in our beloved sports. My supposed-dance-stopping injury occurred when I was a teenager, but I went on to have a 30-year career as a dancer. Both of those young men healed injuries that were supposed to be un-healable; they were supposed to live with that pain for the rest of their lives, but they both went on to lift weights and lead very active lives full of sports, adventure hiking, kayaking, wood chopping, and more.

I have spent nearly my entire life as a dancer and gymnast, stretching and pushing the boundaries of my flexibility, but I have always been fastidious about treating injuries as soon as I could figure out how.

A year before I learned about hEDS, I had closed my dance studio and professional performance company in anticipation of some personal life changes; I barely ever danced during that year. During that time, I was trying to heal my various Joint Injuries and secondary conditions, but I saw little improvement compared to what I experienced in the 6 months after learning about hEDS.

It seemed to me that most of the hyperextending that I was doing for dance was done in a position of strength and control; it had only a slight or negligible effect on my overall health. On the other hand, it seemed that the hyperextending that I was doing in daily life activities — reaching behind myself to pull open a drawer, hyperextending my fingers whenever I worked with my hands, letting my hip pop out when I leaned the laundry basket against it — were causing more pain and Sympathetic Nervous System activation. The serious pelvic displacements and Rib Subluxations, caused mostly by daily activities, that I had lived with for years actually seemed to cause the most pain and Sympathetic Nervous System activation; I should have been more determined to heal those conditions as soon as they occurred.

Recently, when I was working on healing my Rib Subluxations, I had almost succeeded but still had a little bit of pain in one rib. Then for my sister's birthday, the family went to play pickleball. By the end of the hour of play, there was no more pain in my back. After about a week, a little bit of the pain came back every now and then, so I went to play pickleball with my husband, and again, my back became strong, the rib pain disappeared, and I could do anything. I even forgot about my erstwhile rib pain. I could see that continuing to play pickleball on a regular basis would keep my rib cage healthy, and soon it came to be a favorite pastime.

Some of the other sports I have enjoyed participating in in recent months are soccer, swimming, baseball, dancing, croquet, archery, walking, tennis, adventure hiking, kayaking, bicycling, trampolining, and basketball. At this point in my life, I am not joining any teams, playing competitively, or doing physical work professionally. As I have been healing, I have needed to have the control to do just what feels good to me without the pressure to support teammates or fulfill obligations. I've been participating in sports for fun, exercise, fresh air, and sunshine.[764] It feels good to be alive.

Step-By-Step Instructions for Participating in Sports and Hobbies

The kinds of precautions you need to take before participating in sports and hobbies will depend on your physical fitness, joint laxity, overall health, experience, and more. Ask your doctor before trying anything new.

Cautions for Participating in Sports and Hobbies

1. If you have a weak, unstable joint, use a brace, splint, or kinesiology tape on it while you participate.
2. Warm up rather than stretching out. Do Range of Motion exercises. Do not try to force joints to become more flexible.
3. Do not fatigue yourself. Take breaks. Do not try to prove anything to anyone else.
4. Learn to work ambidextrously so that when one hand or foot becomes tired, you can use the other one.
5. Do cross-training to build the strength you need to protect your joints. Also do cross-training to counteract any potential overuse from your specific activities. (For example, if a ballet dancer works with her legs turned out, she also needs to work with her legs turned in.)
6. Choose hobbies that do not produce fumes that you may react to if you have Allergies/MCAS/MCS or Peripheral Neuralgia: wire shaping uses only metal, needle felting uses wool, whittling uses wood, basket and wreath weaving use plant materials, beaded jewelry making uses stones, glass, and natural-fiber cords, crocheting or knitting uses cotton or wool yarn (and special crochet rings or other adaptive tools to make it easier on your hands).
7. Choose alternative supplies that are safer than petroleum-based products. Carpenters can use old-world joinery instead of glue, and natural nut oils instead of varnish and polyurethane. Painters can use watercolors instead of acrylics, and even try making your own paints out of foods and plants. Pastels, pencils, and beeswax crayons are good alternatives to paints and markers. If your craft uses glue, like scrapbooking, try glue dots, stickers, and tapes that will have fewer fumes than liquid glues.
8. Smile and have fun. (People are stronger when they see smiles as compared to frowns. [765])

62

Strength Training

STRENGTH TRAINING OR RESISTANCE TRAINING is one of the most important things that people with hEDS/HSD can do for our health. If we can build up the muscles that support the joints, then we will be much less likely to suffer Joint Injuries and the trauma states that can follow.

Strength Training is a practice of building muscular strength by using free weights, specialized machines, resistance bands, or your own body weight. In addition to being protective of the joints, it improves movement, prevents diabetes, lifts mood, raises metabolism, decreases cardiovascular disease, improves the condition of the arteries, increases bone mineral density, reverses age-related complaints, enhances mental health, and more.[766]

Unfortunately, weight lifting is not the activity that most hypermobile people are drawn to. Most of us have experienced joint pain when we tried to do something that required strength, like carrying a heavy box. Our muscles weren't prepared, and our ligaments weren't strong enough to hold the weight. So, Strength Training is something we will have to do purposefully and carefully.

Fortunately, there are gyms all throughout the world where you can access weight equipment and hire a personal trainer. In my town, at one of the parks, there are areas with exercise equipment with which you lift your own body weight. Inexpensive hand weights and resistance bands are easily available for purchase and take up very little storage room, making them ideal for use at home. And of course, you can use your own body weight for calisthenics, which is completely free and always accessible. Plus, there are now experts posting free videos on YouTube, as well as hosting paid services, such as Whealth and Jeannie di Bon.

https://www.youtube.com/@whealth_

https://www.youtube.com/@JeannieDiBonHypermobility

Note also that tongue posture can affect your strength and posture stability.[767] Keep your tongue pressed to the full length of the roof of your mouth while you are Strength Training. See Chapter 23: Mouth Health.

My Experience with Strength Training

I had done very little Strength Training in my life before I met my husband. I have to admit that it is not something I enjoy or even feel comfortable doing. However, with his guidance, I have discovered that Strength Training is the most important thing I can do to keep my body feeling good. None of my injuries would be healed if I had not built the strength in the muscles around the damaged joints.

I remember that there was a dancer in my professional company who was flawless in her dancing. She could command her body to do anything for the art, and her body would do it. She was dedicated to Strength Training at Crossfit Infinity, and although she was the strongest dancer I'd ever seen, she also had the most feminine, beautiful lines and extensions.

I have also witnessed people who were prone to injuries begin Strength Training and then stop getting injured frequently. It seems that even for the more active of us, our lifestyle is too sedentary and easy for our health. We need to Strength Train.

Step-By-Step Instructions for Strength Training

Ask your doctor before trying anything new.

Strength Train Safely and Effectively

1. Warm yourself up by doing Range of Motion exercises first.
2. If you have POTS, choose Strength Training exercises that are either lying down or upright but not leaning forward.
3. Do not try to do a specific number of "reps" (repetitions). It is better to try to go for a certain amount of time. But even better might be to go until you don't feel quite as strong anymore. You do not want to fatigue your muscles, as you need them to retain their strength to support your fragile joints — training to fatigue may work for other people, but not those with hEDS/HSD.
4. Work one set of muscles briefly and then switch to another. Continue changing which set of muscles you are working, and come back around to them later. The idea is to get a good workout with rest periods built in for the muscles so that they do not fatigue. You also want to try to get to all of the muscle groups in the body at least once a week.
5. Use heavier weights or greater resistance rather than more reps. As soon as an exercise feels easy, increase the weight you use for it.
6. Keep good posture, and especially be sure not to hyperextend nor move your neck in the wrong way. Go slowly in everything you do so that you can be sure of staying safe — going slowly is a good way to build muscle anyway.
7. Drink plenty of water with electrolytes.
8. If you are using any braces or splints, try not to rely on them. Use them for protection, but practice good form so that you will build the strength of your muscles rather than testing the strength of the braces. The eventual goal is to be able to discard the braces and rely on your own strength.
9. If you injure yourself, stop right away and do the recommended treatments from Chapter 9: Joint Instability & Pain.
10. Following the workout session, get a massage or use self-massage to keep the muscles and fascia flexible and keep the fluids moving through the tissues.

11. Do not Strength Train every day. Make sure to include walking and aerobic exercises such as swimming or dancing, as well as rest, in your weekly workout routine.

63

Vagus Nerve Stimulation

THE VAGUS NERVE IS THE LARGEST NERVE in the body and its name means wandering. It wanders directly out of the head instead of descending through the spinal column, and from there it touches everything from the ear to the throat, heart, gastrointestinal system, and all of the organs of the trunk.[768, 769]

As it wanders, the Vagus Nerve takes messages to and from the brain, telling the brain what is going on in the body and then telling the body what to do about it. For this reason, scientists have found that the microbiome in the gut (the bacteria that live in the intestines) can affect the behavior of the Vagus Nerve.

The Vagus Nerve is the main component of the Parasympathetic Nervous System. The Parasympathetic Nervous System controls the rest-and-digest functions of the body (as opposed to the Sympathetic Nervous System that controls the fight/flight response). Some people who experience trauma, stress, or pain end up with their Sympathetic Nervous System so activated that they are always in the fight/flight response and are never able to fully relax, which means their bodies are also unable to effectively digest food, heal injuries, or maintain a state of health.

An overactive Sympathetic Nervous System can cause symptoms like high blood pressure, high blood sugar levels, bowel disease, obesity, inflammation, heart disease, depression, anxiety, and gastrointestinal problems.[770] It can also exacerbate Allergies/MCAS/MCS. For those of us who have been unable to cure Digestive System Problems with probiotics, diet changes, and lifestyle changes, it may be because the problems are neurogenic (coming from the nervous system).[771]

Fortunately, if you stimulate the Vagus Nerve in the right ways, you can help the body return to the parasympathetic state and an anti-inflammatory healing mode.[772] In order for the stimulation techniques to be effective, the Vagus Nerve needs to be in a healthy state, so some of the techniques I will list here include protecting it from damage and nourishing it for repairing itself.

Doctors sometimes stimulate the Vagus Nerve using an electronic device that can be implanted; this is effective for eliminating epilepsy, depression, and other serious conditions. For most of us, these extremes are not necessary. There are handheld electronic Vagus Nerve Stimulation devices available for purchase, but there are also a lot of free, easy, and comfortable ways to stimulate the Vagus Nerve.

If your Vagus Nerve is in a healthy state and is properly activating a parasympathetic state, you will have what is called "good Vagal tone." This can be measured with Heart Rate Variability (HRV). You want your heart rate at rest to be very low and your heartrate when exercising to be much higher. The greater the difference in the heartrate (the greater the HRV), the better the vagal tone (to a point). HRV is a strong predictor of outcome in many critical illnesses.[773, 774] (Of course, POTS can complicate this measurement — the variability seen in POTS episodes does not indicate a healthy HRV.) You can measure your HRV yourself with one of any number of heart rate monitors available for sale.

My Experience with Vagus Nerve Stimulation

For many years, I would try so very hard to relax. It was really a running joke among my close friends. I could tell that my Sympathetic Nervous System was activated and that I needed to stimulate my Vagus Nerve. I have tried all of the different suggestions, and always, they help some...but it wasn't until I stopped hyperextending and started protecting my joints (and added DAO to my personal supplement program) that my nervous system was able to calm down. At that point, I still needed to purposefully stimulate the Vagus Nerve in order for my Parasympathetic Nervous System to start taking some control and it has felt wonderful to finally "rest and digest."

Step-By-Step Instructions for Vagus Nerve Stimulation

Ask your doctor before trying anything new.

Natural Vagus Nerve Stimulation

1. Take Parasym Plus for proper operation of the nervous system (this may be contraindicated if you have Dystonia).[775, 776]
2. Take a probiotic for gut health so that the Vagus Nerve knows that everything is OK.
3. Strengthen your neck so that you will not risk damaging the Vagus Nerve in the neck, which is the location where damage is most likely to occur to the Vagus Nerve. See Chapter 25: Neck Pain & CCI.
4. Do the Valsalva Maneuver.[777] Take a deep breath, close your mouth and pinch your nose, try to breathe out, straining against your throat to increase pressure in the chest. Then release the nose and breathe out as normal.
5. Sing, chant, or hum. This is my favorite way of stimulating the Vagus Nerve to activate the rest-and-digest mode.
6. Shine red light in your ear. I like to do this with my NIR device.[778]
7. Use an electric ear clip stimulator.
8. Take a cold shower or splash cold water on your face. You can use ice cubes or a cold washcloth on your face and neck if you prefer.
9. Do yoga, breathing deeply.[779]
10. Meditate.
11. Make a social connection.
12. Do slow, deep breathing.
13. Laugh!
14. Pray. In particular, learn to live in faith rather than worry.
15. Exercise.
16. Get a massage.
17. Fast. Going without food for a length of time can improve vagal tone.[780, 781]

18. Get acupuncture.
19. Remove as much stress from your life as you possible can.

LINKS FOR PRODUCTS MENTIONED IN THIS CHAPTER

Heart Rate Monitor https://amzn.to/499fbxD
Parasym Plus https://amzn.to/484v0VF
Probiotic https://amzn.to/3HkFUeX
Red Light Therapy https://amzn.to/48ritwy
Ear Clip Vagus Nerve Stimulator https://amzn.to/484v0VF

Section VI

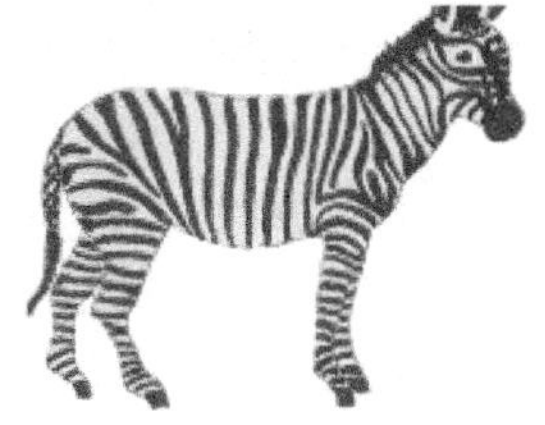

Seek Professional Help

64

Medical Professionals & Complementary-&-Alternative Medical Professionals Who Treat Symptoms of hEDS/HSD

OUR WORLD IS BLESSED WITH AN ABUNDANCE OF professionals who want to help you thrive. They are educated and experienced, and they feel fulfilled and pleased when they see you get better under their care.

However, I caution you to be aware that there are also professionals, both in the medical field and Complementary-and-Alternative (CAM) field, who do not understand hEDS, or who care more about making money than helping their patients, or whose egos will be threatened by the difficult kind of case an hEDS/HSD patient can present. There are countless reports online and in my own social circle of people with hEDS/HSD who have been gaslighted or otherwise mistreated by professionals. It is important that you stand up for yourself and use your own intelligence. If a professional tells you something that doesn't seem right to you or is offensive, don't let it get you down. Get a second opinion.

Standing up for yourself is not only important in the face of a professional who does not have your best interest at heart or is not adequately informed about your condition; standing up for yourself is also the way to get the best results from your time with the really good professionals. Tell them all of the details of what your experience is because of this condition. Tell them what help you really need. If they cannot provide the help you need, ask them for a referral to someone else who might be able to.

Also, keep in mind when you are meeting with a professional that people with hEDS have often gotten used to living with enormous amounts of pain. Do not underreport what you are experiencing or you will not get the help you need. Most of the professionals I have met with have asked me about my pain on a scale of 1 to 10. Think about this before you go in. Remind yourself that the amount of pain a person is supposed to have when they aren't injured is 0.

Acupuncturists and Chinese Medicine Doctors

Many people with hEDS have reported that acupuncture can help with their symptoms, especially reducing pain. However, others like myself are very averse to the pain of needle work. Fortunately, most acupuncturists specialize in other aspects of Traditional Chinese Medicine (TCM) as well. They can provide moxibustion, acupressure, cupping, herbs, meditation, and other treatments that are enjoyable and helpful.

In addition to that, some Chinese medicine clinics also host other healing modalities, such as Herbal Medicine, Functional Release Method Body Work, Craniosacral Therapy, Massage, and Life Constellation Work. (These are some of the offerings at the clinic in my town.)

Ayurveda Practitioners

Ayurveda is the ancient Indian medical tradition, and a session with one of these practitioners is much more thorough than what we are used to when we go to see our Primary Care Physicians. A few days after my 1 ½ hour intake session with the practitioner who worked at my healing center, the practitioner gave me a printout of diet and lifestyle recommendations personalized to me that was 48 pages long. I did not request to be recommended any supplements or other treatments, but Ayurveda practitioners have those at their disposal as well. The recommendations helped me greatly, and I also saw our practitioner's other clients resolve their problems quickly and easily through her help.

Chiropractors

In my experience, Chiropractors give quick fixes that are affordable, and they are easy to find. Even most small towns have a Chiropractor or two. Most of them accept insurance, and if they do not take yours, they will probably offer an affordable price for a session.

Chiropractors often have X-ray machines in their offices, and it can be very helpful to really see what is going on with your joints. They have a lot of experience treating joints that are misaligned, so they will know what to do with your joint problems.

I highly recommend that people with hEDS/HSD request that your Chiropractor use the Activator Tool rather than manual manipulation on your body. Our bodies are a little traumatized by our joints slipping out of alignment so much, and the manual manipulations they typically do can cause the muscles around the joint to freeze up in hypertonicity. The Activator Tool is much gentler and, in my experience, the results last longer.

Even with the Activator Tool, though, Chiropractic adjustments do not usually last as long as Osteopathic or Craniosacral ones. If you have had a sudden injury, Chiropractic is likely to work, but for longer standing conditions, Chiropractic work will also be a long-standing healing method — you may have to return to the office once a week for years. Also, even with the Activator, Chiropractors can be rough and cause pain, so be sure to voice what your specific needs are.

Many Chiropractors' offices also offer other treatments, such as electric muscle stimulation therapy (EMS), massage therapy, exercise recommendations, and more, and all of these options are usually either covered by insurance or fairly inexpensive.

Craniosacral Therapists

Craniosacral Therapy is an exceptionally gentle treatment that results in an adjustment of the bones and membranes of the skull, spine, and pelvis and regulation of the cerebrospinal fluid that circulates throughout the brain and spinal cord.

CST is one of my favorite treatments to receive. During a session, the patient sits or lies on a massage or examination table, usually fully clothed. The therapist uses exceedingly light touch on the head and along the spine or other body parts, usually holding the touch in certain spots for several minutes. When my jaw troubles me, the therapist actually puts her gloved fingers in my mouth to hold certain points. Honestly, it usually feels like the therapist is not doing anything, but while it is happening, a sense of peace, calm, and relaxation descends upon me. Following the session, I move more freely and feel energized.

CST can relieve pain, Migraines, skeletal misalignments, depression, some tongue ties, anxiety, and much, much more. When my baby was a few months old, we started having trouble with breastfeeding, and with one CST appointment for the both of us, the problem was resolved — he started breastfeeding so well that within the next week he grew two clothing sizes!

After receiving training, some people are able to do CST on themselves. During a short workshop I took, I was able to feel the craniosacral rhythm in my own body, but it took intense concentration. I can imagine that if doing CST comes naturally to you, it would be a wonderful tool to have to be able to treat yourself any time you need it.

CST therapists can often be found at holistic healing centers like the one I ran, but they are also at other kinds of locations, like Traditional Chinese Medicine clinics. And, the Osteopath I see uses craniosacral therapy during some of his sessions.

Doctors

Although this book does not encompass the medical treatments available to treat hEDS/HSD and its comorbidities, and although I have not had positive experiences seeking help from the medical establishment, I have heard and read reports from many individuals who have found wonderful doctors who have solved their problems.

I do caution you that some doctors not only do not know what to do for hEDS/HSD patients; they do not want to treat them at all. Some people who have hEDS find it difficult to get the surgery or other treatment they need because the doctors in their area are afraid of the hEDS patient in general. They are afraid of what can go wrong, and they do not know enough to keep it from going wrong. You may be turned away just when you really need help.

Also be aware that many people with hEDS do not respond well to pharmaceutical medications or medical procedures. Find out as much as you can about yourself and the treatment options before you try anything new, whether medical or alternative. There are many medications to be avoided if you have hEDS, MCAS, Peripheral Neuropathy, etc. There are also excipients (additional, inactive ingredients in medications) that you may need to avoid — you may be able to have your medication compounded specifically for your needs at a local pharmacy. The lists of medications and excipients to avoid for specific conditions are frequently updated, so do a thorough online search for these lists as they pertain to you before beginning a medication.

Still, I encourage you to try to find a doctor near you who is knowledgeable about hEDS/HSD and enthusiastic about helping you live the life you want to live.

Fortunately, many doctors now offer telehealth appointments so that you can try out a doctor without risking getting triggered by anything in their clinic.

There is also one clinic in the United States that specializes in hEDS, and I hear that at least one more is planning to open. Perhaps by the time you read this book there will be hEDS specialists near you.

Medical Specialists Who Might Know About hEDS

1. Biologic Dentists — dentists who recognize the connection between dental health and the whole body, mind, and spirit and use more natural techniques.
2. ENTs — doctors who specialize in the Ear, Nose, and Throat.
3. Gastroenterologists — doctors who specialize in the digestive system.
4. Naturopaths — doctors who work from a holistic viewpoint (considering the patient as a whole, looking for root causes rather than focusing on easing specific symptoms) and use an integrative approach (using both medical and alternative treatments such as herbs).
5. Neurologists — doctors who diagnose, treat and manage disorders of the brain and nervous system.
6. Orthopedists — doctors who specialize in injuries and diseases affecting the musculoskeletal system.
7. Primary Care Physicians — doctors who perform regular check-ups, will likely be the first doctor you see about any new symptom or concern, and can make referrals to the specialists you need.
8. Rheumatologists — doctors who specialize in musculoskeletal disease and systemic autoimmune conditions; many patients see them for arthritis symptoms.
9. Pulmonologists — doctors who specialize in lung conditions.

Massage Therapists

Usually, Massage Therapists specialize in certain techniques, so find the one that your body needs at any given time. Some of the helpful therapies are Myofascial Release, deep tissue massage, trigger point therapy, and Lymph Drainage Massage.

I have had very good results from sessions of another kind of massage, Thai Body Work, but I have also had some bad results. This is a massage technique that combines acupressure and passive stretching. I believe that because of the stretching, it is easy for a practitioner to go too far — a lot of yoga enthusiasts get excited when they see our full range of motion.

An assisted stretching technique that I found to be more helpful than Thai Body Work is Strain/Counterstrain, which my Massage Therapist did for me. Again, I caution you to do this only with a professional who is familiar with hypermobility and aware of your condition.

Meditation Guides

At the holistic healing center that I owned for over 10 years, one of my favorite healing modalities that I offered was guided meditations. In some instances, I was able to cure a client of a life-long, debilitating problem in just one session. It is almost miraculous to find such results from a non-invasive, totally safe, easy, empowering exercise.

Be aware that frequently, mediation guides will suggest that you sit upright in a chair with your feet on the ground, which is a position that is very difficult for hypermobile people to relax in. Request an accommodation to sit in a more comfortable position, or be reclined or lying down — supported by pillows and warmed by blankets in whichever position you choose.

Here is a list of my favorite guided meditations. Some of them are simple enough that you can learn to guide yourself through the meditation and use it again and again. However, it is often very nice, if you can afford it, to have a professional accompany you through your meditative journey. These are my favorite meditations that I do for myself or clients:

1. Archangel Michael: ask him to draw out negative, stagnant energy from every part of your body and then fill your body with vibrant, healthy light energy.
2. Body Scan: focusing on one body part at a time, going slowly until the entire body has been examined, notice what is going on in that body part — if there is pain, tension, a desire to move, an emotion that arises when you focus on the body part; just notice it and recognize it. Don't judge it or try to change it during the mediation.
3. Connectedness (or Roots Down, Branches Up): inspired by the prayer in Starhawk's *The Twelve Wild Swans*, connect your body to the world around you and down all of the way to the center of the Earth, and up all of the way to the center of the Universe.
4. Deep Breathing: the breath is extremely important for health, and paying attention to the breath can bring our attention away from our worries and right to our center. Breathing meditations are relaxing and invigorating.
5. *Feeding Your Demons*: turn any health issue into a monster that you can face, and then turn yourself into exactly what that monster is lacking and feed yourself to the monster until it transforms the monster into an ally. This sounds odd, but it is very powerful. Get more information from the book of the same name by Tsultrim Allione.
6. Healing: focus on the specific health concern, encourage the body to make the needed changes.
7. Higher Self: it is difficult to know what is best for ourselves, but our Higher Selves know, and if we can meet them and talk with them, they may give insight.
8. Mediumship with Loved Ones: it is a relief to know that our departed loved ones are OK and watching over us; sometimes, they can give us information we have not found on our own.
9. Muscle Relaxation: there are many different metaphors that can help relax muscles during meditation.
10. Past Life Regressions: with a very specific healing intention in mind, re-examine experiences from past lives to see how they might be affecting your health, behavior, and decisions now so that you can act from a position of understanding.
11. Personalized Meditations: often, spirit guides will want to work with patients, or there are symbols or imagery that are meaningful for a patient to focus on; visualizing problems, solutions, and ideals can be very helpful.

Note that you may also benefit from other meditation forms, such as Transcendental Meditation or Affirmation Meditations. There are many books on the subject, such as *Transcendental Meditation* by Jack Forem, as well as many teachers you can seek out.

Occupational Therapists

I have not had the pleasure of working with an Occupational Therapist, but I have heard wonderful reviews from others who have. Especially if you develop a disability, an Occupational Therapist will have ideas for helping you cope and manage your life that you may never have considered.

Osteopaths

Osteopaths are licensed medical doctors who practice in all areas of medicine but emphasize a whole-person, mind-body-spirit approach. Rather than simply treating symptoms, they give special attention to preventing potential problems and supporting well-being. Their focus is on the musculoskeletal system (muscles, bones, and nerves), which is especially helpful for people with hypermobility.

A Doctor of Osteopathy uses manual body-work techniques to help align the skeleton and mobilize joints. With the hands-on treatments an Osteopath uses, he does not force the joints into alignment but instead encourages the body to align itself. He may also run diagnostic tests, such as blood or urine tests and imaging tests, prescribe medication, perform surgery, and make exercise and lifestyle recommendations.

I highly value my Osteopath, as do my son, mother, and sister. What he does for me is similar to what I used to see the Chiropractor for, but it is more thorough and better for my body. We always feel great after a session with the Osteopath, and I expect that this may be the most important kind of doctor for many people with hypermobility to see frequently.

Personal Trainers

Once you have completed Physical Therapy, you will probably be ready for a personal trainer who can guide you through workouts for strength and stamina building. Personal trainers can be found at gyms and also working independently and traveling to your home or place of work. They often have weights, resistance bands, and other tools that you can use to get exactly the workout you need. Strength and stamina building are extremely important for keeping people with hEDS/HSD healthy — keep your joints in place, prevent POTS episodes, keep lymph and digestion moving, etc.

Unfortunately, it may be hard to find a personal trainer who is familiar with hEDS/HSD, so you will probably need to keep yourself educated about your special needs and be vocal about them. Personal trainers usually spend a lot of their effort motivating, encouraging, and pushing their clients to do more than they thought they could do. You will need to make sure you know the difference between doing more than you were capable of yesterday and doing more than you should do today. It really is helpful to be pushed — especially for someone with hEDS/HSD who is scared because of all of the injuries you have had before. So, find a personal trainer you can trust, and also trust that if you go just a little bit too far, you have the tools to heal yourself and come back as strong as ever.

Jeannie di Bon and some other online hEDS experts have recommended that you not aim to do a certain number of reps but rather to go for a certain amount of time, no matter how slowly you go. This works well for me. What works even better for me is to do as many reps as I can do before it becomes more difficult than it was at first. It is not a good idea for someone with hEDS/HSD to fatigue their muscles.

Also, always be careful to stay within your range of motion. Do not straighten your elbows or knees or fingers past what looks straight. Pay attention to how strong you feel, and if you extend to a point that you feel less strong, that means that you have hyperextended and should reduce your range of motion there.

Physical Therapists

As with doctors, there are PTs who understand hEDS/HSD and those who do not. Be bold about finding a PT who is a good match for you. Try not to spend time with a PT who does not understand your body or hypermobility — more than a waste of time, it may be dangerous. Your PT should understand that your normal range of motion is greater than the average person's, that stretching your joints is almost always a bad idea, and that you need to take extra measures to stabilize your joints.

A good PT will possibly be the most valuable tool in your toolbox for thriving with hEDS/HSD. They have many techniques at their disposal to diagnose and treat your problems. For example, they will do Myofascial Release, trigger point therapy, moist heat, cupping, and more in addition to teaching you exercises and techniques to treat and cope with your condition. One of the commonly used PT techniques to be cautious of is dry needling — although this is effective for some people with hEDS/HSD, I have heard of numerous people with MCAS having bad results from it.

At the end of every session, ask the PT to give you a written list of all of the exercises you have been recommended to do. It is best if the list includes a description of the exercise, drawings or photos of it, and instructions regarding the number of repetitions or amount of time to do the exercises. You can also write your own notes in the margins. Keep these papers in a folder forever. You may need to refer to them years later when an old injury flares up again. Some clinics now provide online videos for their patients to follow, but written notes are a helpful accompaniment to the videos.

One of the most important things to write on your exercise list is what symptoms the exercise will alleviate. I have a list with hand-drawn illustrations that says, "When it hurts here...do this."

These exercises are also a good basis for a personal training regimen — even when you move on to different workouts, it is a good idea to keep rotating a few of these exercises along with the new ones.

The PT will also make recommendations such as to take a warm bath with Epsom salts. Do not hesitate to ask for their advice about ways in which the injury they are addressing is affecting your life.

Pilates Teachers

A series of private sessions on a reformer with a Pilates Teacher can be extremely beneficial. The reformer is a brilliantly designed machine that will support your body as you move in precise ways. A good Pilates Teacher will listen to you describe any pain in your body and will know how to strengthen your body to reduce the pain, and the reformer will help keep your body supported so that you don't injure it.

Pilates studios sometimes also offer reformer classes and mat classes, all of which are helpful once you are ready for the next step. Pilates is among the best forms of exercise for people with hEDS/HSD.

Reiki Practitioners and Teachers

At the holistic healing center that I owned for 10 years, this was our most popularly requested healing treatment. It is energy healing — laying on of hands as mentioned in The Bible — working with the divine to bring about what is in your highest good. Reiki can heal physical ailments, emotional pain, and even situational problems.

During a Reiki session, the client lies fully clothed, usually on a massage table or other comfortable surface, and the Reiki practitioner directs healing energy through her hands toward the client. Depending on preferences, the practitioner may or may not touch the client. Even when the practitioner does laying on of hands, she does not manipulate the body at all; the hands lie still while the energy pours out of them.

A Reiki session usually feels very calming and warming, but many different sensations and experiences can occur. It is common for Reiki to cause tingling, emotional release, and more, but sometimes clients do not even feel it happening. Sometimes clients fall asleep on the table and wake well rested but unaware of the healing that happened during the session. (You can ask your practitioner to keep you awake if you do not want to sleep.)

Reiki has been shown to help relax you as compared to a placebo treatment,[782, 783, 784, 785] whether it is performed in person or from a distant location.[786, 787, 788] Scientists have also found that the electromagnetic wavelengths that radiate from a Reiki Master's hands when giving Reiki are different from their normal wavelengths, and that they change depending on whom and which part they are working on.[789] Some of these wavelengths are the same as those of the ultrasound machines used at hospitals to speed healing.

In all large cities and some small towns, you will be able to find a Reiki healer. You will probably also be able to find classes in which you can learn to do Reiki. It is very easy for most people, though it does take a lot of training, experience, and dedication to get the kind of results that some Reiki Masters can get.

I strongly recommend that you learn to do Reiki on yourself. The military teaches Reiki to their fighters who are at risk of being captured so that they can heal themselves while they are in a prisoner of war camp.[790] On bad days, when you're stuck in bed, you can do Reiki on yourself so that you feel better faster. On other days, you can do Reiki on yourself during a break so that you keep feeling good.

Reiki also can be sent and received across distances. I offer long-distance Reiki sessions, and you can choose whether you are present via Zoom or text, or not at all. One of the really effective ways of receiving a Reiki treatment is to request that it be sent from a long distance while you are napping or otherwise relaxing.

Section VII

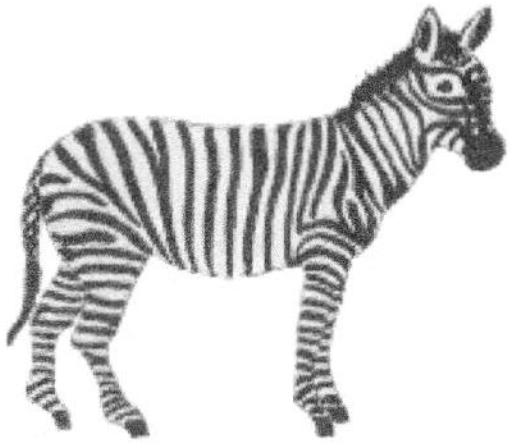

Be Well

65

Hypermobile and Happy Review

THE PREMISE OF NATURALLY HEALING THE symptoms of hEDS/HSD is simple: stop harm.

Stop the Harm Caused by Hypermobility

1. **Protect your joints from hyperextending and dislocating.** In order to do this, adjust movement patterns, increase muscular strength, take nutritional supplements, and use adaptations like braces and tools. *While you are healing Joint Injuries and the secondary conditions they cause, treat symptoms in natural ways to reduce Sympathetic Nervous System overactivity.*
2. **Protect your body from toxins and stressors,** to which it will be more susceptible than the general population. Avoid petrochemicals and your personal allergens or triggers in foods, cleaning products, scents, building materials, etc. *While you are healing sensitivities and the secondary conditions they cause, treat symptoms in natural ways to reduce immune system overactivity.*
3. **Interrupt the feedback loops.** The symptoms of hEDS/HSD and their secondary conditions and common comorbidities serve as feedback loops for each other. You will need to treat all of the conditions and comorbidities concurrently so that you can feel better while you are healing and heal faster. *Interrupt the feedback loops everywhere you can.*
4. **Focus on individual steps.** You cannot do everything at once. *Add only 1-3 new things at a time so that you can analyze how they affect you.*
5. **Don't give up.** Keep going, even when it's hard, even when you mess up, even when the answers are not clear. *You've got this!*

> Stop the Harm Caused by Hypermobility
>
> 1. Protect your joints from hyperextending and dislocating.
> 2. Protect your body from toxins and stressors.
> 3. Interrupt the feedback loops.
> 4. Focus on individual steps.
> 5. Don't give up.
> 6. Celebrate successes.
>
> Ask your doctor before trying anything new.

6. **Celebrate successes.** Even while you are healing, enjoy your life. Look on the bright side whenever you can. *Every little bit of improvement is something to celebrate.*

66

Health Maintenance

MY PRAYER IS THAT ONCE YOU HAVE GONE through the steps in this book for whatever combination of symptoms you have, you will be well on your way to good health. As symptoms subside, instead of an overwhelming misery, you will start to find the patterns, reasons, and solutions for each set of symptoms.

My hope is that eventually you will calm and strengthen your body to the point that you can turn off the syndrome, but there may be a period before that happens (maybe for the rest of your life), when you are mostly well but still getting stronger.

Continue Trials

During this time, you will probably need to keep taking certain supplements or medications and doing certain exercises or lifestyle behaviors. Be faithful to the program and protocols you have developed for yourself. When you are doing well, you don't want to mess anything up of your own accord — plenty of outside influences and experiences will occur to change things without your help.

However, there will come a time when you are strong enough and calm enough to try letting go of some of your program. If you want to stop taking a supplement, do not wait until you get to the end of the bottle; if it turns out that it was a bad idea to stop, you will have to wait until you can purchase more. Instead, stop with a week or two worth of the supplement left so that if you need to go back on it, you can do so immediately. If you don't need to go back on the supplement, then it provides you an opportunity to try it again in a few months to see if it makes a difference and should come back into rotation.

Just as in the beginning, do your trials with just one or a small number of supplements and exercises at a time. Keep a diary so you know what's working. Trust your body to know what it needs. Also, try to plan your trials for times when you have a little leeway in your schedule, just in case things don't go as well as you hope.

Cascade of Symptoms

When you are in the health maintenance stage, you may feel great most days but still be vulnerable to injuries and setbacks. We can't prevent every injury in our future, so the trick is to know your own probable cascade of symptoms and your own likely cures for it. Try to stop the cascade as early as possible. In the figure at the end of this chapter, I have included a sample of the most common cascade of symptoms that I experience.

This cascade starts with a Joint Injury and ends with MCAS and POTS activation. These conditions are considered the hEDS triad because they are the most common combination of conditions. The cascade could, however, start with MCAS and develop to cause POTS episodes and Joint Injuries. Sometimes, the cascade starts with POTS, but for me, now that I have gotten practiced at recognizing the signs of a POTS episode starting, I can quickly halt the cascade before it gets going by lying down with my legs up and drinking electrolytes or caffeine.

You can also think of the cascade of symptoms as a feedback loop. We have heard the screeching sound when a microphone picks up the output from an audio speaker in a feedback loop. When one system in the body has a problem, it can instigate a problem in a second system; then, the problem in the second system can exacerbate the problem in the first system, and the loop continues and the problems intensify. In fact, numerous systems can be involved, amplifying and multiplying the problems. But it also works the other way: a condition of calm and health in one system can inform another system and help it calm down and heal.

Whatever your symptom cascade starts with, if you notice the symptoms of the first step happening, you might be able to treat that condition quickly, prevent a feedback loop from developing, and halt the progression of symptoms completely. That is always my goal, but I give myself grace when I'm not successful, whether I did everything I know to do or I messed up. If you miss the signs or aren't successful at Step 1, try to stop the symptoms at Step 2.

It is very important, as soon as you recognize that an injury or trigger has occurred, to begin avoiding all of your potential triggers. Now that you're healthier and stronger, you probably can eat some things that used to make you sick or go into stores where the fragrance used to give you an MCAS flare, or do some exercises that used to be guaranteed to knock a joint out of place. When you are injured, you need to go back to your old methods of caution.

Avoid triggers and try to stay calm until healing has occurred. Staying calm can be especially challenging if your symptoms are getting worse. I find it very stressful and even frightening when I can't stop the cascade — I remember what it was like when I was debilitated by similar symptoms, and I dread returning to that state. But my stress and fear only make the cascade stronger and more complete. Try not to get caught in this cycle. Relax and reset.

Reset

Sometimes when I have gotten caught in the cycle, I can do a reset by taking a hot shower, going for a walk in the woods, or taking a nap (or all 3). Figure out what your reset activities or treatments are, and use them to calm your body and mind down so that the cascade of symptoms can begin to diminish down to something manageable. Keep in mind that your reset activities may change over time – showers used to be one of my worst triggers, but now it is a reset.

After all of my years with hEDS/HSD, I can handle a little pain if I understand that it is part of the healing process. I know that I'll be better soon, and I turn to my loved ones to help me out until then.

Rest and reset, accept the circumstance, continue your treatments, and soon, you will be back on your feet again, feeling good and more grateful than ever for your health and all of the wonderful things in your life.

Step-by-Step Instructions for Health Maintenance

Health maintenance is easier than healing, but it still takes dedication. Ask your doctor before trying anything new or stopping anything you've been doing.

Be Well

1. **Maintain the health program you have developed for yourself.** Every morning, start with your Range of Motion exercises, take your needed supplements, and say your personalized Affirmations and prayers. Write down your list of things to do, and set all of your supplies out together where they are easy to see and access. *Keep to your daily, weekly, and yearly rhythms, and continue to find more joys and things to be grateful for every day.*
2. **Trial removing supplements or behaviors from your personal health program.** As you get healthier and stronger, your self-care plan can get easier and simpler. Use your intuition to know when to trial removing things from your program. *Eventually, you will not need to spend so much time, money, or mental energy taking care of your health; you will feel normal.*
3. **Halt the cascade of symptoms when injury or triggering occurs.** Do not hesitate, even though you haven't had a problem like this happen in a really long time. Take it seriously and attend to your needs so that it won't escalate and start an even worse cascade with a feedback loop that is hard to stop. *Always stand up for your needs.*
4. **Rest and reset to get back on track.** Find the activities that can reset your nervous system and give you the nourishing rest your body needs for healing. *Remind your body that you know how to be well.*

BE WELL

1. Maintain the health program you have developed for yourself.
2. Trial removing supplements or behaviors from your personal health program.
3. Halt the cascade of symptoms when injury or triggering occurs.
4. Rest and reset to get back on track.

Ask your doctor before trying anything new.

SAMPLE CASCADE OF SYMPTOMS FOLLOWING INJURY

Step 1. Joint Injury or other injury can create:

- a. muscular tightness at the site of injury and surrounding areas, leading to:
  - i. further misalignment of joints.

Step 2. Misalignment of joints can create:

- a. nerve compression or stretching, leading to:
  - i. pain, tingling, numbness, and itching along the path of the nerve, possibly in both directions.
  - ii. more muscular tightness at the affected sites and further sites.
- b. blood vessel compression, leading to:
  - i. swelling
    - 1. in nearby body parts, resulting in:
      - a. pain and itching.
      - b. loss of mobility, leading to more tightness in more sites.
    - 2. in the brain, causing:
      - a. Ataxia and Dystonia.
      - b. brain fog and Insomnia.
      - c. Migraine attack.
  - ii. loss of blood flow, potentially to the:
    - 1. gut, causing:
      - a. gastrointestinal distress.
    - 2. brain, causing:
      - a. Ataxia and Dystonia.
      - b. Migraine attack.
      - c. nausea and weakness.
      - d. brain fog, dizziness, and anxiety.

Step 3. As the nerve heals, the symptoms get worse, which tends to create:

- a. more severe pain.
- b. stress.

Step 4. The pain and stress get the immune system activated, which was already been primed by the initial injury, causing:

- a. MCAS flares and POTS episodes, with all of their associated symptoms, such as hives, flushing, itching, swelling, sore throat, watery eyes, coughing, bloating, vomiting, diarrhea or constipation, headache, anger, fatigue, brain fog, and racing heart.

Step 5. Then, each of these symptoms can amplify other symptoms and conditions.

67

Additional Health Topics for Further Investigation

HEALING, LEARNING, AND DISCOVERING NEVER STOP. Life continues and changes, and our needs evolve. With that in mind, here is a list of other topics that have been beneficial to me in the past or that I may investigate further in the future. If you have tried the ideas in this book and are still in need of help, you might benefit from researching these topics.

Note that one of the obstacles to healing can be emotional or psychological trauma. As one of my massage therapists told me, the body is a recording device; whatever you experience will be stored in your cells and can affect your health. Some of the techniques described earlier in this book as well as some of the additional health topics listed here can be effective means of addressing and resolving emotional trauma. Speaking with a counselor can be of great benefit as well.

I pray that you continue to heal and thrive in your life.

- Aborted fetus genetic material in products, supplements, and vaccines — Some scientist and doctors are concerned that this genetic material affects people in unexpected ways.
- Adaptogens — Herbs that balance hormones and especially offer support during stressful times. Ashwagandha is used effectively by many people I know; I have had good results using Rhodiola and Maca Root (separately) to balance hormones.
- ASEA Redox Molecules — This may simply be expensive salt water sold through a multi-level-marketing (MLM) program, but I have known people who have experienced enhanced health by using them.
- Beef Tallow as moisturizer — This is a natural, scent-free oil that is solid at room temperature and is purported to be very good for the skin.
- Biofeedback — Practitioners can use machines to determine the state of health of each body system.
- Breath Work — There are many methods of breathing for health, and one that has been highly recommended is called Breath Work.
- Castor Oil Packs — Apply castor oil in a flannel pack to the stomach or to injured parts for quick healing.
- CBD Oil — Cannabidiol has been found to relieve pain, inflammation, and Insomnia; some people with hEDS have commented on social media that it helps them. It has become readily available, but many brands have been found to be contaminated. There are unanswered questions regarding the safety of CBD oil regarding reproduction.[791, 792]

(I personally have not investigated because I am so happy with comfrey oil, which has the same benefits, is less expensive, smells better (in my opinion), plus helps repair collagen structures to promote the healing of injuries.)

- Constellation Work — Practitioners help you heal the problems and diseases that have been handed down your ancestral line.
- Cromolyn Sodium — This medicine is a mast cell stabilizer that is available over the counter and is prescribed by many doctors for MCAS. Some patients have wonderful results from it but then are required to take it indefinitely; other patients have bad reactions to it. For MCAS, it is recommended to be taken orally; spraying it in the nose can cause harm for hEDS/HSD.
- Crystal Healing — This is the use of stones to enact healing based on the qualities of the stones. Practitioners offer private sessions and classes in the modality; it is also possible to wear jewelry made with natural crystals for a constant effect.
- Dance Therapy — With the guidance of a teacher, clients use a variety of movements to explore, express, and release emotions. If there are emotional blocks to physical healing, this can be very helpful, and I have witnessed clients with frozen joints or stiffness of movement regain fluid range of motion during these sessions.
- EFT Tapping — Emotional Freedom Technique is easy to learn for free through YouTube videos to heal your own physical, emotional, and psychological problems with specific mantras and tapping with your fingers on your body.
- EMDR (Eye Movement Desensitization and Reprocessing) — This is a program of eye exercises led by a practitioner that can serve as psychotherapy.
- Essential Oils — This is a convenient form of herbal medicine that can be stored much longer than fresh or dried plant materials. It is very powerful; depending on the plant, one drop of the oil can be equivalent to 40-100 cups of herbal tea.[793] For example, peppermint essential oil is antibacterial, anti-inflammatory, antiviral, antiparasitic, antitumor, antifatigue, antioxidant, neuroprotective, and immune moderating.[794] This is of benefit when it is used safely, but dangerous otherwise. Also, an incredible amount of plant material is required to make a tiny bottle of essential oil, so it is not the most environmentally friendly health product. At my holistic healing center, for some time we had an aromatherapist who was highly intelligent and very careful; her blends helped many people, but ultimately, we decided that so many of our customers were reactive to the oils that we had to stop carrying them in the store except at special aromatherapy events. Many people with Allergy/MCAS/MCS and Migraine are triggered by essential oils.
- Eurythmy Therapy — Eurythmy is a form of spiritual dance that was developed by Rudolf Steiner (who also created anthroposophy, biodynamic farming, and the Waldorf/Steiner education method). Specific Eurythmy movements can be used in repetition to enact specific healing. A teacher at a workshop I attended had seen children be cured of allergies and ADHD using Eurythmy. A friend of a friend turned to Eurythmy for painfully impacted wisdom teeth, and the teeth grew in into their proper, pain-free alignment — no surgery necessary after all.
- Herbs — Herbalists can treat virtually any condition with plants. Some herbalists believe that when you need specific health help, herbs will spontaneously begin growing in your yard; so, you can go outside from time to time, identify the "weeds" that are growing in your lawn or landscaping, and if they have healing properties that apply to your needs, try using them, under the guidance of an herbalist and your doctor.
- HIIT (High Intensity Interval Training) workouts — This exercise method might work well for you because it puts you in charge and prevents overexertion. Whatever exercise you are doing, you do it as hard as you can for a short amount of time (you can choose when to stop), and then you rest (however long you want). There are variations on the timing of activity, rest, and repetition, but for people with hypermobility, doing what feels right is probably better than following a prescribed plan.

- Hugging Workshops — I have known two people who attended different hug workshops, and they gave the best hugs. Previously, I would never have imagined a person could be taught how to hug better. Hugs are very healing, especially when done really well.
- Intermittent Fasting — This meal timing method is really popular among people who want to lose weight, but it can also be beneficial for people who have Digestive System Problems. It gives the digestive system a chance to rest and repair in between meals.
- Iridology — Experts are able to see the history of your body and the state of its health based on signs in the iris of your eyes.
- Mold Illness — Exposure to mold in the home or workplace may exacerbate the symptoms of other conditions or create problems of its own in all of the body's systems.
- Muldowney Protocol — This is a Physical Therapy plan specifically designed for people with hEDS, and it is highly respected among people in the social media groups. It is available as a book but is designed to be used with the supervision and guidance of a Physical Therapist.
- Neural Retraining Programs — There are a lot of these programs, the two most famous being Gupta and DNRS, that use meditation and/or hypnosis to retrain the brain not to react to benign substances like food allergens. Some people get wonderful results, but there have been cases of patients dying when they believed they were no longer allergic to something and then, unprepared, had a severe anaphylactic reaction to it.
- Organic Foods — Avoid GMOs and foods that have been grown with poisonous pesticides.
- Ozone for Eliminating VOCs — Be careful because ozone is dangerous when inhaled in great quantity, but ozone machines are useful for eliminating fragrances, smoke, mold, etc. from rooms, cars, and belongings, and the ozone breaks down into oxygen quickly.
- Parasite Cleanses — If you get grumpy or have a hard time sleeping around the time of the full moon, this is a sign you might have parasites, which are usually more active at the time of the full moon. Parasites can also cause other changes in behavior, as well as many symptoms of illness.
- Post Traumatic Stress Disorder — PTSD is more common among hypermobile people than the general population. If you have experienced a trauma, it may be indirectly responsible for some of the conditions you are suffering with now. There are a lot of effective methods for overcoming PTSD, especially psychotherapy, but many of the treatments in this book may help as well.
- Raw Milk — Find a good, careful, local dairy farmer through the Weston A. Price Foundation, and enjoy the benefits of raw milk, including increased energy, improved gut biome, and decreased illness.
- Retained Reflexes — Read *The Symphony of Reflexes: Interventions for Human Development, Autism, ADHD, CP, and Other Neurological Disorders* by Bonnie Brandes, and do any of the exercises that might apply to you.
- Root Cause Protocol Developed by the Magnesium Advocacy Group (MAG) — Balance minerals like iron and magnesium.
- Saunas — Full-spectrum infrared saunas, especially when combined with a niacin protocol and/or cold plunging, can enhance health in many ways, and they are especially good for detoxing the body.
- Sciatica — This common condition can cause severe pain in the back, buttocks, and/or legs and can be treated the same way as other Joint Injuries.
- Seed Oils — Many people say that oils from seeds like canola, sunflower, corn, and soybean, found in most processed foods, are bad for you. Some people suggest that they are inherently bad, but others say that they are bad because they are almost assuredly rancid when in processed food.
- Sleep — Obviously, sleep is extremely important, as it is the best opportunity for the body to heal itself. Avoid bright lights and screens in the evening, preserve your sleep environment for sleeping only, and go to bed and wake up at the same time each day.

- Sound Healing — Practitioners and performers can work wonders for health with sound waves, using their voice, tuning forks, crystal bowls, drums, and other instruments.
- Structured Water — Stir or swirl your water before you drink it to align the molecules for easier absorption in the body. There are machines and waterfall structures sold for this purpose also.
- Tea and Coffee — There is great disagreement regarding the health impacts of tea and coffee. People with POTS should avoid caffeine most of the time, but it is probably fine to have decaffeinated versions, but only if they are either CO^2 or Swiss Process, organic, and not using paper bags or filters. Tea should be made with a stainless-steel strainer; coffee is easily made in a glass-and-stainless-steel coffee press.
- Tick-Borne Illnesses — Lyme Disease can cause many disruptions to the body's systems, including affecting collagen, upsetting the digestive system, and causing swelling and dislocation of joints; Alpha Gal can cause Allergy/MCAS/MCS-like symptoms; and there are many other tick-borne illnesses as well, some of which, like ehrlichiosis, that can be active for years while undetected.
- Trigger Point Therapy — Pain radiates from small knots in the muscles but can sometimes be relieved by applying pressure to the knots. I have heard that the knots can hold chemicals and that releasing them sometimes aggravates MCAS/MCS (though storing the chemicals in the knots also can cause symptoms).
- Ubiquinol — This is a form of CoQ10. Many people in hEDS social media groups have said that when they told their doctor that they were going to try PQQ, per the Cusack Protocol, their doctors recommended using CoQ10 also because the combination would give them energy. I did not experience an energy boost from it, nor did I experience any noticeable difference from taking it alone previously. It is purported to have a number of different health benefits, including improving fertility.
- Underlying infections — Infections like Guillain-Barre Syndrome, h pylori, SIBO, and others can exacerbate the symptoms of hEDS. If you treat your hypermobility-induced problems but don't treat an underlying infection, you will not achieve full healing.
- Viome — This company offers testing of the microbiome and personalized recommendations for diet and supplements.
- Weston A. Price diet — Dentist Dr. Price developed this diet based on his observations of traditional, indigenous communities around the world whose mouth health and overall health was far superior to those of modernized communities.

68

Encouragement & Inspiration

I REALIZED RECENTLY THAT NOW WHEN I READ articles or social media posts written by someone struggling with chronic illness, I don't feel the same solidarity that I used to, I don't have the same understanding of what they're going through. I feel some guilt about this — it is hard to believe that I have forgotten so quickly what it is like to be chronically ill. But what a blessing!

I look at my mother as my inspiration. She has hypermobility, and although she has never suffered with the severe symptoms my sister and I have had, she has had a number of the conditions in this book (more than I have mentioned)...but she has also heeded the advice in this book and been rewarded for it. In her 70s, she still dances ballet and tap, goes on adventure hikes, plays pickleball, kayaks, snorkels, and gets into whatever kind of active fun her spirited grandchildren suggest.

My mother lived with chronic pain in her knees and hips for years, but when I started my dance studio, she began, at age 46, taking the teen and adult classes and soon her pain was gone. She went on to become a dance teacher herself, and at 68 became a professional performer, too! She suffered with stomach pain for years, but dedication to an organic, whole-food, plant-based diet and the *L-rhamnosus GG* probiotic has made that a thing of the past. She has treated numerous injuries with diligent Physical Therapy work. She uses many of the supplements, tools, techniques, and exercises listed in this book every day.

In short, when hypermobility problems have arisen, my mother has devoted herself to curing them with natural methods, even when that has required a lot of effort on her part. Perhaps her strongest healing tool, though, has been her positive attitude and belief that loving family and friends is the reason for living. She stood in my house not long ago and gestured with her hands from her head toward her feet and exclaimed, "I love my body!"

Multiple times I have seen stories on social media of hypermobile grandmothers in their 80s or 90s walking long distances for exercise every day. I've even seen videos of dancers and gymnasts performing their arts at those ages. Perhaps we can all find our paths to vitality, longevity, and the freedom that wellness brings.

Keep in mind that healing takes a lot of focus and energy. It will feel really difficult sometimes, but it will be worth it. And, in time, as you get better, you will be able to stop doing some of the things you used to have to do. That's why I started writing this book, after all — I could see that some things would become so habitual that I wouldn't even remember that I was doing them, and other things would not need to be continued and would be forgotten once I stopped them.

Remember, it takes time to heal. In this computerized world, we have gotten used to having things happen instantly on demand, but our bodies are not computerized. Give yourself grace and time to heal.

In the time that I have written this book, I have found the book itself to be surprisingly useful. All of the information that I had previously been carrying in my head was now written down, organized, and easy to access. I was suddenly able to take even better care of myself because if I experienced a trigger and couldn't remember what to do because of brain fog, I could look in the book to see the treatment options that would help heal the symptoms I was having at the time. I am feeling great! I hope that this book will do the same for you.

It has been a lifelong journey to gather this information — a lot of trial and error. I have felt fulfilled in my work because I have been able to help clients heal, and I am grateful that I can help my son. I hope to hear many success stories from you in coming days.

Share the Health

Share this book with your loved ones so that they can begin to understand your experience. Let this be a jumping off point for loving conversations about how you can help each other.

If you have any friends or acquaintances who might be suffering from a hypermobility-related condition, tell them about my website, www.shannonegale.com and encourage them to read this book.

If you know any doctors or medical research scientists, please tell them about this book. Seeing the lists of what has worked for me and people I know might inspire their clinical treatments and, perhaps more importantly, give them hints about where to look next as they seek better treatments and even a cure.

Look to the Future

As I have been completing this book, I have continued to learn more – too much to put into one book. So, I am planning to write many more books, develop video demonstrations, create a Hypermobile and Happy App, and maybe even invent a new dance genre specifically for people with hypermobility. Please follow me on social media and subscribe to my email list so that you will be kept up to date on these offerings. Visit my website at shannonegale.com or scan the QR code below.

With your renewed health, what are you planning to do?

Be Well

I pray for you to experience long-lasting, robust health and to enjoy a long and joyful life.

Further Resources

Appendix A
Recipes: Personal Care, Symptom Relief, & Nontoxoic Cleaning

Adrenal Cocktail

From Chapter 11: Allergy, MCAS, & MCS

4 ounces orange juice
¼ teaspoon cream of tartar
¼ teaspoon salt

Mix together in a glass and drink.

Chlorine Neutralizer

From Chapter 31: Scoliosis

½ cup filtered water
½ teaspoon powdered ascorbic acid

Mix together in a spray bottle and spray on skin before and after swimming in a chlorinated pool.

Cleaning and Disinfecting Spray

From Chapter 44: Detox

1 orange's peel
White vinegar

Put the orange peel into a jar. Pour on enough vinegar to cover the peel. Put the lid on the jar and leave it sitting in a cool dark place for 2 weeks.

After 2 weeks, pour the liquid through a strainer into a spray bottle. Add an equal amount of water.

To clean surfaces, spray it on, let it sit for a minute, and then wipe it off.

Cooked Comfrey Oil

For pain relief and speedy healing of injuries.

1 comfrey leaf or 1 piece of comfrey root
6 oz organic olive oil

Cold pressed comfrey oil, which can be purchased online or made with a cold pressing machine, may retain more of the beneficial constituents of comfrey than cooking it does. However, the cooked comfrey oil is still effective as a healing aid and pain reducer for injuries.

Comfrey plants grow easily on sunny hillsides (in my region, at least). The leaves are large, but they have stinging hairs on them, so you should not touch it with your hand until it has been cooked.

If using a leaf, hold a basket below a leaf and clip it with scissors so that it falls into the basket. Without touching the leaf, clip it into small pieces, then pour it out of the basket into preheated oil in a saucepan or skillet on the stove at low/medium temperature.

If using a piece of root, chop the root into tiny pieces and then place into preheated oil in a saucepan or skillet on the stove at low/medium temperature.

Cook for half an hour. Strain into a glass jar and put on the lid.

Elderberry Syrup

This is a bonus recipe not mentioned previously in this book. It supports the immune system to fight off colds and flus or minimize their severity. Many people with Allergy/MCAS/MCS have overactive immune systems and may not get the intended results from this syrup. Still, even for them, it may be beneficial during the emerging stages of an illness.

This syrup can be a valuable part of your Health Maintenance. Whereas other Elderberry Syrup recipes use honey (I prefer honey for allergies and topical antiseptic), maple syrup has constituents that strengthen you against winter illnesses. You can grow elderberry bushes, purchase them at a local health food store, or buy them at the link in Appendix B.

⅔ cup dried elderberries
3 ½ cups water
1 Tablespoon ground cinnamon
½ teaspoon ground cloves
⅓ teaspoon ground ginger
1 cup real maple syrup

Put all ingredients except syrup into a medium pot. Bring it to a boil on the stove, and then reduce the heat to simmer for 45 minutes. Allow the mixture to cool, then strain the liquid into a jar. Discard the berries. Add maple syrup to the jar, put on the lid, and shake to combine.

Store in the refrigerator. Take one spoonful a day when you have been or will be exposed to contagious illnesses. Take as much as you like if you feel an illness coming on.

To make a tea, put one or two spoonfuls of the elederberry syrup into a tea cup, add hot water until the cup is full, and stir. You can chill the tea if desired.

You can also use this as a syrup for pancakes, biscuits, yogurt, etc. For this purpose, you may choose to add more maple syrup, to taste.

Face Mask

From Chapter 54: Oil Cleansing Method

1 part bentonite clay

1 part water — more or less

Drops of jojoba oil (optional)

Put bentonite clay and water into a small jar, put the lid on, and shake. Leave sitting overnight, and the next day, check the consistency of the paste. Add more water or clay if necessary.

If you desire, stir in some jojoba oil. If you do not stir it into the mask, you can apply it to your face after removing the mask.

Using your fingertips, spread the mask onto your face. Allow to dry (about 15 minutes). Splash face with water and then gently scrub mask off with a warm wet washcloth.

Face Oil

From Chapter 54: Oil Cleansing Method

3 parts organic extra virgin olive oil

1 part organic castor oil

¼ teaspoon diatomaceous earth (optional)

Mix together in a 3-ounce bottle.

When you need more moisturizing effect, increase the ratio of olive oil. When you need an astringent effect to reduce acne, increase the ratio of castor oil. When you need extra exfoliation, add the diatomaceous earth to the mixture.

Rather than mixing the diatomaceous earth into the bottle of oil, I usually add the diatomaceous earth only on days when I need it by sprinkling ⅛ teaspoon of it into the oil that I have already poured onto my hand. Be careful not to agitate the diatomaceous earth into the air because it is bad for you to breathe it in.

Pour the face oil into your hands and rub it onto your face for one minute, massaging all of your face gently with your fingertips. Keep your facial muscles relaxed during the massage.

Put a hot, wet washcloth on your face, and allow it to steam your skin for one minute.

Gently scrub the oil off with a hot wet washcloth.

When your skin is too dry, moisturize it by applying the face oil again after having cleansed your face, sparingly this time, and do not wash it off. This may be necessary when you first begin using the Oil Cleansing Method but will probably be needed only rarely once your skin adjusts.

Fresh Comfrey Poultice

For pain relief and speedy healing of injuries.

2-inch piece of comfrey leaf
1 cup of hot water

Comfrey plants grow easily on sunny hillsides (in my region, at least). The leaves are large, but they have stinging hairs on them, so you should not touch it with your hand until it has been cooked.

Hold a basket below a leaf and clip it with scissors so that it falls into the basket. The leaf can be refrigerated for use over the next week.

Cut off a 2-inch square piece of leaf, put it in a cup and pour boiling water over it. Let it steep until it has cooled enough to handle comfortably.

Remove the leaf piece from the cup and apply it like a compress to the wounded area. Tie it on with a cloth, or use medical tape. You can keep the compress on for up to 6 hours at a time.

Do this once or twice daily.

(Large quantities of comfrey are toxic, so it is recommended not to drink it.[795] However, I have been told by herbalists that if the tea tastes good to you, that is a sign that your body will make good use of it; if it begins to taste bad, that is your sign that you have had enough. Proceed with great caution, or forego drinking comfrey tea altogether.)

Magnesium Oil

For relief of cramping and pain from injuries, tight muscles, and nerve damage.

1-ounce spray bottle almost full of filtered water
A generous pinch or two of Ancient Minerals magnesium flakes

Shake the bottle well to combine. Spray onto skin to relieve nerve, fascia, and muscle pain, tightness, and cramping. Allow to air dry.

Skin Spray for Rashes

From Chapter32: Sensitive Skin

1-ounce spray bottle almost full of water
¼ teaspoon borax

Combine ingredients, then shake the bottle for up to 10 minutes to get the borax to dissolve into the water.

If it is a cold time of year, you can put the spray bottle into a bowl of hot water for a few minutes so that it will be more comfortable when you spray it on your skin.

Spray onto skin rashes, especially those caused by yeasts or fungi. Allow to air dry. Repeat up to 3 times per day until rash disappears.

Tooth Powder

From Chapter 23: Mouth Health

¼ cup bentonite clay
3 Tablespoons calcium carbonate
1 Tablespoon baking soda
1 teaspoon cinnamon
1 ½ Tablespoons xylitol powder (or 1 Tablespoon stevia powder)

Put all ingredients into a jar, apply the lid, and shake. Pour into smaller jars for individuals' 1-2-week use. Wet the toothbrush, and then dip it into the toothpowder, and brush teeth. Some people prefer to pour the powder onto the brush or pour it into the palm of their hand and dip their brush there.

Underarm Mask

From Chapter 43: Deodorant

1 part bentonite clay
1 part water — more or less

Put bentonite clay and water into a small jar, put the lid on, and shake. Leave sitting overnight, and the next day, check for the consistency of the paste. Add more water if necessary.

Using your fingertips, spread the paste onto your underarms. Allow to dry, about 10-15 minutes. Wash off with soap and water.

Appendix B
Annotated List of Recommendations: Books, Experts, & Products

Please note that I am an Amazon affiliate and so I may receive a commission for any purchases you make on Amazon shortly after clicking one of the Amazon links.

These links are also available on my website, so that you can easily click them: shannonegale.com . Or, scan the QR code:

Books

Accessing the Healing Power of the Vagus Nerve by Stanley Rosenberg https://amzn.to/3T3rfdE

Anxiety: A Quick Immersion by Antonio Bulbena https://amzn.to/3KtuerR

The Bates Method for Better Eyesight Without Glasses by William Bates https://amzn.to/48VlXac

Cure Tooth Decay: Remineralize Cavities and Repair Your Teeth Naturally with Good Food by Ramiel Nagel https://amzn.to/3NWMKuW

Earthing (2nd Edition): The Most Important Health Discovery Ever! by Clinton Ober, Dr Stephen T Sinatra M.D., et al. https://amzn.to/3O9jfpP

Feeding Your Demons: Ancient Wisdom for Resolving Inner Conflict by Tsultrim Allione https://amzn.to/3TRTHky

It Starts with the Egg: The Science of Egg Quality for Fertility, Miscarriage, and IVF by Rebecca Fett https://amzn.to/3wPDPWk

The Mercury Detoxification Manual: A Guide to Mercury Chelation by PE Rebecca Rust Lee and Andrew Hall Cutler https://amzn.to/3HtiO66

The MindFit Method: The Collision of Exercise and STEM That's Driving Innovation, Creativity, and Learning by Michael Fancher https://amzn.to/4572BhV

No-Drama Discipline: The Whole-Brain Way to Calm the Chaos and Nurture Your Child's Developing Mind by Daniel J. Siegel and Tina Payne Bryson https://amzn.to/3S0SvsG

Older Yet Faster: The Secret to Running Fast and Injury Free by Keith Roland Bateman, Heidi Jones, et al. https://amzn.to/428dluS

The Symphony of Reflexes: Interventions for Human Development, Autism, ADHD, CP, and Other Neurological Disorders by Bonnie Brandes https://amzn.to/4b6qFUv

Transcendental Meditation by Jack Forem https://amzn.to/3SDrZXY

The Twelve Wild Swans by Starhawk https://amzn.to/4dfr5cy

Zero Limits: The Secret Hawaiian System for Wealth, Health, Peace, and More by Joe Vitale and Ihaleakala Hew Len https://amzn.to/3xdKwC6

Experts

Action For ME — Myalgic Encephalomyelitis. https://www.actionforme.org.uk/

The AIM Center for Personalized Medicine — this is the website for the clinic at which famed MCAS expert, Dr. Lawrence Afrin, is currently working; the website includes information in the form of podcasts, blogs, and links. https://drtaniadempsey.com/

American Migraine Foundation — https://americanmigrainefoundation.org/

Dr. Paul Anderson — he shares helpful information about MCAS on his website and YouTube channel. https://dranow.com/about/

Arthritis Foundation — https://www.arthritis.org/

Bates Method — this is an online repository of information from William Bates's book about seeing better without eyeglasses. https://www.seeing.org

Deborah Cusack — she developed the Cusack Protocol, which is supplement recommendations for people with EDS. https://www.youtube.com/@deborahcusack8782

Jeannie di Bon — a brilliant, calming, and encouraging Pilates Teacher who specializes in hypermobility. https://www.youtube.com/@JeannieDiBonHypermobility

EDS Awareness — https://www.chronicpainpartners.com/

Ehlers-Danlos News — https://ehlersdanlosnews.com/

Ehlers-Danlos Research Foundation — https://www.edsrf.org/

The Ehlers-Danlos Society — https://www.ehlers-danlos.com/

Ehlers-Danlos Support UK — https://www.ehlers-danlos.org/

Fibromyalgia Care Society of America — https://www.fibro.org

Shannon E. Gale, Author — this is my website, where you can find the list of links and end notes for easy clicking, information about future books and other products that I offer, and links to my social media pages, where I intend to post videos giving demonstrations and more information about hypermobility and healing symptoms naturally. shannonegale.com

Haka Tours New Zealand — this page shares information and a video about the Haka war dance of the Māori people. https://hakatours.com/blog/haka-meaning/

Healing Histamine — https://www.healinghistamine.com/

Histamined — this is a link to the list of medications to avoid if you have MCAS https://www.histamined.com/post/medications-to-avoid-with-mcas .

Dr. Ross Houser of Caring Medical — he has a lot of fascinating videos, mostly about how Craniocervical Instability (CCI) causes a host of symptoms and how he can cure CCI with prolotherapy. https://www.youtube.com/@CaringmedicalProlotherapy

Hyperemesis Foundation — I do not agree with everything on this website, but it is the only one I know of that focuses on Hyperemesis Gravidarum in pregnancy. www.helpher.org

Hypermobility Syndromes Organization — https://www.hypermobility.org/

Michelle Kenway — on her YouTube channel, she gives helpful information about and exercises for pelvic organ prolapses, bathrooming, and sex. https://www.youtube.com/@michellephysio

Dr. Ben Lynch — a doctor specializing in treating symptoms from folate deficiency caused by MTHFR. https://mthfr.net/mthfr-c677t-mutation-basic-protocol/2012/02/24/

Mast Attack — educating people about life with mast cell disorders. https://www.mastattack.org/

The Mast Cell Disease Society. https://tmsforacure.org/

Melt Method — a gentle self-care technique based on neurofascial science using balls and foam rollers to relieve pain and restore range of motion. https://meltmethod.com/

Drs. John and Mike Mew — the inventors of orthotropics and mewing. https://www.youtube.com/@Orthotropics

Migraine Foundation interview with Dr. Vincent Martin about POTS. https://www.youtube.com/watch?v=Lf_3rD7BtR4

Motivational Doc — this link goes directly to the video with the suboccipital muscle stretch, but this optimistic guy has a lot of great videos. https://www.YouTube.com/watch?v=gj0luiN422Q&list=LL&index=

MSK Neurology — innovative rehabilitation of musculoskeletal and neurological disorders by Kjetil Larsen. https://mskneurology.com/

My Chemical Free House. https://www.mychemicalfreehouse.net/

Paradiso and Rasamayi Sound Healing. https://www.youtube.com/channel/UC4iovRaHYs0MLHgQkMXNoJg

Standing Up To POTS — includes information about POTS plus The POTScast podcast. https://www.standinguptopots.org/

The TMJ Association. https://tmj.org

Trauma Prevention — a website about Dr. David Berceli's Trauma Release Exercises that use shaking (TRE). https://traumaprevention.com/

Wellness Mama — a great blog from a woman in my state that offers information about natural healing and motherhood. https://wellnessmama.com/

Whealth — energetic, fun-loving personal trainers who specialize in hEDS and paint the muscles, veins, and nerves on their bodies or clothing so that you can see what is happening inside the body when you're moving. https://www.youtube.com/@whealth_

Yoga International — Bunion relief exercises. https://yogainternational.com/article/view/9-poses-to-prevent-Bunions-relieve-Bunion-pain/

The Zebra Network — awareness, education, and advocacy for patients with Ehlers-Danlos Syndrome. https://thezebranetwork.org/

Products

Most of these products are the specific brands that I have used and liked. In a few cases, the brand I used is not available anymore, so I included one that appears to be identical. However, even the ones that I have liked might have changed in quality, price, or other attributes since when I purchased. So, this list may serve as a starting-off point for shopping, but my hope is that it allows you to get what you need quickly and easily.

Activated Charcoal: Zen Hardwood Activated Charcoal Powder — absorbs toxins, including excess hormones. It can be helpful when taken immediately after exposure to a trigger or allergen, but it is dehydrating, so drink extra water. https://amzn.to/3S6Vgc7

Allergy-Preventing Herb Tea: AllergEase Tea by Health King — I have relieved myself and many clients of seasonal allergies by prescribing them to drink a cup of this tea each day with a spoonful of local, same-season honey. I find it also to diminish MCAS. It includes the herbs scute, astragalus, polygonatum, angelica daburica, polygala, eleuthro, green tea, and jasmine. https://amzn.to/4aaIQHh

Aloe Juice: George's Aloe Vera Distilled Liquid — an option on the Cusack Protocol to tighten joints. This has been the most helpful supplement for me in strengthening my joints. https://amzn.to/3Uzvz6h

Antacid: Alka Seltzer Gold — reduces MCAS/MCS reactions and indigestion. https://amzn.to/48GafAO

Aspirin: Bayer Baby Aspirin — taking just one every 12 or every 24 hours reduces inflammation because it is a COX inhibitor. https://amzn.to/3Snl7Of

Astragalus Capsules: Oregon's Wild Harvest, Certified Organic Astragalus Capsules — an immune system regulator, included on the Cusack protocol. https://amzn.to/4di1Nu8

Astragalus Tea: Health King Astragalus Immunity Tea — a delicious way to balance the immune system and improve lymph flow. https://amzn.to/3Qpsaoh

B Vitamins: Seeking Health B-Minus – this blend contains bioavailable versions of B vitamins that should be better absorbed and tolerated by people with the conditions addressed in this book, but it does not contain B12 or folate, so that you can be more precise with your dosages of those two that may make people feel worse at times or may be needed in higher doses by other people. The B vitamins are important in treating MCAS, Cerebellar Ataxia, and Neuralgia/Neuropathy symptoms. https://amzn.to/3wmXBsz

B1: Pure Encapsulations BenfoMax 90's - 200 mg Benfotiamine - Vitamin B1 Thiamin Supplement. https://amzn.to/3WjNHT6

B12: Methylcobalamin — this is a vegan sublingual spray version of B12 that is safe for people with MTHFR. It increases energy, especially when taken with methylfolate. https://amzn.to/422EaRi

B6: Pure Encapsulations P5P 50 - Active Vitamin B6. https://amzn.to/3QoP8vP

Baking Pan: GreenLife Bakeware Healthy Ceramic Baking Pan — these pans scratch easily, but I still love them. The food slides right off, and there is almost never any scrubbing to clean them. Other sizes and shapes are available, too. https://amzn.to/3SrqvA3

Barefoot Shoes: Carets — barefoot dress shoes for men. www.carets.com

Barefoot Shoes: PedTerra — a website that carries numerous brands of barefoot shoes and offers free shipping and free returns. www.pedterra.com

Barefoot Shoes: Vivobarefoot — barefoot shoes and boots. www.vivobarefoot.com

Barefoot Shoes: Xero Shoes — we especially like their barefoot sandals. www.xeroshoes.com

Bentonite Clay: Aztec Secret Indian Clay — useful in Remineralizing Tooth Powder, Face Mask, Underarm Mask, and more. https://amzn.to/4aetcut

Berberine: Thorne Berberine — a mast cell stabilizer that gave me energy when I first started taking it. https://amzn.to/3WbJrF9

Bioplasma Cell Salts: Hylands Naturals — let one tiny sugar pill melt under your tongue each day to encourage your body to absorb and use minerals more effectively. https://amzn.to/493krT2

Book Opener: TILISMA Book Page Holder - Handmade Natural Walnut Thumb Bookmark — put your thumb through the hole of the simple wooden design, and it will hold the book's pages open for you without taxing your fingers. https://amzn.to/3Umrl2j

Book Support: The Most Comfortable Way to Read, Hands Free! https://amzn.to/4bqRUt6

Broom: Vietnamese Grass Fan Broom — this broom requires very little effort to use and will keep your pelvis and back safe when they are weak or injured and you still have to clean the floor. You hold the broom with one hand and swing your arm, so you still may need to be cautious of unstable shoulder joints. The brooms don't last very long, but if you find an Asian store in your town, you will likely find these brooms for just a couple dollars apiece. https://amzn.to/43k26A4

Caffeinated Beverage: Ale 8 One — this is a tasty soda similar to ginger ale, created and sold in Kentucky. It is not the healthiest of my health treatments, but I appreciate that I can drink it as needed; a small bottle contains only 22 mg of caffeine, which is usually the maximum I need for ending a POTS episode. Sometimes I have a little before exercising and then finish the bottle when I have completed my exercise routine. https://amzn.to/4b5yoCf

Caffeine with Electrolytes and L-Theanine: Hydrant Energy 30 Stick Pack, Caffeine & L-Theanine Rapid Hydration Mix. https://amzn.to/3wcdIcm

Cake Pans: P&P CHEF 9½-inch Round Cake Pan Set of 2, Stainless Steel Bakeware Tier Cake Pan Set — you do not want to cook with aluminum, Teflon, or any other material that will leach poisons into your food. I love how the cakes slide right out of these pans. https://amzn.to/3S914Sa

Chelating and Detoxifying Spray: TRS — Toxin Removal System contains nano-zeolites that are able to cross the blood/brain barrier. Thus, it can chelate heavy metals out of the brain, as well as detoxing the entire body. It does not have the risk of redistributing heavy metals within the body the way that most chelation therapies do. However, it is possible for it to create healing crises, so it is wise to join a TRS social media group for thorough advice. https://www.ledamedical.com/product-page/copy-of-saccharomyces-boulardii-60-c

Chi Machines: Daiwa Felicity Original Chi Swing Machine USJ-201 Passive Aerobic Exerciser — get lymph flowing and exercise the body while lying down. I have not used one of these, but I have friends who love them. https://amzn.to/3TwD2m2

Chinese Skullcap: Nutricost Baikal Skullcap — purported to be a mast cell stabilizer and beneficial during some viral infections such as Covid. https://amzn.to/4aUg9PT

Coffee Maker: Cafe Du Chateau Stainless Steel French Press Coffee Maker — this is not the exact brand or style of French Press that I was gifted, but I appreciate that it is all stainless steel and glass, with no plastic. There are many different options available, for making 1 cup of coffee up to 4 cups, and some with very pretty designs and made with different metals, like copper. It is very easy to pour in coffee grounds and boiling water — easier, I think, even than running a typical electric coffeemaker, and easy to clean in the dishwasher. I prefer the taste of the coffee made this way as well. https://amzn.to/48VG7Rd

Collagen: Orgain Hydrolyzed Collagen Peptides Powder — although taking collagen does not cure hEDS, it is typical for people to make less collagen as they age. Since our collagen is already faulty, it doesn't help us to get depleted. The collagen supplement is really just proteins, which your body will break down in order to use them for making new collagen or whatever else the body deems most important. I do not take a full dose of this collagen, usually just ½ teaspoon or so, and it gives me energy, especially when my diet is low in protein. https://amzn.to/3SqgTp2

Comfrey Oil: Earth Elements Organic Comfrey Oil — I keep a bottle of this by my bed and a bottle in my purse, and sometimes a bottle in the living room. It relaxes muscles, relieves pain, and speeds healing. https://amzn.to/3y5ZsSP

Compression Socks: NEWZILL Cotton-Rich Compression Dress Socks. https://amzn.to/4bhcqvy

D-Ribose: Bulk Supplements D-Ribose Powder — on the Cusack Protocol to reduce fatigue and pain. https://amzn.to/4dx0WWP

DAO (see also Histamine Degrading Enzyme): NaturDAO Enzyme Supplement — helps the body reduce histamine, which may be responsible for Allergy/MCAS/MCS symptoms. It is especially helpful for some people if they take it 5 minutes before a meal, immediately after exposure to an environmental trigger, and at bedtime. https://amzn.to/3QQKpDi

Diatomaceous Earth (DE): Nature's Wisdom Food Grade Diatomaceous Earth — an optional exfoliator to use with the Oil Cleansing Method. DE is also useful as a safe pesticide, but be careful not to inhale the dust. It is also part of the Cusack Protocol to help with yeast, gastrointestinal symptoms, and more. https://amzn.to/3JZTIgt

Digestive Help: Papaya Enzyme — assists with digestion. https://amzn.to/3UeJONY

Dryer Balls: Handy Laundry Wool Dryer Balls — I have not used this particular brand; many brands are available. You can also felt your own with raw wool. If you are allergic to wool, you may want to try plastic dryer balls or balls of aluminum foil; both of those options may contain poisonous chemicals, but they are not as bad as dryer sheets or liquid fabric softener. You only need dryer balls if you are washing synthetic fabrics or down-filled items; if you are washing only natural fabrics like cotton, you will not get static cling. https://amzn.to/4azJxL9

Ear Plugs: Vibes High Fidelity Earplugs and FLARE Calmer Soft Earplug Alternative — I have not tried these. There are many different types of noise-filtering ear plugs and a variety of other earplugs that have differing effects as to how they fit and what noises they diminish and to what extent. These would be among the first I would try. https://amzn.to/42qkGWP and https://amzn.to/3SJoEXp

Earthing Therapy Patches: Earthing Grounding Patches — products for making an electrical connection between your body and the ground. Apply one directly to an injured area to decrease inflammation. https://amzn.to/4aFvdjY

Earthing Tester: Grounding Continuity Tester with 15 Foot Cord — use this to make sure that your earthing product works, or when earthing outside, make sure that you are in effective contact with the ground. https://amzn.to/43YH0aZ

Elderberries: Frontier Co-Op Organic Dried Elderberries — use these in the bonus recipe for Elderberry Syrup in Appendix A. https://amzn.to/3wYYIPi

Electric Shock Wristband: EmeTerm Fashion Electrode Stimulator Wrist Bands — reduces nausea from any cause. https://amzn.to/48B2ko4

Electrolytes: Body-Bio Electrolytes — I used this for many years, appreciating that they do not have flavor added. However, their blend of electrolytes is not ideal for me, and I don't love that it is a liquid stored in a plastic bottle. https://amzn.to/3HoFt38

Electrolytes: Hydrant Hydrate, Individual Hydration Electrolyte Powder Stick Packets — these are currently my favorite electrolytes. I do not love that they contain either sugar or xylitol (depending on which flavor you choose), but they make me feel so much better that I have decided to use them. At first, I did not love their flavors, but I have come to enjoy them, especially Fruit Punch. I drink one every day. https://amzn.to/3SJgLAZ

Epsom Salts: Amazon Basics Epsom Salt Soak — Epsom salts are also readily available at your local grocery store, but be careful because sometimes Epsom salts are fragranced and the scent is not always written predominantly on the bag. Use these to relax muscles and prevent acne on the body. https://amzn.to/3S4Y1KQ

Evening Primrose Oil: Cliganic Organic Evening Primrose Oil — popularly used by women to reduce wrinkles, evening primrose oil (EPO) is also beneficial to the nervous system. EPO is also sold in capsules to be taken internally, but I have not tried that yet. I apply this oil to joints where a nerve compression or strain has occurred and to the path of the nerve where I am experiencing neuropathic symptoms, and it quickly reduces the symptoms. https://amzn.to/3UxiEBW

Eye Mask: Mulberry Silk Sleep Eye Mask & Blindfold with Elastic Strap/Headband. https://amzn.to/3UEnBIY

Fertility Monitoring: Fairhaven Health Fertile Focus Ovulation Test Kit — use saliva to find out when you are about to ovulate. This lipstick-sized microscope with a built-in light is an easy, inexpensive, non-intrusive way of keeping track of your ovulation cycle. https://amzn.to/3VhXCrG

Finger Protectors: Medsuo 2pcs Stainless Steel Finger Guards for Cutting — useful for chopping vegetables when you are feeling clumsy. https://amzn.to/3Hlviwv

Floss Picks: Bambo Earth Natural Dental Floss Picks. https://amzn.to/3JfcyQ9

Floss Picks Individually Wrapped: Floss Guys Premium Unflavored Compostable Floss Picks — these are great for keeping in your purse, backpack, or vehicle. https://amzn.to/4cQmOfg

Folate: Methylfolate — these are delicious and give me energy. It is safe for and recommended for people with MTHFR. https://amzn.to/3U3sSdy

Food Storage: Pyrex Meal Prep Simply Store Glass Rectangular and Round Food Container Set. https://amzn.to/3U8wQBr

Fulvic and Humic Acid: Fulvic Humic Acid Ionic Trace Minerals with Electrolytes Liquid Supplement — this liquid is easily added to tea and actually improves the taste of it, or it can simply be dropped into the mouth. The biggest difference I noticed while using fulvic and humic acid with trace minerals was significantly healthier skin, fingernails, and hair. https://amzn.to/3xNZIFY

Gua Sha: Sinikoro Gua Sha Facial Tool - Natural Jade Stone — a tool for scraping the skin according to the Traditional Chinese Medicine practice. It will increase blood flow. https://amzn.to/3Hrd9gQ

Glucosomine/Chondroiton: 21st Century Glucosamine Chondroitin 500/400mg — on the Cusack Protocol for the teeth. https://amzn.to/44nh4G2

Hairspray: AZ's Own Hairspray — the ingredients are simply distilled water, prickly pear plant extract, and citric acid (and you can ask for it without the citric acid if you are sensitive to it). It gives the hair a nice texture. You can spray on the hairspray and then brush your hair, and it looks beautiful with no fly-aways. However, in my experience in a humid environment, it lasts for only a couple hours before it needs to be reapplied. http://azsungoldsoaps.com/mobile/order/samples/products_hairspray.html

Handkerchiefs: 100% Cotton Handkerchiefs with Scalloped Edges and Floral Print. https://amzn.to/44chpuZ

Hayaluronic Acid: Amazing Formulas Hyaluronic Acid — on the Cusack Protocol to support the eyes. https://amzn.to/4dfsGyN

Headache Relief: Zok Device — regulates pressure in the head and helps the ear to drain. https://amzn.to/3HnmRAO

Heart Rate Monitor: Polar H10 Heart Rate Monitor Chest Strap — I have not used this before; it has good reviews both on Amazon and in articles online. There are a variety of styles of heart-rate monitors available, including sleeves and watches. https://amzn.to/499fbxD

Heating Pad: Sunbeam XL Heating Pad with Sponge for Moist Heating Option — this is not exactly the model I have, but I have been using my Sunbeam heating pad for about 30 years. I have not tried the moist heat sponge; I would imagine that one of the cotton canvas moist heat pads that you boil on the stove would work better, though be inconvenient. https://amzn.to/4dcOzi8

Herbal Healing Oil: Earth Elements Organic Comfrey Oil — comfrey, also known as "bone knit," is effective at quickly healing and reducing pain in body tissues. Apply it to the skin at the site of the injury. It is meant to be used daily during healing, but not typically for daily use. https://amzn.to/3TDV4D9

Histamine Degrading Enzyme (see also DAO): Histamine Digest – these pills contain the Diamine Oxidase (DAO) enzyme that helps the body rid itself of excess histamine; taken 15 minutes before a meal, immediately after an environmental trigger, and at bedtime, they can potentially prevent or reduce MCAS symptoms. https://amzn.to/3WvIqHY

Homeopathic Remedies: Boiron Homeopathic Remedies — these pills are safe and helpful. They come in little bottles that dispense one pill at a time with a twist of the lid. These do contain dairy, so if you need vegan, search and you will find a dairy-free version. https://amzn.to/49S8LTS

Overexertion, physical or emotional trauma, bumps, bruises, scratches, emotional shock, hurt feelings, sore muscles from working out, pain: *Arnica montana*. https://amzn.to/48ryZwi

Bee or wasp sting: *Apis mellifica*. https://amzn.to/4aOV2ic

Itchy bug bites, prevention of bug bites: *Ledum palustre*. https://amzn.to/3RT4OqV

Difficulty breathing, fatigue, exposure to poisonous chemicals, food poisoning: *Arsenicum album*. https://amzn.to/3HawrH9

Sinus pressure, sneezing, colds: *Pulsatilla*. https://amzn.to/3vv0832

Body aches and exhaustion: *Chamomilla*. https://amzn.to/4b1KpJ0

Motion Sickness: *Cocculus indicus* https://amzn.to/48jxvUW

Stiff neck, tension headache, stage fright, fever, muscle tension: *Gelsemium sempervirons*. https://amzn.to/3tLaTO3

Allergic reaction initial stage and anxiety: *Ignatia amara*. https://amzn.to/48QcuRP

Inflamed mucous membranes, sore throat, Sinus Congestion, fever: *Belladonna*. https://amzn.to/3NVDR4M

Cough and chest congestion: *Phosphorous*. https://amzn.to/47xYESO

Hopelessness, overwhelm, menstrual cramps, mood swings, sense of being overworked at home: *Sepia*. https://amzn.to/3RRVN1t

Poison ivy rash, itchy rashes: *Poison ivy and oak*. https://amzn.to/3HdjU5C

Nausea, Motion Sickness, Insomnia caused by worry: *Nux vomica*. https://amzn.to/3vAOKT3

Deep-seated fear: *Stramonium*. https://amzn.to/428imU9

Muscle tension and anxiety: *Magnesium phosphorica*. https://amzn.to/3TVPhJw

Sores in mouth, sore throat: *Mercurius solubus*. https://amzn.to/3TTMArP

Swelling in face, sneezing, coughing, allergen exposure: *Histaminum hydrochloricum*. https://amzn.to/3tOerPO

Exposure to petroleum products like synthetic fragrances and gasoline, skin rashes: *Petroleum*. https://amzn.to/3Scgllx

Motion sickness: *Tabacum*. https://amzn.to/427IKxH

Social stress, nervousness about talking in front of a crowd, bloating, gas: *Lycopodium clavatum*. https://amzn.to/4aS57La

Fatigue: *Silicea*. https://amzn.to/3Scn4wX

Nerve pain: *Hypericum perforatum*. https://amzn.to/3S7CC4V

Indigestion: *Carbo vegetabilis*. https://amzn.to/41TiQNP

Vomiting, nausea: *Ipecacuanha*. https://amzn.to/3Scgllx

Sunburn, blisters, urinary tract infection: *Cantharis*. https://amzn.to/3vAPWG1

Prevention of flu or cold if taken immediately at onset of symptoms: *Aconitum napellus*. https://amzn.to/48LnkZ5

Colds: *ColdCalm*. https://amzn.to/3tNJA5Q

Flu, Motion Sickness: *Oscillococcinum*. https://amzn.to/3SbegqU

Diarrhea: *Diaralia*. https://amzn.to/47tGzFm

Insoles: Cork Insoles for Men and Women — they absorb sweat and scents and provide just a little bit of natural cushioning. I like to buy them a size too big and cut them with scissors down to the shape of my shoe. These are flat, do not have arch supports, and are flexible, so they are appropriate for barefoot/minimalist shoes. https://amzn.to/3PYfpAD

Ionizer: Wein AS300 Personal Air Purifier - Rechargeable — Ionizers neutralize fragrances, other Volatile Organic Compounds (VOCs), and even bacteria and viruses that are in the air. This one is easily wearable and creates a little atmosphere of safe air around your face. It is indispensable for me when I am sensitive to fragrances and desire to go into public. https://amzn.to/3OmbfSo

Jars: Cornucopia 2oz Cobalt Blue Glass Jars w/Metal Lids — I use these for a lot of the little potions I mix up, like the bentonite clay face mask or underarm mask. I also use them for carrying with me small amounts of refined organic shea butter and remineralizing tooth powder. https://amzn.to/49oQlua

Jar Opener: 5 in 1 Multi Function Can Opener Bottle Opener Kit with Silicone Handle. https://amzn.to/3Sz2S8I

Jojoba Oil: Handcraft Blends Organic Jojoba Oil — I actually do not like jojoba oil, but scientific studies have shown that it is one of the more effective oils for repairing the skin barrier. https://amzn.to/3VkZUEY

Kinesiology Recovery Tape: KT Tape — this cotton-and-elastic kinesiology recovery tape can be used in place of a brace or on body parts that cannot be braced to stabilize joints. Physical Therapists are trained to apply KT Tape correctly. If you have some experience with it, you may be able to follow YouTube videos to tape yourself. Before using it to stabilize a joint, test for skin sensitivity to the adhesive by applying a small piece of tape for a short amount of time and then increasing the time. https://amzn.to/47YF0zy

L-Arginine: THORNE L-Arginine Sustained Release — on the Cusack Protocol, may reduce fatigue and improve the health of the lungs, heart, eyes, and ears. https://amzn.to/3UH63fG

Lion's Mane Mushroom: Host Defense Lion's Mane Mushroom — on the Cusack Protocol to reduce stress and social anxiety. https://amzn.to/3UEQuFh

Lymph Supporting Herbs: Cedar Bear Lymphatic Cleanse Immune Support Supplement — these drops contain Red Root Bark, Echinacea Purpurea Root, Elderberry, Plantain Leaf, Graviola Leaf, Blue Vervain Herb, Yarrow Leaf/Flower, Myrrh Oleo-Gum-Resin, Thyme Leaf, USP Grade Vegetable Glycerin and Purified Water; the glycerin is said to be made from palm oil. https://amzn.to/3TS76aW

Magnesite Stones: Natural Magnesite Rough Stones — these are an inexpensive, comfortable, and safe way of getting magnesium and reducing muscle tension, cramps, spasms, and twitches. Place a stone inside your sock so that it is against your skin. According to numerous clients at my holistic center, it can also help with restless leg syndrome. Place a stone inside your underwear, bra, or a sweatband, and your body can absorb the amount of magnesium it needs all throughout the day. If you do crystal healing, these stones offer a very calming and purifying sensation. https://amzn.to/42pdkD5

Magnesium: BodyBio - Liquid Magnesium — this worked really well for me when I needed magnesium without other minerals. It is easy to control your dose, it is nearly tasteless but makes water taste a little bit sweet (when you need magnesium), and it is gentle. https://amzn.to/4bawDms

Magnesium Flakes: Ancient Minerals Magnesium Bath Flakes — these are wonderfully powerful; I always feel my muscles relax and my anxiety melt away after a bath with magnesium flakes. For me, they are worth the greater expense than Epsom salts. Also, you can mix a small amount of them with a tiny bit of water in a jar to make Magnesium Oil, which you can rub on your skin when you have tight muscles or stress. Be aware that if you are severely deficient in magnesium, the Magnesium Oil will make your skin burn, and it is hard to wash off, so test with a very small amount at first; you will need to supplement with oral magnesium to get your levels up first. If you are not deficient in magnesium, Magnesium Oil sprayed on the skin feels like a mist of water that relaxes you. https://amzn.to/3HrNIvn

Magnesium Malate: Source Naturals Magnesium Malate — a form of magnesium that is well absorbed, reduces pain, and is gentle on the digestive system. https://amzn.to/44mPmZO

Maitake Mushroom: Host Defense Maitake Mushroom Capsules — an option on the Cusack Protocol. https://amzn.to/3WldYQT

Milk Thistle Extract: Lean Neutraceuticals Organic Milk Thistle 12000 Mg — supports the liver. https://amzn.to/48LdF4S

Motion Sickness Glasses: Initio Anti Motion Sickness Glasses — a pair like these cured my Motion Sickness. Now my son wears them when we are on long, winding car rides. https://amzn.to/3U8VMZF

Motion Sickness Wristbands: Sea Bands — wrist bands that use acupressure to reduce nausea https://amzn.to/3tT4hND

Multivitamins: Smarty Pants — these are not necessarily the best vitamins for you to take because they contain synthetic vitamins and sugar and they are gummies, which can stick to the teeth, but everything else about them is good — including their taste. I can't make myself take most vitamins — even whole-food vitamins bother me — but I enjoy these and they make me feel better, whereas all of the other vitamins have stuck in my throat and/or upset my stomach. (I have recently discovered some new brands of whole food organic gummy vitamins to try, and I will update the vitamin link on my website if I find a product I like better than Smarty Pants.) This link is for the prenatal version, but they also have other types. https://amzn.to/3OaHYdw

Neti Pot: Into the Scented Garden Aromatic Salt Premium Ceramic Neti Pot. https://amzn.to/4aLpskj

NIR Light Therapy: Hooga Red Light Therapy Box — This is the light box that both my mother and I use. We have gotten great results with healing injuries and improving how our skin looks. https://amzn.to/3S8vLXG

Olive Leaf Extract: Gaia Herbs Olive Leaf for Immune Support — Olive leaf extract supports the immune system so that you can fight off infections from viruses, bacteria, yeast, and other fungi. It also regulates blood pressure and blood glucose levels and prevents cancer. It is very powerful, and in many cases, it will only be needed for 10 days; it is not recommended to take it for more than 3 months at a time. https://amzn.to/3OxpILh

Oven Mitts: DoMii Professional Silicone Oven Mitts Baking Gloves Elbow Length with Cotton Lining — these are elbow length, silicon mitts that protect well for those days when you are feeling clumsy but still need to cook or bake. https://amzn.to/48YbZoQ

Olive Oil: Sky Organics Organic Extra Virgin Olive Oil for Cooking, 100% Pure & Cold Pressed. https://amzn.to/3VwrYqh

Oxygen: Boost Oxygen Pocketsize Canister — conveniently carry this for any time you are exposed to an environmental allergen or trigger. It is less expensive to buy it in larger bottles if you want some to keep at home. https://amzn.to/3UdO9kR

Pans: Lodge 10.25 Inch Cast Iron Pre-Seasoned Skillet — Lodge cast iron comes in many shapes and sizes. https://amzn.to/3U8eCjz

Peppermint Tea: Davidson's Organics, Peppermint Loose Leaf Tea. https://amzn.to/44sybWX

PQQ: Health Thru Nutrition Pyrroloquinoline Quinone — a supplement from the Cusack Protocol which is intended to reduce MCAS sensitivity and improve the health of the gastrointestinal system. https://amzn.to/4aXP1iU

Probiotic: Culturelle Probiotic — recommended on the Cusack protocol to help the digestive system https://amzn.to/3HkFUeX

Quercetin: Pure Encapsulations Quercetin — recommended for MCAS patients because it stabilizes mast cells and can reduce reactions to sensitivities. It also supports the cardiovascular system and immune system. It is a mild supplement that most people can tolerate. https://amzn.to/49oLrgE

Reading Angle Glasses: Lazy Glasses Horizontal High Definition Prism Periscope Lie Down Eyeglasses — for reading without tilting your head. https://amzn.to/3vUcdyP

Rebounder/Mini Trampoline: BCAN 40/48" Foldable Mini Trampoline https://amzn.to/4b14wH2

Red Ball: GoSports Playground Balls for Kids — these balls work well for the Red Ball Exercises. I bought these because I like the variety of colors (the ball doesn't *actually* have to be red for the exercises), and I wanted to give one to all of my family members so that they could keep their necks healthy, too. https://amzn.to/4bgpYXU

Resistance Bands: THERABAND Resistance Bands Set, Professional Non-Latex Elastic Band For Upper & Lower Body Exercise — I use these for doing Shoulder External Rotation exercises and other resistance training. https://amzn.to/48ZtftQ

Resistance Bands with Handles: WHATAFIT Resistance Bands Set, Exercise Bands with Door Anchor, Handles — these work great for doing pull overs (but make sure you hook it onto the doorway according to directions or else it will come down on your face and it hurts, don't ask me how I know). https://amzn.to/3OawB5k

Riboflavin: Thorne Riboflavin 5'-Phosphate — this is a bioactive form of Vitamin B2, supportive of nervous system health. https://amzn.to/49srRQ1

Ring Splints: Arthritis EDS finger splint adjustable — I bought this one because it was affordable and adorable, with a little heart on it. It is adjustable and has really been doing the trick to protect my finger joint. I am sure there are other designs and makers of good quality ring splints, and this link will get you to Etsy where they will be shown to you. Ring splints are available through other sites as well. You may also be able to have a Physical Therapist fit you in ring splints that will be paid for by your health insurance, and with the PT's help, you can be assured that you are choosing a design and fit that helps and doesn't harm. https://www.etsy.com/listing/752986696/splint-ring-silver-925-sterling-silver?ga_order=most_relevant&ga_search_type=all&ga_view_type=gallery&ga_search_query=heart+ring+splint&ref=sr_gallery-1-20&pro=1&frs=1&content_source=d4f2402a0901ddea1fcbeda34cc62a375ba16aee%253A752986696&search_preloaded_img=1&organic_search_click=1

Rolling Chair: Saddle Stool Chair with Backrest and Foot Ring, Ergonomic Rolling — rolling chair for working in the kitchen; I haven't tried it but I have heard that people with hEDS love it. https://amzn.to/3HJiS1p

Rose Geranium Hydrosol: Skincare Guardian Rose Geranium Hydrosol — useful as an insect repellant (ticks, mosquitoes, chiggers), as well as for toning the skin of the face. It has a nice smell that isn't too strong, and the sale page indicates that it has many more healing benefits as well. https://amzn.to/3x0Flp3

Salt: REDMOND Real Sea Salt - Natural Unrefined — this is the salt I use for all my cooking. It contains trace minerals and is not contaminated like many sea salts can be https://amzn.to/3vAoNDd

Shea Butter: Mountain Rose Organic Refined Shea Butter — this organic refined shea butter has no scent and is a very nice moisturizer for hands, lips, face, and body. https://mountainroseherbs.com/refined-shea-butter

Soap: Arizona Sungold Level H High Suds Liquid Soap Shampoo — I use this soap for everything, including washing hands, bodies, dishes, floors, and anything soap is used for. I love it for all of those purposes. I also use it for shampoo because I haven't found a better option for myself, but I do not really like it for that purpose. http://azsungoldsoaps.com/mobile/order/liquid/products_shampoo.html

Snow Boots: Manitobah Mukluks — this brand is high quality, very comfortable and warm, available in children's, women's and men's sizes in a variety of styles. I have the Waterproof

Snowy Owls and can't imagine better boots for wearing to forest school all winter. https://amzn.to/3W7zFnu

Stinging Nettle: FGO Organic Nettle Leaf Loose Tea https://amzn.to/3Unh6Jt

Sunblock: Badger Reef Friendly Sport Mineral Sunscreen — although it can be difficult to rub this in all the way, it works very well and is very safe. My mother adds a little glycerin, and then it rubs in easily. https://amzn.to/3TAtUNw

Tea Strainer: Teablee Stainless Steel Extra-Fine Mesh Brew-in-Mug Basket — use this with looseleaf tea to avoid the poisons that might be in the paper of tea bags. https://amzn.to/4aa7TKG

Therapy Balls: MELT Hand & Foot Therapy Ball Kit — these help loosen up your feet when you are transitioning into barefoot shoes or if you are treating Plantar Fasciitis. https://amzn.to/3u481vV

Toe Separators: Star Han Yoga Gym Sports Five Toe Separator Massage Foot Alignment Socks — these can help release tight muscles and fascia in the feet and help heal Bunions. There are many other toe separating socks, shoes, and devices available, but these are the only ones I tried and they were sufficient and comfortable for me. https://amzn.to/3ICd3Dn

Toilet Stool: Squatty Potty Original Bathroom Stool — a stool that goes around your toilet so that you can sit in the best position for evacuating the bowels. Although a wood one is nice in an adult's bathroom, the plastic stool is probably easier to clean. https://amzn.to/4aRQjvg

Tongue Scraper: HealthandYoga SteloSwipe Tongue Cleaner — made of stainless steel. https://amzn.to/4cMp5bv

Toothbrushes: Bass Toothbrushes — these have a small number of soft bristles and short handles to help you brush your teeth gently to prevent damaging the gums. Although I usually want everything to be all-natural, plastic-free, I found that my oral mucosa was too fragile to use the bamboo version of these toothbrushes. https://store.orawellness.com/products/bass-toothbrush?variant=31237245841

Trace Minerals: ION* Gut Support — just take a drop or two a day, and this expensive bottle will last a long time. https://amzn.to/49Dzaoj

Vagus Nerve Stimulator: Ear Clip Electrode Wire for TENS Vagus Stim and CES Device — I have not used this, though I have heard people get good results with ear clip stimulation. You hook this up to a TENS unit for the electrical power; the TENS unit is not included. https://amzn.to/4cpH3jQ

Vagus Nerve Supporting Nutritional Supplement: Parasym Plus — This supplement contains acetylcholine, which is integral to the operation of the nervous system, including the Vagus Nerve. It was recommended to me by Sterling Cooley of Vagus Nerve Stimulation and Repair. When I started taking it, I felt that it did make a difference, but I soon hit a plateau in improvement and did not notice any problems when I stopped taking it. I do take it whenever a Joint Injury causes strain or compression of a nerve, as recognized by symptoms of pain, weakness, and itching along the nerve pathway, and my experience is that the injury seems to heal more quickly than without the supplement. However, it may exacerbate Dystonia, which can be caused by overactive nerves, since this supplement will increase the nerves' power. You can measure the Vagus Nerve's health by measuring your Heart Rate Variability (the difference in heart rate between resting and exercising — the greater the difference, the better) — see the link for Heart Rate Monitor. https://amzn.to/484v0VF

Vibrating Massager: Wahl Deep Tissue Corded Long Handle Percussion Massager — this is a really powerful massager that my muscles love. You may need a gentler one for some purposes, though. https://amzn.to/3U5y4xm

Vibration Plate: LifePro Hovert 3D Vibration Plate Machine — get lymph flowing and develop an exercise routine that gets faster results, especially for building core strength. Although these can be dangerous for particularly vulnerable joints, I have read that Physical Therapists get great results for their patients with them. My mother and a friend have used this one. https://amzn.to/3UxvHmT

Vitamin C: Revitalize Wellness Fine Powder Ascorbic Acid — you can mix this into a drink to take it. It is a high quality ascorbic acid; the company also has other Vitamin C offerings. https://revitalizewellness.org/products/vitamin-c-as-ascorbic-acid-16oz-fine-powder

Vitamin C Sucker: YumEarth Organic Vitamin C Pops — for the times when I've taken more pills than I can stand. Vitamin C suckers travel well, are easy and enjoyable to take, are appropriate for children, and slightly help reduce Allergy/MCAS/MCS reactions for me. https://amzn.to/4a06BBz

Vitamin C With Bioflavanoids: THORNE Vitamin C - Blend of Vitamin C and Citrus Bioflavonoids from Oranges. https://amzn.to/4bisYmX

Water Bottle: Lifefactory 16-Ounce BPA-Free Glass Water Bottle with Classic Cap and Protective Silicone Sleeve — https://amzn.to/3TDiW9N

Water Filter: Aquasana SmartFlow Reverse Osmosis Water Filter System — This is an under-sink system that stores the water in a stainless-steel tank, and the dispensing spout is stainless steel as well. The filter (which is not made of coconut like most water filters) removes up to 99.99% of fluoride, arsenic, chlorine, and lead, and it comes with a remineralizer so that you get what you need out of your water. There is also a Water for Life subscription so that your replacement filters will be sent to you automatically when it is time to replace them. There is some plumbing required for installing this filter. It is a little bit difficult to change the filters until you get the hang of it, but the customer service is very good. This company also offers a number of other water filtration options. https://amzn.to/43m3qSZ

Water Flosser: Waterpik Aquarius Water Flosser. https://amzn.to/3RTLidI

Weights: Amazon Basics Neoprene Coated Hexagon Workout Dumbbell Hand Weights. https://amzn.to/3VlXvuR

Yoga Ball: THERABAND Exercise Ball, Professional Series Stability Ball —I lean backwards over this ball to stretch my chest and relieve Thoracic Outlet Syndrome and Rib Subluxations. You may need a different size depending on the size and flexibility of your body. Be careful not to instigate a POTS episode when you lean back. You can also sit on this ball and bounce if you're not able to stand on a mini-trampoline and jump. https://amzn.to/3O79qbZ

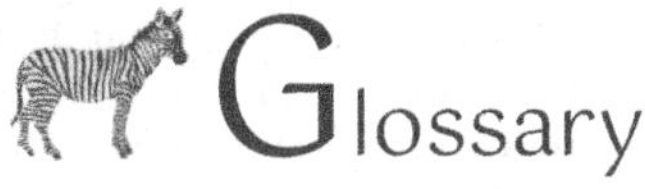

Glossary

Abhyanga Oil Massage — a tradition from India that helps to remove toxic chemicals from the body.

Acupressure — a therapy that presses on energy points in the body, hands, feet, or energy meridians, corresponding to other parts or conditions of the body.

Acupuncture — a Traditional Chinese Medicine therapy that applies tiny needles into the skin along energy meridians. This should be conducted by a certified TCM doctor.

Acute — happening quickly and lasting for a short time.

Adrenal Cocktail — a beverage you can make at home with kitchen staples to support your body when you are feeling adrenal fatigue, which can be caused by chronic stress or illness. See Appendix A.

-algia — a suffix from Greek meaning pain.

Amalgam Filling — the silver-colored tooth fillings that contain mercury, which is poisonous.

Analgesic — pain reducing.

Anaphylaxis — illness that develops in reaction to a food, airborne chemical, or substance that has touched the skin and that includes two or more body systems. Severe anaphylaxis can be fatal because it constricts airways, but there are three less severe levels of anaphylaxis that include many possible symptoms.

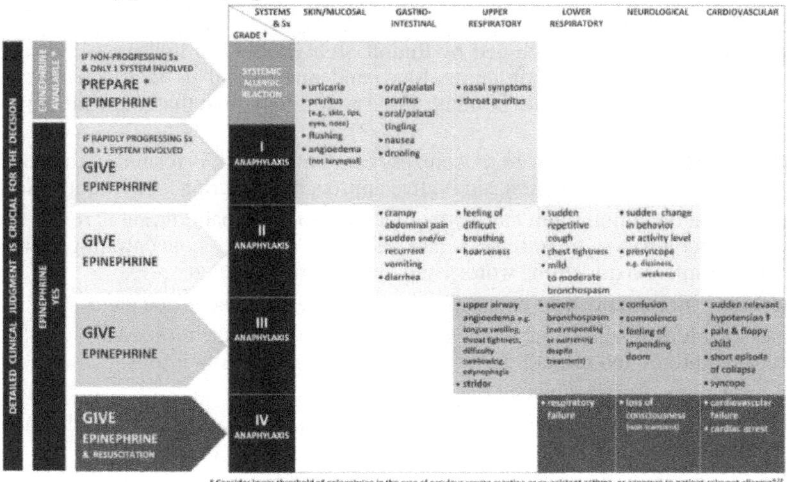

Reprinted with permission from Błażowski, Łukasz & Majak, Pawel & Kurzawa, Ryszard & Kuna, Piotr & Jerzyńska, Joanna. (2021).[796]

Andy Cutler Chelation Protocol — a method of removing heavy metals such as mercury and lead from the body. This method is very effective and safe, but it takes dedication.

Anthroposophy — a philosophy of spiritual science developed by Rudolf Steiner that offers guidance on every aspect of life, including accessing the spirit worlds, and has led to the birth of Biodynamic farming and Waldorf schools.

Antiseptic — prohibiting infection by killing bacteria, viruses, and fungi.

Anxiety Disorder — A condition in which a patient detects a worry- or fear-inducing stimulus at a lower threshold than normal; experiences biological, emotional, and cognitive responses that are more extreme than normal; and enacts preventive measures that are more restrictive than normal. Many of the physiological symptoms of anxiety are similar to symptoms of hEDS (and its common secondary conditions), such as racing heart, breathlessness, dizziness, prickling sensations, restlessness, trembling, muscle tension, fatigue, insomnia, and irritability.

Aphasia — inability to remember and speak words or form proper sentences.

Atlantoaxial Instability (AAI) — instability between the topmost vertebra (Atlas or C1) and the one right below it (Axis or C2). Frequently, this condition is lumped in with Cranio-Cervical Instability under the umbrella term CCI.

Auditory Processing Disorder — a neural disorder in which sounds are not processed as they should be. It can lead to overwhelm in noisy environments and difficulty understanding speech, especially if carried or amplified over electronic equipment.

Aura — the phase of a Migraine attack immediately preceding the headache, usually consisting of seeing lights.

Ayurveda — the ancient Indian tradition of medicine that looks to the mind, body, and spirit and uses natural diet, lifestyle, and herbs to bring about holistic health.

Bates Method — a method of improving eyesight and eye health, developed by William Bates. It is most famous for the practices of Sunning and Palming, but many other exercises can release the hypertonicity in the eyeball and surrounding muscles and bring about desired improvements.

Benign — harmless, not dangerous.

Bio- — a prefix from Greek meaning life.

Biodynamic Farming — developed by Rudolf Steiner, this is a holistic, ecological, and ethical approach to farming, gardening, food, and nutrition. This is a step beyond the requirements of certified organic farming, and it is so productive that many farmers in my area practice it.

Biologic Dentist — a dentist who recognizes that dental health is related to the condition of the entire body and uses natural, alternative approaches to caring for the teeth and gums.

Brain Fog — a condition often caused by inflammation and pain during flares of chronic illnesses, it encompasses forgetfulness, lack of focus, difficulty concentrating, confusion, slow thinking, aphasia (forgetting words), and being scatter-brained.

Buccal Tie — abnormally tight mucosal tethers between the cheek and gums.

Bunion — a misalignment of the joint where the big toe meets the foot, usually causing pain and other symptoms and sometimes involving misalignment of other toes.

CCI — see Cranio-Cervical Instability.

Cerebellar Ataxia — clumsiness or lack of coordination caused by a problem in the cerebellum, which is located at the back of the brain just above the neck.

Cervico- — a root word from Latin meaning neck (cervix = neck of the uterus).

Cervical Spine — the vertebrae (spinal bones) of your neck.

Chelate — remove heavy metals from the body using chemicals or herbs.

Chiari Malformation — a structural abnormality in which part of the Cerebellum (lowest part of the brain) extends down through the base of the skull into the spinal canal, where it can interfere with the flow of cerebrospinal fluid and create a wide variety of symptoms, some life-threatening. It is thought to be very rare but has been diagnosed in 4.7% of hEDS patients.[797]

Chiropractor — a doctor who treats the musculoskeletal system, generally using manipulation, tools, and exercises to align joints properly.

Chronic — persistent and long-lasting; usually describes a disease that lasts for more than 3 months.

Clinical — happening in the clinic with real patients. Clinical experience is often different from what happens during non-clinical research studies.

Collagen — a connective tissue made of protein. It provides structural support to the skin, ligaments, bones, and other tissues.

Collagen Peptides — a protein supplement powder.

Community Supported Agriculture (CSA) — a subscription arrangement in which the consumer pays for farm products up front and then receives them periodically throughout the growing season, according to an arrangement developed by the specific farmer.

Comorbidity — a condition occurring simultaneously with another condition. Some of the comorbidities that are common with hEDS are thought to be caused by hEDS, but others are not caused by it.

Connective Tissue — tissue that provides a framework, supporting and connecting other types of tissues in the body, such as muscles, organs, skin, nerves, etc. It is made mostly of collagen.

Constellation Work — This work is led by a certified practitioner and heals the generational problems that you have inherited from your ancestors. It is fascinating and fun to participate in.

Cranio- — having to do with the cranium or skull.

Cranio-Cervical Instability (CCI) — unnatural movement of the first and second vertebrae in the neck (C1 and C2 or Atlas and Axis). It can cause injury to the nerves in the neck and to the brain. Pain, inflammation, and a host of other symptoms can be expected.

Craniosacral Therapy (CST) — a gentle, hands-on method of aligning the movement of the skull, spine, and hips and regulating the pulse and flow of the craniosacral fluid in the brain and spinal cord.

Cranium — skull.

Crepitus — noises that emanate from joints when they are moved. The noises may sound like cracking, popping, snapping, grinding, sparkling, crunching, creaking, etc. Crepitus can also apply to sounds emanating from the lungs.

Cross Training — exercising to strengthen, activate, stretch, or increase stamina in a way that is opposing to your main form of working out. This keeps the body balanced, especially when you focus on stabilizing a joint by giving exercise attention to all of the different muscles that support and move the joint in all of its different types of movement.

CSA — See Community Supported Agriculture.

CST — See Craniosacral Therapy.

Cusack Protocol — a supplement protocol developed by Deborah Cusack to treat many of the symptoms of hEDS.

Degranulate — the process through which mast cells release numerous immunomodulatory substances such as histamine, tryptase, prostaglandins, and cytokines to activate an immune response to pathogens, stress, or injuries.

Detox — remove toxins from the body.

-dynamic- — a root word from Greek meaning full of activity or change.

Dysphagia — difficulty swallowing which may cause pain or discomfort.

Earthing or Grounding — connecting to the Earth's electric field to heal the body.

Edema — swelling.

EHS — see Electromagnetic Hypersensitivity.

Electrolytes — minerals, such as sodium, potassium, and magnesium, that carry an electric charge and are necessary for our health.

Electromagnetic Frequency (EMF) — the wavelengths emitted from every object. EMFs generally refers to the frequencies released from electronics, cell phones, cell towers, WiFi routers, etc. They are thought to be harmful to biological bodies, and many people must take measures to protect themselves from them, either by avoidance or by using shielding and grounding technologies.

Electromagnetic Hypersensitivity (EHS) — sensitivity to certain electromagnetic frequencies (EMFs), especially those emanating from technological devices, manifesting with a variety of symptoms in multiple body systems such as Insomnia, fatigue, anxiety, difficulty concentrating, and headaches.

Elimination — urination (peeing) and defecation (pooping).

Elimination Diet — a diet in which you eliminate a suspected allergen from your meals for a certain amount of time (often 3 weeks) and then reintroduce it to discover if your body reacts to it in a negative way. Sometimes a larger number of suspect foods are eliminated at once and then added back one at a time.

EMFs — see Electromagnetic Frequencies.

Endocrine System – hormone secreting organs of the body.

Endogenous — originating from within the body rather than caused by an outside factor.

Epigenetics — from the Greek *epi*, meaning in addition to; it is the changing nature of genetic expression affected by environmental factors such as toxins, viruses, experiences, hormones, foods, and more.

Excipient — ingredients in medications that are not the active ingredient but aid in the delivery or effectiveness of the medication.

Eye Strain — pain of the eyes, often caused by looking at computer and cell phones screens. It is generally caused by hypertonicity of the eye muscles, though other facial and skull muscles may be involved.

Faraday Cage — an enclosure that blocks EMFs.

Forest Bathing — spending time in a forest or other natural setting for the enjoyment and healing benefits.

Fragrance — a term used on ingredient labels that can refer to one or more of over 3,500 chemicals, 95% of which are toxic petrochemicals that endanger our health and the environment.

Gaslighting — Named for the movie *Gaslight*, in which a man tries to make his wife think she is crazy by dimming and flashing the gas lights but telling her that they did not dim or flash. For example, when a diagnosis cannot be determined, a patient may be told that her symptoms are all in her head or caused by psychological problems.

Goniometer — a ruler with two pivoting lengths that measures angles and is used to measure the range of motion of joints.

Green Washing — the act of deceptively calling something "green" or "non-toxic" when it is not.

Grounding — see Earthing.

Growing Pains — unexplained pains that children get, usually in the arms and legs. It is now believed that they are often caused by Joint Injuries or other soft-tissue injuries.

Gua Sha — a practice of Traditional Chinese Medicine that uses a smooth tool (usually made of jade) to scrape the skin rather roughly to release stagnant blood and other fluids. When this is done, the skin over areas that have a lot of stagnation (which are usually the areas of pain or other complaints) tends to turn bright red as compared to the other areas.

Haka — the traditional war dance of the Māori people of New Zealand. It contains elements such as shaking, stomping, thumping, and yelling that can relieve and prevent stress and trauma.

Healing Crisis — unpleasant surge of new symptoms or exacerbation of pre-existing symptoms caused by healing. For example, the die-off of overabundant candida yeast can cause flu-like symptoms and rashes.

Heart Rate Variability — A measurement that is sometimes used as an indicator of health for the heart, veins, autonomic nervous system, and Vagus Nerve. The larger the difference between resting and active heart rates, the better.

hEDS - see Hypermobile Ehlers-Danlos Syndrome.

Herxheimer Reaction — unpleasant, usually flu-like symptoms created by the killing of spirochete bacteria (such as Lyme). This most often occurs when a new supplement or technique is implemented.

Hip Upslip — a misalignment of the hip in which the pelvis moves too high in relation to the sacrum along the sacroiliac joint. It is very painful.

Histamine — a hormone that acts as part of the immune system to incite inflammation in response to threats.

Holistic — having to do with all of the components of the body, as well as the mind and spirit, all together.

Homeopathic Remedies — products made from sugar and plant, mineral, or animal components that are so diluted they cannot be measured scientifically. As an inexpensive treatment for an enormous variety of symptoms, they are a safe way of communicating with the body so that it can heal itself.

Hopi — a Native American tribe from eastern Arizona.

HSD — see Hypermobility Spectrum Disorder.

Hyper- — a prefix from Greek that means excessive.

Hyperemesis Gravidarum — extreme nausea and vomiting during pregnancy.

Hyperextension — extending a joint beyond its normal range of motion, sometimes causing pain and injury.

Hypermobile Ehlers-Danlos Syndrome (hEDS) — a connective tissue disorder described by Dr. Ehlers and Dr. Danlos in 1901. Not long ago, it was thought that 1 in 5,000 people have hEDS, but it is now considered to be much more common.

Hypermobility — an unusually large range of movement in one or more joints.

Hypermobility Spectrum Disorder (HSD) — a connective tissue disorder with the same treatments and symptoms as hEDS, but that does not reach the current clinical diagnostic criteria of hEDS. There are several HSDs, including Generalized, Peripheral, Localized, and Historical.

iGE-Mediated Allergies — a reaction to a protein mediated by Immunoglobulin-E in the body. These are the typical, recognizable allergies and include symptoms such as sneezing, watery eyes, hives, vomiting, etc. These reactions usually occur immediately upon exposure to the allergen. They sometimes cause severe anaphylaxis, a potentially fatal acute condition in which a person's airway may swell closed.

Hypertonicity — tension in muscles beyond what is normal. Often it feels like the muscle is hard or frozen. See also -ton-.

Iatrogenic — from the Greek *iatro* for physician and *genesis* for origin; causing harm through medical treatment, diagnosis, neglect, or mistakes.

Idiopathic — of unknown origin. Doctors put this in front of a diagnosis when they do not know what caused it.

in utero — in the uterus, as in what happens to a fetus before birth.

Incontinence — loss of control of urination.

Insomnia — inability to sleep through the night.

Interoception – your conscious or subconscious sense of the condition within your body, such as feeling your heart beat or feeling hungry. (People with hEDS often have heightened interoception.)

Interstitial Cystitis — interstitial means the spaces between cells, and cystitis means inflammation of the urinary bladder. Sometimes a result of MCAS, it can cause bladder pain and other pelvic pain, as well as urinary frequency and urgency.

Invisible Illness — a chronic illness that has periodically or chronically debilitating symptoms but does not feature an appearance of illness; sufferers tend to stay home when they are at their worst, and when they appear in social venues, they look healthy, whether they feel good or not.

-itis — suffix from Greek that means inflammation.

Laxity — looseness, lack of firm control.

Leaky Gut — a condition in which the small intestines are more permeable than they should be and molecules leak out of the gut into the bloodstream.

LEDs — Light Emitting Diodes are the most common of the new types of light bulbs, and they power some cell phone and computer screens. LEDs flicker imperceptibly during normal operation, and it is thought that this flicker can trigger Migraine attacks and other health issues in sensitive people.

Lhermitte's Sign — sudden pain, tingling, and loss of sensation in the neck and radiating out from it; it usually lasts for only seconds or minutes.

Ligament — a band of fibrous connective tissue made of collagen that connects bones to other bones and stabilizes the joint.

Light Sensitivity — discomfort caused by the apparent brightness of light. Related conditions are Photo Sensitivity, in which the skin may react to sunlight, and Visual Disturbances such as Aura, which may happen during Migraine attacks.

Logos — Greek root word meaning reason, idea, or word.

Lyme Disease — a tickborne illness that might increase symptoms for hEDS/HSD patients because it affects the joints and damages collagen.

Lymph — a fluid that carries nutrients to cells and waste and harmful substances like toxins and pathogens away from them. It travels through the Lymphatic System, which consists of vessels in the skin, some organs, and lymph nodes.

Lymph Congestion — a buildup of lymph fluids in the body due to poor lymph flow. It can cause headache, bloating, weight gain, fatigue, muscle and joint pain, and more.

Lymph Drainage Massage — a gentle massage that helps move the lymph fluid through the Lymphatic System.

Maple Syrup — pure maple syrup is the boiled sap from a maple tree and it contains many constituents that are good for your health. It is also delicious and lower in glycemic load than most sweeteners. This is not the same as the pancake syrup that is commonly sold on grocery store shelves, which is mostly corn syrup, does not have the same healing properties as maple syrup, and can actually be bad for you if you eat very much of it.

Mast Cell Activation Syndrome (MCAS) — mast cells are an important part of the immune system, protecting us from invaders like viruses, bacteria, and parasites; in this condition, they get overly activated and/or activated by things that are not true threats. This creates an allergy-like reaction with symptoms in any or all of the body's systems; it also runs a risk of severe anaphylaxis, a life-threatening condition in which the throat can swell shut.

MCAS — see Mast Cell Activation Syndrome.

MCS — see Multiple Chemical Sensitivity.

Mediumship — transmitting communications from the spirits of deceased people to their living loved ones.

Meridian — in Traditional Chinese Medicine, these are pathways through which vital energy moves. The acupuncture points are located along these pathways.

Methylenetetrahydrofolate Reductase Single Nucleotide Polymorphism (MTHFR SNP) — this is a very common variation of the genetic code which can cause a reduction in the effectiveness of the body's detox systems. It is treated primarily with avoidance of folic acid and supplementation of methyl folate.

Methylcolbalamin — a form of Vitamin B12 that is more often safe and bioavailable for people with hEDS and its comorbidities than are other forms of B12.

Methyl Folate — biologically active form of folic acid that is more readily bioavailable for people with MTHFR.

Mewing — advocated for by John and Mike Mew, this is a popular name for a resting tongue posture in which the tongue is pressed with suction against the roof of the mouth, possibly resulting in benefits like better facial formation, sleep, neck tensegrity, and much more.

Migraine — not just a bad headache, Migraine is a disabling neurological disease with 4 distinct phases and a long list of symptoms.

Military Neck — loss of the normal curvature in the cervical spine.

Mobile — able to move.

Mobility — ability to move.

Morning Sickness — nausea during pregnancy, considered to be normal.

Motion Sickness — nausea and possibly vomiting, dizziness, and malaise that occurs when moving in a vehicle, boat, airplane, etc.

MTHFR — See Methylenetetrahydrofolate Reductase Single Nucleotide Polymorphism.

Multiple Chemical Sensitivity (MCS) — referred to also by other names like TILT (Toxicant Induced Loss of Sensitivity), CI (Chemical Intolerance), and EI (Environmental Illness). This condition causes sensitivity to environmental and food allergens; many people believe that people with these sensitivities are like canaries in the coal mines, being noticeably harmed by poisonous chemicals (such as fragrances and food additives) before other people notice their effects. Doctors are not in agreement about what causes these conditions nor how to treat them.

Mutagenic —can permanently change DNA.

Myofascial Release — a variety of techniques for releasing adhesions among the fascia, a connective-tissue framework that provides structure and separates and connects components of the body.

Near Infrared and Red Light Therapy (NIR) — the use of light bulbs that emit red and near-infrared wavelengths of light to trigger changes in cells and mitochondria and generate ATP (adenosine triphosphate), which provides necessary energy for cellular metabolism.

Neuralgia — pain, inflammation, and other sensations that occur in a damaged nerve.

Neuromodulating — exerting control over or changes in the behavior of the nervous system.

Neuropathy — pain, numbness, cramping, weakness, itching, or tingling along the route of an injured nerve.

Neurotoxic — harmful to the nerves and brain.

Nociception — the ability of the nervous system to sense, anticipate, and react to threats before they occur. Nociceptive nerve fibers can recognize noxious chemical substances, near-hyperextension (mechanical strain), and dangerous temperatures (such as heat from a hot stove). Signals are sent from the small nerve endings to the central nervous system, inciting defensive actions, emotional experience, and pain, even though damage has not yet occurred to the body. Nociception can activate the fight/flight response in order to protect the body from potential harm.

Non-iGE-Mediated Allergies — a reaction to a substance that is not mediated by Immunoglobulin-E but by other immune system components. These reactions often do not appear immediately upon an exposure to an allergen; it may take days for recognizable symptoms to occur. Symptoms can include diarrhea, constipation, eczema, headache, acne, mouth sores, and many other symptoms. Doctors and scientists have not yet learned as much about these kinds of allergies as the iGE-Mediated Allergies. See also MCAS and MCS.

Normobaric Oxygen Therapy — breathing oxygen through a mask or nasal cannula from an oxygen condensing machine, tank, or canister to treat symptoms.

Noxious – poisonous or otherwise harmful.

Occipital Neuralgia — damage to the occipital nerve that runs from the eye to the back of the neck, causing headaches, eye pain, neck pain, and more.

Occupational Therapist — similar to a Physical Therapist in the way they work, an Occupational Therapist will help a patient find ways to manage and regain skills for managing daily life.

Oil Pulling — a treatment for the teeth and gums in which you swish approximately one tablespoon of organic sesame or olive oil in your mouth for twenty minutes. Spit the oil into the trash can (so it won't clog the sink) and then rinse your mouth with water. This can be part of a regimen to heal and prevent cavities and abscesses.

-ology — a suffix from Greek meaning a science or branch of study.

Orthotropics — developed by John Mew, unlike orthodontics that moves the teeth and can damage the facial structure, orthotropics guides facial development and tongue posture to eliminate the underlying structural causes of crooked teeth and make a more attractive and healthy facial structure.

Osteo- — a prefix from Greek meaning bone.

Osteopathy — a branch of medicine that uses massage, craniosacral therapy, Physical Therapy, and many other techniques to manipulate joints and address problems such as pain, digestive upset, and more.

Osteopenia — a loss of bone density that is a precursor to Osteoporosis.

Parasympathetic Nervous System — controls the rest-and-digest response, whereas the Sympathetic Nervous System is active during the fight-or-flight response.

Past Life Regression — a form of meditation that allows a client and the practitioner to envision events from past lives that are having an impact on the client in this lifetime.

-pathy — suffix from Greek meaning disease, method of treating disease, or feeling.

Pathogenesis — the process of how a disease develops and progresses.

Pathology — the underlying cause(s) of an injury, disease, or other medical condition.

Pathophysiology – the changes that occur in the body as the result of an injury, disease, or other medical condition.

Pelvic Dysfunction — improper behavior or condition of the joints, muscles, fascia, and ligaments in the pelvis, causing symptoms like pain, incontinence, urinary frequency, and more.

Pelvic Organ Prolapse — condition in which the vagina, cervix, uterus, bladder, urethra, and/or rectum drop out of position due to the connective tissues being too weak to hold the organs in place, resulting in pain, discomfort, and/or sometimes trouble with elimination and/or sex.

Pelvic Torsion — a twisted misalignment of the pelvic bones, causing pain and possibly other symptoms.

Peripheral Neuropathy — damaged nerve(s) in the peripheral nervous system, which is all of the nerves outside of the spinal cord and brain. Peripheral Neuropathy can cause pain, tingling, numbness, burning, or itching; sometimes these symptoms are felt in body parts distant from the damaged nerves.

Personal Trainer — a trained coach who guides clients through workouts, including Strength Training, aerobic activities, stretching, and whatever is beneficial for the client.

Petroleum Products or Petrochemicals — products made from petroleum or crude oil, which is poisonous to humans, such as plastic, synthetic fragrances, and polyester.

Physical Therapy — a form of treatment that uses bodywork, exercise, and lifestyle recommendations to restore function and comfort following an injury or surgery and to address factors that can prevent future injuries, increase abilities, improve athletic performance, prepare patients for surgery, and more.

Pilates — a form of low-impact exercise developed by Joseph Pilates that aims to strengthen muscles while improving postural alignment and flexibility.

Plantar Fasciitis — inflammation and pain in the connective tissues in the sole of the foot and heel.

Postdrome — a phase of Migraine following the headache that has a long list of potential symptoms.

Postural Orthostatic Tachycardia Syndrome (POTS) — racing and sometimes erratic heart rate due to dysautonomia and causing many possible symptoms, like headache, dizziness, heart pain, and nausea.

POTS — see Postural Orthostatic Tachycardia Syndrome.

Present — used as a verb in the medical world to mean showing signs and symptoms.

Prodrome — a phase of Migraine following a trigger that occurs before the headache and has a long list of potential symptoms.

Progressive — used to describe a condition that gets worse over time.

Prolotherapy — a regenerative therapy in which a natural irritant solution is injected into a joint to stimulate new growth following an injury. (In one of his videos, Dr. Hauser said that the irritant solution is cells taken from the patient's own body and then injected near the concerned ligament(s); other irritant solutions can be used instead.)

Prophylactic — a preventative action or substance.

Proprioception — your sense of where your body is and how it is moving in relation to itself and the space and items around it. (People with hEDS often have reduced proprioception.)

Psychosomatic — a condition of the body that is created in the mind.

Pubic Symphysis — a cartilaginous joint in the front of the pelvis; it usually opens for childbirth and then closes again.

Range of Motion — the comfortable expanse through which a joint can move without damaging it.

Rebounding — jumping on a trampoline, usually a mini trampoline.

Red Light Therapy — red light bulbs can be used for treating skin conditions without including near infrared light. See also Near Infrared and Red Light Therapy.

Referred Pain — pain that is felt at a distant location from the site of injury or disfunction that is causing the pain.

Reiki — energy that is from the divine and directed through the hands of the practitioner to heal physical, emotional, mental, spiritual, and situational problems.

Reverse Osmosis — a water filtration method that removes contaminants, including fluoride, more effectively than other filters, in most cases. It is often used in conjunction with a remineralizing element to provide some of the healthiest water available for drinking.

Self-Agency — the sense of being in control of what happens to you or the actual ability to control what happens to you by controlling your own decisions, physical movements, and environment.

Signs and Symptoms — diagnostically, signs are observable evidence of a condition, including visible rashes, cuts, discolorations, or malformations, as well as the results of blood tests, urine tests, X-ray or MRI images, etc.; symptoms are conditions reported by the patient but not visible to the doctor or clinician, such as pain or fatigue. Practically, in many circumstances and in this book, the word symptom(s) is used to encompass signs as well.

Spectrum Disorder — an illness in which the symptoms vary widely from person to person.

Somatic — biological, of the body, as opposed to of the mind, spirit, or environment.

Sound Healing — using the power of sound waves from musical instruments, the voice, or tuning forks to heal physical and emotional complaints.

Sound Sensitivity — discomfort created by sounds, whether due to their pitch, volume, or complexity. Some people are particularly bothered by sound that is amplified through an electrical speaker, including a telephone. This is sometimes caused by a neural processing disorder and can be somewhat relieved or eliminated by doing The Basic Exercise. See also Auditory Processing Disorder.

Strain/Counterstrain Technique — a method of increasing range of motion, usually instigated by a Massage Therapist or done on yourself. It uses passive body positioning of hypertonic muscles and dysfunctional joints to move them into positions of comfort. This technique is an alternative to stretching for people with hypermobility.

Stroke — death of brain cells due to a blockage or break in a blood vessel in the brain. Depending on where in the brain the problem occurs, it can affect the body in a variety of ways.

Subchorionic Hematoma (SCH) — a bleed or pocket of blood beneath the placenta during pregnancy.

Subluxation — partial dislocation of a joint.

Suboccipital Muscles — the muscles that run from the eyebrow, over the top of the head, to the first two vertebrae in the neck.

Substance P — P is for preparation, a term used by the scientists, Euler and Gaddum, who originally discovered it. It is a neuropeptide that is released by neurons and mast cells; it enhances nociception (nervous system sensing and processing of physical threats and dangers), pain sensations, and sensitivity.

Tailor's Bunion — a Bunion of the pinky toe. It often appears as a bump on the side of the foot near the pinky toe, and sometimes the pinky toe twists and/or bends toward the other toes.

Teflon — a synthetic chemical coating applied to pots and pans for cooking. When scratched, it can release poisonous chemicals into the air, killing pet birds, and into the food that is being cooked on it.

Temporomandibular Joint Disorder (TMJ or TMJD or TMD) — a painful condition of the joints and muscles of the jaw that can cause the jaw to have reduced range of motion.

Tendon — a band of fibrous connective tissue made of collagen that connects a muscle to a bone.

Tennis Elbow — pain in the forearm that is often caused by improper use of the arm due to weakness in the back or instability in the shoulder.

Tensegrity — the balance of tension among the soft tissues in the body.

Terminal — condition that leads to death.

Thai Body Work — a form of massage using acupressure and assisted stretching.

Thoracic Outlet Syndrome (TOS) — a compression of the nerves and veins behind the clavicle. The condition can cause symptoms both above and below the compression point(s) in the chest, including swelling in the shoulders and neck, pain along the sides of the rib cage, and pain and numbness in the shoulders, arms, and hands.

Thymus — a small gland in the upper chest that is shaped like a thyme leaf and is responsible for activating and moderating the immune system. It shrinks as we age, but it can be activated if the skin at that point is tapped or thumped.

Tinea Versicolor — a discoloration of the skin caused by overgrowth of the Malassezia that normally is present on the skin in lower numbers. It is usually not uncomfortable, but it can be unsightly.

Titrate — to adjust the dosage of a medicine or supplement to get the desired results.

TMJ — see Temporomandibular Joint Disorder.

-ton- — (pronounced with a long O sound), a root word from Greek that means tightness. (This originally applied to stretching a string tightly on a musical instrument, so it has been used for "tone of voice" as well as "muscular hypertonicity".)

Tongue Tie — a shortness or tightness of the frenulum that stretches between the tongue and the floor of the mouth. A tongue tie in a baby can cause difficulty with breastfeeding. In children and adults, it can cause Insomnia, headaches, crowded teeth, and numerous symptoms. It can be released with Craniosacral Therapy, Occupational Therapy, and medical intervention, but it should be handled only by very knowledgeable providers.

Traditional Chinese Medicine (TCM) — a long-existing form of medicine that is best known for acupuncture but also utilizes many other techniques and herbs.

Trauma Release Exercises (TRE) — a means of initiating an instinctive shaking in body parts to help release any trauma memories that have been stored there and inhibit proper function of that part.

TRE — See Trauma Release Exercises.

Trigger Finger — the temporary freezing of a finger joint, very common in hEDS patients.

Trigger Point Therapy — a special massage technique to relieve painful knots in the muscles.

Tumor Necrosis Factor — a protein that can be released by mast cells and that triggers and focuses inflammation in areas of injury or infection; it can be responsible for creating pain.

Turf Toe — pain beneath the first joint of the big toe caused by straining the ligaments there or by a stress fracture of a sesamoid bone. The sesamoid bones are similar to knee caps, but under the toes. This condition is called Turf Toe because it is common among football players running and changing direction on artificial turf. It is also a potential complication of Plantar Fasciitis.

Upper Crossed Syndrome — a condition in which the muscles of the chest, upper back, and neck are out of balance and may have become deformed. This causes or is caused by poor posture, and the most commonly affected muscles are the trapezius and levator scapula. This condition causes pain in the neck and back and contributes to improper forward head posture.

Urinary Frequency — the need to urinate more frequently than normal.

Urinary Urgency — an abrupt, unusually strong, and overwhelming need to urinate.

Vagus Nerve — the longest and most complex nerve of the body. It originates in the brain, serves much of the torso, and moderates the parasympathetic control of the heart, lungs, and digestive tract.

Vocal Cord Dysfunction — a condition in which the vocal cords become hypertonic and close partly or completely. When they close all of the way, the patient is unable to breathe in or out or to talk. This can sometimes happen in response to certain MCAS triggers.

Whole Foods — foods that have been minimally processed before being used for cooking at home or in a restaurant. They are generally in the form in which the farmer harvested them.

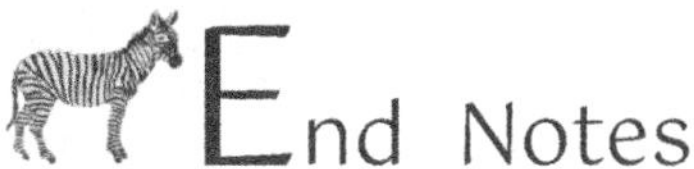

End Notes

These notes can be found online for easy link clicking at shannonegale.com.

1 Hakim, A. (2004). Hypermobile Ehlers-Danlos Syndrome. In Adam, M. P., et. al. (Eds.), *GeneReviews®*. University of Washington, Seattle.

2 Baeza-Velasco, C., Gély-Nargeot, M. C., Pailhez, G., Vilarrasa, A., & Hakim, A. (2004). Hypermobile Ehlers-Danlos Syndrome. In Adam, M. P., et al. (Eds.), *GeneReviews*®. University of Washington, Seattle.

3 Baeza-Velasco, C., Gély-Nargeot, M. C., Pailhez, G., & Vilarrasa, A. B. (2013). Joint hypermobility and sport: a review of advantages and disadvantages. *Current sports medicine reports*, *12*(5), 291-295. https://doi.org/10.1249/JSR.0b013e3182a4b933 .

4 Tinkle, B., Castori, M., Berglund, B., Cohen, H., Grahame, R., Kazkaz, H., & Levy, H. (2017). Hypermobile Ehlers-Danlos Syndrome (a.k.a. Ehlers-Danlos Syndrome Type III and Ehlers-Danlos Syndrome Hypermobility Type): Clinical description and natural history. *American Journal of Medical Genetics. Part C, Seminars in Medical Genetics*, *175*(1), 48-69. https://doi.org/10.1002/ajmg.c.31538 .

5 Bulbena, A. (2022). *Anxiety: A quick immersion*. Tibidabo Publishing, Inc.

6 Aubry-Rozier, B., Schwitzguebel, A., Valerio, F., Tanniger, J., Paquier, C., Berna, C., Hügle, T., & Benaim, C. (2021). Are patients with Hypermobile Ehlers-Danlos Syndrome or Hypermobility Spectrum Disorder so different? *Rheumatology International*, *41*(10), 1785-1794. https://doi.org/10.1007/s00296-021-04968-3 .

7 Hakim, A., & Grahame, R. (2004). Non-musculoskeletal symptoms in joint hypermobility syndrome. Indirect evidence for autonomic dysfunction? *Rheumatology* (Oxford, England). 43. 1194-5. 10.1093/rheumatology/keh279.

8 Ricard-Blum, S. (2011). The collagen family. *Cold Spring Harbor Perspectives in Biology*, 3(1), a004978. https://doi.org/10.1101/cshperspect.a004978 .

9 Tinkle, B., Castori, M., Berglund, B., Cohen, H., Grahame, R., Kazkaz, H., & Levy, H. (2017).

10 Demmler, J. C., Atkinson, M. D., Reinhold, E. J., Choy, E., Lyons, R. A., & Brophy, S. T. (2019). Diagnosed prevalence of Ehlers-Danlos yndrome and hypermobility spectrum disorder in Wales, UK: a national electronic cohort study and case-control comparison. *BMJ Open*, -*9*(11), e031365. https://doi.org/10.1136/bmjopen-2019-031365

11 Kidder, L. (2018, May 22). Ehlers-Danlos Syndrome: When collagen goes bad. *Loma Linda University*. https://drayson.llu.edu/about-news/drayson-news/ehlers-danlos-syndrome-when-collagen-goes-bad

12 Pearce, G., Bell, L., Pezaro, S., & Reinhold, E. (2023). Childbearing with Hypermobile Ehlers-Danlos Syndrome and Hypermobility Spectrum Disorders: A large international survey of outcomes and complications. *International Journal of Environmental Research and Public Health*, *20*(20), 6957. https://doi.org/10.3390/ijerph20206957 .

13 Bulbena, A. (2022). *Anxiety: A quick immersion*. Tibidabo Publishing Inc.

14 Libre Texts Medicine. Lymphatic Vessel Structure. https://med.libretexts.org/Bookshelves/Anatomy_and_Physiology/Anatomy_and_Physiology_(Boundless)/19:_Lymphatic_System/19.2:_Lymphatic_Vessels/19.2A:_Lymphatic_Vessel_Structure .

15 Hardy, D. (2022, October). What is lymphoedema? *The Lymphoedema Support Network.* https://www.lymphoedema.org/information/what-is-lymphoedema/ .

16 National Heart, Lung, and Blood Institute. (2022, May 18). What Is metabolic syndrome? https://www.nhlbi.nih.gov/health/metabolic-syndrome .

17 Oliver, G., et al. (2020, July). The Lymphatic Vasculature in the 21st Century: Novel functional roles in homeostasis and disease. *Cell*, 182. https://doi.org/10.1016/j.cell.2020.06.039

18 Lindberg, G., & Mohammadian, G. (2023). Loose ends in the differential diagnosis of IBS-like symptoms. *Frontiers in Medicine, 10*, 1141035. https://doi.org/10.3389/fmed.2023.1141035 .

19 Lopetuso, L. R., Scaldaferri, F., Bruno, G., Petito, V., Franceschi, F., & Gasbarrini, A. (2015). The therapeutic management of gut barrier leaking: the emerging role for mucosal barrier protectors. *European Review for Medical and Pharmacological Sciences, 19*(6), 1068-1076.

20 Bascom, R., Dhingra, R., & Francomano, C. A. (2021). Respiratory manifestations in the Ehlers-Danlos Syndromes. *American Journal of Medical Genetics. Part C, Seminars in Medical Genetics, 187*(4), 533-548. https://doi.org/10.1002/ajmg.c.31953 .

21 Tinkle, B., Castori, M., Berglund, B., Cohen, H., Grahame, R, Kazkaz, H., & Levy, H. (2017). Hypermobile Ehlers-Danlos Syndrome (a.k.a. Ehlers-Danlos Syndrome Type III and Ehlers-Danlos Syndrome Hypermobility Type): Clinical description and natural history. *American Journal of Medical Genetics. Part C, Seminars in Medical Genetics, 175*(1), 48-69. https://doi.org/10.1002/ajmg.c.31538.

22 Hamonet, C., Schatz, P. M., Bezire, P., Ducret, L., Brissot, R. (2018). Cognitive and Psychopathological Aspects of Ehlers-Danlos Syndrome - Experience in a Specialized Medical Consultation. *Research Advances in Brain Disorders and Therapy.* DOI: 10.29011/ RABDT-104. 100004 . https://www.gavinpublishers.com/assets/articles_pdf/1525934180article_pdf97661175.pdf

23 Deodhar, A. A., & Woolf, A. D. (1994). Ehlers Danlos Syndrome and osteoporosis. *Annals of the Rheumatic Diseases, 53*(12), 841-842. https://doi.org/10.1136/ard.53.12.841-c .

24 Tinkle, B., Castori, M., Berglund, B., Cohen, H., Grahame, R., Kazkaz, H., & Levy, H. (2017).

25 Rachapudi, S. S., Laylani, N. A., Davila-Siliezar, P. A., & Lee, A. G. (2023). Neuro-ophthalmic manifestations of Ehlers-Danlos Ssyndrome. *Current Opinion in Ophthalmology, 34*(6), 476-480. https://doi.org/10.1097/ICU.0000000000001002 .

26 Voermans, N. C., van Alfen, N., Pillen, S., Lammens, M., Schalkwijk, J., Zwarts, M. J., van Rooij, I. A., Hamel, B. C., & van Engelen, B. G. (2009). Neuromuscular involvement in various types of Ehlers-Danlos Syndrome. *Annals of Neurology, 65*(6), 687-697. https://doi.org/10.1002/ana.21643 .

27 Thwaites, P.A., Gibson, P.R., & Burgell, R.E. (2022, September). Hypermobile Ehlers-Danlos Syndrome and disorders of the gastrointestinal tract: What the gastroenterologist needs to know. *J Gastroenterol Hepatol, 37*(9):1693-1709. https://doi.org/10.1111/jgh.15927 .

28 Demmler, J. C., Atkinson, M. D., Reinhold, E. J., Choy, E., Lyons, R. A., & Brophy, S. T. (2019). Diagnosed prevalence of Ehlers-Danlos Syndrome and Hypermobility Spectrum Disorder in Wales, UK: a national electronic cohort study and case-control comparison. *BMJ Open, 9*(11), e031365. https://doi.org/10.1136/bmjopen-2019-031365 .

29 Herzberg, S.D., Motu'apuaka, M.L., Lambert, W., Fu, R., Brady, J., & Guise, J-M. (2017). The effect of menstrual cycle and contraceptives on acl injuries and laxity: A systematic review and meta-analysis. *Orthopaedic Journal of Sports Medicine*, 5(7). https://doi:10.1177/2325967117718781 .

30 On the other hand, numerous transgender men have commented on social media that when they began taking testosterone as part of their gender transition, their hEDS symptoms significantly abated.

31 Tinkle, B., Castori, M., Berglund, B., Cohen, H., Grahame, R., Kazkaz, H., & Levy, H. (2017).

32 Tinkle, B., Castori, M., Berglund, B., Cohen, H., Grahame, R., Kazkaz, H., & Levy, H. (2017).

33 Rogers, B. A., Chicas, H., Kelly, J. M., Kubin, E., Christian, M. S., Kachanoff, F. J., Berger, J., Puryear, C., McAdams, D. P., & Gray, K. (2023). Seeing your life story as a hero's journey increases meaning in life. *Journal of Personality and Social Psychology, 125*(4), 752—778. https://doi.org/10.1037/pspa0000341 .

34 Bulbena-Cabré, A., Baeza-Velasco, C., Rosado-Figuerola, S., & Bulbena, A. (2021, November 9). Updates on the psychological and psychiatric aspects of the Ehlers-Danlos syndromes and hypermobility spectrum disorders. *American Journal of Medical Genetics.* https://doi.org/10.1002/ajmg.c.31955 .

35 Cueto, I. (2022, December 12). Revenge of the gaslit patients: Now, as scientists, they're tackling Ehlers-Danlos Syndromes. *STAT*. https://www.statnews.com/2022/12/12/ehlers-danlos-syndrome-patients-turned-researchers/ .

36 Kobayasi, T., Oguchi, M., & Asboe-Hansen, G. (1984). Dermal changes in Ehlers-Danlos Syndrome. *Clinical Genetics*, *25*(6), 477-484. https://doi.org/10.1111/j.1399-0004.1984.tb00490.x.

37 Weill Cornell Medicine. Ehlers-Danlos Syndrome (EDS). (2021, April). https://neurosurgery.weillcornell.org/condition/ehlers-danlos-syndrome-eds

38 It is theorized that the biosynthesis of connective tissues does not function correctly in the bodies of people with hEDS, leading to insufficient quantities of collagen. This error can be rectified, at least somewhat, with supplements like polysaccharides that act as growth signaling factors to stimulate the cells to produce colalgen: Liu, L. Y., Chen, X. D., Wu, B. Y., & Jiang, Q. (2010). Influence of Aloe polysaccharide on proliferation and hyaluronic acid and hydroxyproline secretion of human fibroblasts in vitro. *Journal of Chinese integrative medicine*, *8*(3), 256-262. https://doi.org/10.3736/jcim20100310 . https://pubmed.ncbi.nlm.nih.gov/20226148/

39 This is the premise upon which the Cusack Protocol is based. An explanation of her theory can be found at https://www.facebook.com/groups/edsandaloe

40 Narcisi, P., Richards, A. J., Ferguson, S. D., & Pope, F. M. (1994). A family with Ehlers-Danlos Syndrome Type III/Articular Hypermobility Syndrome has a glycine 637 to serine substitution in type III collagen. *Human Molecular Genetics*, *3*(9), 1617-1620. https://doi.org/10.1093/hmg/3.9.1617 .

41 Courseault, J., Kingry, C., Morrison, V., Edstrom, C., Morrell, K., Jaubert, L., Elia, V., & Bix, G. (2023). Folate-dependent hypermobility syndrome: A proposed mechanism and diagnosis. *Heliyon*, *9*(4), e15387. https://doi.org/10.1016/j.heliyon.2023.e15387 .

42 Lyme Disease was indicated by Justin Kerbyson in the private Facebook group he founded: Rib Syndromes Connective Tissue Weakness and Hidden Autoimmune Disorders. Damage to the connective tissues of the joints by Lyme Disease is confirmed by Czupryna, P., Moniuszko, A., Czeczuga, A., Pancewicz, S., & Zajkowska, J. (2012). Ultrasonographic evaluation of knee joints in patients with Lyme disease. *International Journal of Infectious Diseases : IJID : Official publication of the International Society for Infectious Diseases*, *16*(4), e252-e255. https://doi.org/10.1016/j.ijid.2011.12.004 , among others.

43 Feced Olmos, C. M., Fernández Matilla, M., Robustillo Villarino, M., de la Morena Barrio, I., & Alegre Sancho, J. J. (2016). Joint involvement secondary to Epstein-Barr virus. *Reumatologia Clinica*, *12*(2), 100-102. https://doi.org/10.1016/j.reuma.2015.05.014 .

44 Estrella, E., & Frazier, P. A. (2024). Healthcare experiences among adults with Hypermobile Ehlers-Danlos Syndrome and Hypermobility Spectrum Disorder in the United States. *Disability and Rehabilitation*, *46*(4), 731-740, https://doi.org/10.1080/09638288.2023.2176554 .

45 Bulbena, A., Baeza-Velasco, C., Bulbena-Cabré, A., Pailhez, G., Critchley, H., Chopra, P., Mallorquı-Bague, N., Frank, C., & Porges, S. (2017). Psychiatric and psychological aspects in the Ehlers-Danlos Syndromes. *American Journal of Medical Genetics Part C Seminar on Medical Genetics* 175C:237-245.

46 Bennett, S. E., Walsh, N., Moss, T., & Palmer, S. (2022). Developing a self-management intervention to manage Hypermobility Spectrum Disorders (HSD) and Hypermobile Ehlers-Danlos Syndrome (hEDS): An analysis informed by behaviour change theory. *Disability and rehabilitation*, *44*(18), 5231-5240. https://doi.org/10.1080/09638288.2021.1933618 .

47 Baeza-Velasco, C., Hamonet, C., Montalescot, L., & Courtet, P. (2022). Suicidal behaviors in women with the Hypermobile Ehlers-Danlos Syndrome. *Archives of Suicide Research : Official Journal of the International Academy for Suicide Research*, *26*(3), 1314-1326. https://doi.org/10.1080/13811118.2021.1885538.

48 These assertions of attractiveness are based upon my experience and the opinions of people I know in person and in social media groups. It might be more accurate to say that people with hEDS find people with hEDS to be attractive, but beauty is always subjective and many successful fashion models and performing artists have the physical attributes of someone with hEDS (or actually have the condition).

49 In social media groups for hEDS, people often play games of posting their own pictures and guessing how old they are — usually, for ages approximately 20-50, faces are guessed to be younger and hands are guessed to be older than their actual age.

50 Halverson, C. M. E., Clayton, E. W., Garcia Sierra, A., & Francomano, C. (2021). Patients with Ehlers-Danlos Syndrome on the diagnostic odyssey: Rethinking complexity and difficulty as a hero's journey. *American Journal of Medical Genetics. Part C, Seminars in Medical Genetics*, *187*(4), 416-424. https://doi.org/10.1002/ajmg.c.31935 .

51 Afrin, L. B., Self, S., Menk, J., & Lazarchick, J. (2017). Characterization of Mast Cell Activation Syndrome. *The American Journal of the Medical Sciences, 353*(3), 207-215. https://doi.org/10.1016/j.amjms.2016.12.013 .

52 On social media and on many hEDS support websites, patients report that their experience of suffering with hEDS symptoms has increased their ability to feel empathy; some have suggested that people with hEDS are more empathetic to start with.

53 Hamonet C, Schatz PM, Bezire P, Ducret L, & Brissot R (2018) Cognitive and psychopathological aspects of Ehlers-Danlos Syndrome - Experience in a specialized medical consultation. *Research Advances in Brain Disorders and Therapy.* RABDT-104. https://doi.org/10.29011/ RABDT-104. 100004 .

54 Bulbena, A. (2022). *Anxiety: A quick immersion.* Tibidabo Publishing, Inc.

55 Bulbena, A. (2022).

56 Bulbena, A. (2022).

57 Hamonet C, Schatz PM, Bezire P, Ducret L, & Brissot R (2018)

58 Bulbena-Cabré, A., Baeza-Velasco, C., Rosado-Figuerola, S., & Bulbena, A. (2021, November 9). Updates on the psychological and psychiatric aspects of the Ehlers-Danlos Syndromes and Hypermobility Spectrum Disorders. *American Journal of Medical Genetics.* https://doi.org/10.1002/ajmg.c.31955 .

59 Halverson, C. M. E., Clayton, E. W., Garcia Sierra, A., & Francomano, C. (2021).

60 Baeza-Velasco, C., Hamonet, C., Montalescot, L., & Courtet, P. (2022). Suicidal behaviors in women with the Hypermobile Ehlers-Danlos Syndrome. *Archives of suicide research : official journal of the International Academy for Suicide Research, 26*(3), 1314-1326. .

61 Atwell, K., Michael, W., Dubey, J., James, S., Martonffy, A., Anderson, S., Rudin, N., & Schrager, S. (2021, July). Diagnosis and management of Hypermobility Spectrum Disorders in primary care. *The Journal of the American Board of Family Medicine, 34*(4) 838-848. http://doi.org//10.3122/jabfm.2021.04.200374 .

62 Casanova, E. L., Baeza-Velasco, C., Buchanan, C. B., & Casanova, M. F. (2020). The Relationship between autism and Ehlers-Danlos Syndromes/Hypermobility Spectrum Disorders. *Journal of Personalized Medicine, 10*(4), 260. https://doi.org/10.3390/jpm10040260 .

63 Malfait, F., Francomano, C., Byers, P., Belmont, J., Berglund, B., Black, J., Bloom, L., Bowen, J. M., Brady, A. F., Burrows, N. P., Castori, M., Cohen, H., Colombi, M., Demirdas, S., De Backer, J., De Paepe, A., Fournel-Gigleux, S., Frank, M., Ghali, N., Giunta, C., ... Tinkle, B. (2017). The 2017 international classification of the Ehlers-Danlos Syndromes. *American Journal of Medical Genetics. Part C, Seminars in Medical Genetics, 175*(1), 8-26. https://doi.org/10.1002/ajmg.c.31552 .

64 Halverson, C. M. E., Cao, S., Perkins, S. M., & Francomano, C. A. (2003). Comorbidity, misdiagnoses, and the diagnostic odyssey in patients with Hypermobile Ehlers-Danlos Syndrome. *Genetics in Medicine Open, 1*(1). https://doi.org/10.1016/j.gimo.2023.100812.

65 Halverson, C. M. E., Cao, S., Perkins, S. M., & Francomano, C. A. (2003).

66 Diagnostic Criteria for Paediatric Joint Hypermobility: from Tofts, L.J., Simmonds, J., Schwartz, S.B., et al. (2023). Pediatric joint hypermobility: A diagnostic framework and narrative review. *Orphanet Journal of Rare Diseases*, 18(104). https://doi.org/10.1186/s13023-023-02717-2.

67 Cueto, I. (2022, December 12). Revenge of the gaslit patients: Now, as scientists, they're tackling Ehlers-Danlos Syndromes. *STAT.* https://www.statnews.com/2022/12/12/ehlers-danlos-syndrome-patients-turned-researchers/ .

68 Wozniak-Mielczarek, L., Osowicka, M., Radtke-Lysek, A., Drezek-Nojowicz, M., Gilis-Malinowska, N., Sabiniewicz, A., Mielczarek, M., & Sabiniewicz, R. (2022). How to distinguish marfan syndrome from marfanoid habitus in a physical examination-comparison of external features in patients with marfan syndrome and marfanoid habitus. *International Journal of Environmental Research and Public Health, 19*(2), 772. https://doi.org/10.3390/ijerph19020772 .

69 The Marfan Foundation. What are the signs of marfan syndrome. https://marfan.org/expectations/signs/ .

70 Hypermobility Syndromes Foundation. Types of HMS. https://www.hypermobility.org/types-of-hms

71 Siegel, C., Berman, J., Barbhaiya, M., & Sammaritano, L. (2022, March 1). Undifferentiated connective tissue disease — In-depth overview. *Hospital for Special Surgery.* https://www.hss.edu/conditions_undifferentiated-connective-tissue-disease-overview.asp#diagnosed .

72 The Ehlers-Danlos Society. What is HSD? https://www.ehlers-danlos.com/what-is-hsd/

73 Atwell, K., Michael, W., Dubey, J., James, S. Martonffy, A. Anderson, S., Rudin, N., & Schrager, S. (2021, July). Diagnosis and management of Hypermobility Spectrum Disorders in primary care. *The Journal of the American Board of Family Medicine, 34*(4) 838-848. https://doi.org/10.3122/jabfm.2021.04.200374 .

74 The International Consortium on Ehlers-Danlos Syndromes and Related Disorders in Association with the Ehlers-Danlos Society. Diagnostic criteria for Hypermobile Ehlers-Danlos Syndrome (hEDS). https://www.ehlers-danlos.com/heds-diagnostic-checklist/

75 Tofts, L.J., Simmonds, J., Schwartz, S.B., et al. (2023). Pediatric joint hypermobility: A diagnostic framework and narrative review. *Orphanet Journal of Rare Diseases* 18, 104. https://doi.org/10.1186/s13023-023-02717-2 .

76 Mathews L. (2011). Pain in children: Neglected, unaddressed and mismanaged. *Indian Journal of Palliative Care, 17*(Suppl), S70-S73. https://doi.org/10.4103/0973-1075.76247 .

77 The International Consortium on Ehlers-Danlos Syndromes and Related Disorders in Association with the Ehlers-Danlos Society.

78 Weinhold B. (2006). Epigenetics: The science of change. *Environmental Health Perspectives, 114*(3), A160-A167. https://doi.org/10.1289/ehp.114-a160 .

79 Punzi, L., Galozzi, P., Luisetto, R., Favero, M., Ramonda, R., Oliviero, F., & Scanu, A. (2016). Post-traumatic arthritis: Overview on pathogenic mechanisms and role of inflammation. *RMD Open, 2*(2), e000279. https://doi.org/10.1136/rmdopen-2016-000279 .

80 Lepley, A. S., Ly, M. T., Grooms, D. R., Kinsella-Shaw, J. M., & Lepley, L. K. (2020). Corticospinal tract structure and excitability in patients with anterior cruciate ligament reconstruction: A DTI and TMS study. *NeuroImage: Clinical, 25*, 102157, ISSN 2213-1582, https://doi.org/10.1016/j.nicl.2019.102157.

81 Lepley, A. S., Ly, M. T., Grooms, D. R., Kinsella-Shaw, J. M., & Lepley, L. K. (2020).

82 Todorovic, M. (2022, April 22). *Pain vs nociception | In 2 minutes!!* [Video]. Dr. Matt and Dr. Mike (YouTube). https://www.youtube.com/watch?v=RD6QY5KWiko .

83 Some people call this the Fight/Flight/Freeze/Fawn Mode, lumping friending and fornicating into the category of fawning, but others feel that it is important to point out that fawning can look drastically different in different circumstances.

84 Wang, L. X., & Wang, Z. J. (2003). Animal and cellular models of chronic pain. *Advanced Drug Delivery Reviews, 55*(8), 949-965. https://doi.org/10.1016/s0169-409x(03)00098-x .

85 Bass, E. (2012). Tendinopathy: Why the difference between tendinitis and tendinosis matters. *International Journal of Therapeutic Massage & Bodywork, 5*(1), 14-17. https://doi.org/10.3822/ijtmb.v5i1.153 .

86 Nakama, L. H., King, K. B., Abrahamsson, S., & Rempel, D. M. (2007). Effect of repetition rate on the formation of microtears in tendon in an in vivo cyclical loading model. *Journal of Orthopaedic Research : Official Publication of the Orthopaedic Research Society, 25*(9), 1176-1184. https://doi.org/10.1002/jor.20408 .

87 Hodgson, R. J., O'Connor, P. J., & Grainger, A. J. (2012). Tendon and ligament imaging. *The British Journal of Radiology, 85*(1016), 1157-1172. https://doi.org/10.1259/bjr/34786470 .

88 Caring Medical Florida. Chronic muscle spasms and tightness can indicate you have a ligament problem, not a muscle problem. https://www.caringmedical.com/prolotherapy-news/chronic-muscle-spasms-tightness-can-indicate-ligament-problem-muscle-problem/ .

89 Cleveland Clinic. (2022, May 19). Endorphins. https://my.clevelandclinic.org/health/body/23040-endorphins .

90 Sutton, J. (2023, March 21). Best sleeping positions for a good night's sleep. *Healthline.* https://www.healthline.com/health/best-sleeping-position#on-your-back .

91 The Cusack Protocol has not been evaluated through a scientific trial; however, Deborah Cusack has shared the scientific reasons for having chosen the supplements on the protocol. Furthermore, numerous people with hEDS have been helped by this protocol. However, it has not helped all of those who have tried it.

92 Toulabi, T., Delfan, B., Rashidipour, M., Yarahmadi, S., Ravanshad, F., Javanbakht, A., & Almasian, M. (2022). The efficacy of olive leaf extract on healing herpes simplex virus labialis: A randomized double-blind study. *Explore (New York, N.Y.), 18*(3), 287-292. https://doi.org/10.1016/j.explore.2021.01.003 .

93 Salamanca, A., Almodóvar, P., Jarama, I., González-Hedström, D., Prodanov, M., & Inarejos-García, A. M. (2021). Anti-influenza virus activity of the elenolic acid rich olive leaf (Olea europaea L.) extract Isenolic®. *Antiviral Chemistry & Chemotherapy*, 29, 20402066211063391. https://doi.org/10.1177/20402066211063391 .

94 Abdelgawad, S. M., Hassab, M. A. E., Abourehab, M. A. S., Elkaeed, E. B., & Eldehna, W. M. (2022). Olive leaves as a potential phytotherapy in the treatment of covid-19 disease; A mini-review. *Frontiers in Pharmacology*, *13*, 879118. https://doi.org/10.3389/fphar.2022.879118 .

95 Brazier, Y. (2017, July 25). Hot or cold: Which therapy works best? *Medical News Today*. https://www.medicalnewstoday.com/articles/29108 .

96 Ruiz-Sánchez, F. J., Ruiz-Muñoz, M., Martín-Martín, J., Coheña-Jimenez, M., Perez-Belloso, A. J., Pilar Romero-Galisteo, R., & Gónzalez-Sánchez, M. (2022). Management and treatment of ankle sprain according to clinical practice guidelines: A PRISMA systematic review. *Medicine*, 101(42), e31087. https://doi.org/10.1097/MD.0000000000031087 .

97 Staiger C. (2012). Comfrey: A clinical overview. *Phytotherapy Research: PTR*, 26(10), 1441-1448. https://doi.org/10.1002/ptr.4612 .

98 Brazier, Y. (2017, July 25).

99 Proksch, E., Nissen, H.-P., Bremgartner, M., & Urquhart, C. (2005). Bathing in a magnesium-rich Dead Sea salt solution improves skin barrier function, enhances skin hydration, and reduces inflammation in atopic dry skin. *International Journal of Dermatology*, 44: 151-157. https://doi.org/10.1111/j.1365-4632.2005.02079.x .

100 International Sports Sciences Association. (2023, March 25). Magnesium for muscle recovery: How it works & how to use it. https://www.issaonline.com/blog/post/magnesium-for-muscle-recovery-how-it-works-how-to-use-it .

101 Haleem, Z., Philip, J., & Muhammad, S. (2021). Erythema ab igne: A rare presentation of toasted skin syndrome with the use of a space heater. *Cureus*, *13*(2), e13401. https://doi.org/10.7759/cureus.13401.

102 Aria, A. B., Chen, L., & Silapunt, S. (2018). Erythema ab igne from heating pad use: A report of three clinical cases and a differential diagnosis. *Cureus*, *10*(5), e2635. https://doi.org/10.7759/cureus.2635.

103 Bervoets, D. C., Luijsterburg, P. A., Alessie, J. J., Buijs, M. J., & Verhagen, A. P. (2015). Massage therapy has short-term benefits for people with common musculoskeletal disorders compared to no treatment: A systematic review. *Journal of Physiotherapy*, *61*(3), 106-116. https://doi.org/10.1016/j.jphys.2015.05.018 .

104 Bass, E. (2012). Tendinopathy: Why the difference between tendinitis and tendinosis matters. *International Journal of Therapeutic Massage & Bodywork*, *5*(1), 14-17. https://doi.org/10.3822/ijtmb.v5i1.153 .

105 Ruiz-Sánchez, F. J., Ruiz-Muñoz, M., Martín-Martín, J., Coheña-Jimenez, M., Perez-Belloso, A. J., Pilar Romero-Galisteo, R., & Gónzalez-Sánchez, M. (2022).

106 Ruiz-Sánchez, F. J., Ruiz-Muñoz, M., Martín-Martín, J., Coheña-Jimenez, M., Perez-Belloso, A. J., Pilar Romero-Galisteo, R., & Gónzalez-Sánchez, M. (2022).

107 Li, W. H., Seo, I., Kim, B., Fassih, A., Southall, M. D., & Parsa, R. (2021). Low-level red plus near infrared lights combination induces expressions of collagen and elastin in human skin in vitro. *International Journal of Cosmetic Science*, *43*(3), 311-320. https://doi.org/10.1111/ics.12698 .

108 Leyane, T. S., Jere, S. W., & Houreld, N. N. (2021). Cellular signalling and photobiomodulation in chronic wound repair. *International Journal of Molecular Sciences*, 22(20):11223. doi:10.3390/ijms222011223.

109 Wan, Z., Zhang, P., Lv, L., & Zhou, Y. (2020). NIR light-assisted phototherapies for bone-related diseases and bone tissue regeneration: A systematic review. *Theranostics*, *10*(25), 11837-11861. https://doi.org/10.7150/thno.49784 .

110 Oschman, J. L., Chevalier, G., & Brown, R. (2015). The effects of grounding (earthing) on inflammation, the immune response, wound healing, and prevention and treatment of chronic inflammatory and autoimmune diseases. *Journal of Inflammation Research*, *8*, 83-96. https://doi.org/10.2147/JIR.S69656 .

111 Zhang, J., Zhang, B., Zhang, J., Lin, W., & Zhang, S. (2021). Magnesium promotes the regeneration of the peripheral nerve. *Frontiers in Cell and Developmental Biology*, *9*, 717854. htt*ps://doi.org/10.3389/fcell.2021.717854 .

112 Wachholtz, A. B., Malone, C. D., & Pargament, K. I. (2017). Effect of different meditation types on migraine headache medication use. *Behavioral Medicine (Washington, D.C.), 43*(1), 1-8. https://doi.org/10.1080/08964289.2015.1024601 .

113 Halverson, C. M. E., Cao, S., Perkins, S. M., & Francomano, C. A. (2003). Comorbidity, misdiagnoses, and the diagnostic odyssey in patients with Hypermobile Ehlers-Danlos Syndrome. *Genetics in Medicine Open, 1,* 1. https://doi.org/10.1016/j.gimo.2023.100812.

114 Tinkle, B., Castori, M., Berglund, B., Cohen, H., Grahame, R., Kazkaz, H., & Levy, H. (2017). Hypermobile Ehlers-Danlos Syndrome (a.k.a. Ehlers-Danlos Syndrome Type III and Ehlers-Danlos Syndrome Hypermobility Type): Clinical description and natural history. *American Journal of Medical Genetics. Part C, Seminars in Medical Genetics, 175*(1), 48-69. https://doi.org/10.1002/ajmg.c.31538 .

115 Hoskin, J., & Rowe, V. The Gut-brain-hypermobility connection with autoimmunity. *Rowe Neurology Institute*. https://www.neurokc.com/back-pain-neck-pain/gut-brain-hypermobility-connection-autoimmunity/ .

116 Jones, J. G., Minty, B. D., & Royston, D. (1982). The physiology of leaky lungs. *British Journal of Anaesthesia, 54*(7), 705-721. https://doi.org/10.1093/bja/54.7.705-a .

117 University of Zurich. (2021, May 6). Defective epithelial barriers linked to two billion chronic diseases. *ScienceDaily*. www.sciencedaily.com/releases/2021/05/210506105352.htm .

118 Afrin, L. B., Self, S., Menk, J., & Lazarchick, J. (2017). Characterization of Mast Cell Activation Syndrome. *The American Journal of the Medical Sciences, 353*(3), 207-215. https://doi.org/10.1016/j.amjms.2016.12.013 .

119 Błażowski, Ł., Majak, P., Kurzawa, R., Kuna, P., & Jerzyńska, J. (2021). A severity grading system of food-induced acute allergic reactions to avoid delay of epinephrine administration. *Annals Of Allergy, Asthma & Immunology: Official Publication of The American College Of Allergy, Asthma, & Immunology*. 127. 10.1016/j.anai.2021.04.015.

120 Błażowski, Ł., Majak, P., Kurzawa, R., Kuna, P., & Jerzyńska, J. (2021). A severity grading system of food-induced acute allergic reactions to avoid delay of epinephrine administration. *Annals of allergy, asthma & immunology : official publication of the American College of Allergy, Asthma, & Immunology*. 127. 10.1016/j.anai.2021.04.015.

121 Galant, S. P. (1989). Allergy shots for hay fever. *Postgraduate Medicine, 85*(6), 203-209. https://doi.org/10.1080/00325481.1989.11700701 .

122 Sato, S., Yanagida, N., & Ebisawa, M. (2015). Oral immunotherapy and potential treatment. *Chemical Immunology and Allergy, 101,* 106-113. https://doi.org/10.1159/000371697 .

123 The Mast Cell Disease Society. Overview, Diagnosis, Definitions and Classification. https://tmsforacure.org/overview/ .

124 Molderings, G.J., Brettner, S., Homann, J., et al. (2011). Mast cell activation disease: A concise practical guide for diagnostic workup and therapeutic options. *Journal of Hematology and Oncology, 4,* 10. https://doi.org/10.1186/1756-8722-4-10 .

125 Marshall, T. J., & Piller, A. (2022, July 19). Ehlers-Danlos Syndrome and its comorbidities as a co-occurring health issue in autistic people. *Autism Spectrum News.* https://autismspectrumnews.org/ehlers-danlos-syndrome-and-its-comorbidities-as-a-co-occurring-health-issue-in-autistic-people/ .

126 Kempuraj, D., Selvakumar, G. P., Thangavel, R., Ahmed, M. E., Zaheer, S., Raikwar, S. P., Iyer, S. S., Bhagavan, S. M., Beladakere-Ramaswamy, S., & Zaheer, A. (2017).

127 Seneviratne, S. L., Maitland, A., & Afrin, L. (2017, March 6). Mast cell disorders in Ehlers-Danlos Syndrome. https://doi.org/10.1002/ajmg.c.31555 .

128 Australasian Society of Clinical Immunology and Allergy. (2024, March). Mastocytosis and other mast cell disorders. https://www.allergy.org.au/patients/allergy-testing/mastocytosis .

129 Monaco, A., Choi, D., Uzun, S., *et al.* Association of mast-cell-related conditions with hypermobile syndromes: a review of the literature. *Immunologic Research, 70,* 419–431 (2022). https://doi.org/10.1007/s12026-022-09280-1

130 Kempuraj, D., Selvakumar, G. P., Thangavel, R., Ahmed, M. E., Zaheer, S., Raikwar, S. P., Iyer, S. S., Bhagavan, S. M., Beladakere-Ramaswamy, S., & Zaheer, A. (2017). Mast cell activation in brain injury, stress, and post-traumatic stress disorder and Alzheimer's disease pathogenesis. *Frontiers in Neuroscience*, 11, 703. https://doi.org/10.3389/fnins.2017.00703 .

131 Monaco, A., Choi, D., Uzun, S., Maitland, A., & Riley, B. (2022). Association of mast-cell-related conditions with hypermobile syndromes: A review of the literature. *Immunologic Research, 70*(4), 419-431. https://doi.org/10.1007/s12026-022-09280-1 .

132 Afrin, L. B., Self, S., Menk, J., & Lazarchick, J. (2017). Characterization of Mast Cell Activation Syndrome. *The American Journal of the Medical Sciences*, *353*(3), 207-215. https://doi.org/10.1016/j.amjms.2016.12.013 .

133 Carnahan, J. (2018, March 12). Mold is a major trigger of mast cell activation syndrome. *Dr. Jill.* https://www.jillcarnahan.com/2018/03/12/mold-is-a-major-trigger-of-mast-activation-cell-syndrome/ .

134 Boyden, S. E., Desai, A., Cruse, G., Young, M. L., Bolan, H. C., Scott, L. M., Eisch, A. R., Long, R. D., Lee, C. C., Satorius, C. L., Pakstis, A. J., Olivera, A., Mullikin, J. C., Chouery, E., Mégarbané, A., Medlej-Hashim, M., Kidd, K. K., Kastner, D. L., Metcalfe, D. D., & Komarow, H. D. (2016). Vibratory urticaria associated with a missense variant in ADGRE2. *The New England Journal of Medicine*, 374(7), 656-663. https://doi.org/10.1056/NEJMoa1500611 .

135 Jennings, S., Russell, N., Jennings, B., Slee, V., Sterling, L., Castells, M., Valent, P., & Akin, C. (2014). The Mastocytosis Society survey on mast cell disorders: patient experiences and perceptions. *The Journal of Allergy and Clinical Immunology in Practice*, *2*(1), 70-76. https://doi.org/10.1016/j.jaip.2013.09.004 .

136 Hall, C. (2023, January 4). How can a dietitian help support those with Mast Cell Activation Syndrome? *The British Dietetic Association*. https://www.bda.uk.com/resource/how-can-a-dietitian-help-support-those-with-mast-cell-activation-syndrome.html .

137 Mast Cell 360. Start. https://mastcell360.com/start-here/ .

138 Smolinska, S., Winiarska, E., Globinska, A., & Jutel, M. (2022). Histamine: A mediator of intestinal disorders — A review. *Metabolites*, *12*(10), 895. https://doi.org/10.3390/metabo12100895 .

139 De Sutter, A. I., Eriksson, L., & van Driel, M. L. (2022). Oral antihistamine-decongestant-analgesic combinations for the common cold. *The Cochrane Database of Systematic Reviews*, *1*(1), CD004976. https://doi.org/10.1002/14651858.CD004976.pub4 .

140 Mandola, A., Nozawa, A., & Eiwegger, T. (2019). Histamine, histamine receptors, and anti-histamines in the context of allergic responses. *LymphoSign Journal*. *6*(2), 35-51. https://doi.org/10.14785/lymphosign-2018-0016 .

141 Gannage, J. (2022, February 2). Medications to avoid with MCAS. *Histamined.* https://www.histamined.com/post/medications-to-avoid-with-mcas .

142 Thomas, L. (2019, Septe,ber 11). Long term effects of taking allergy medications. *News Medical Life Sciences.* https://www.news-medical.net/health/Long-Term-Effects-of-Taking-Allergy-Medications.aspx .

143 Kempuraj, D., Selvakumar, G. P., Thangavel, R., Ahmed, M. E., Zaheer, S., Raikwar, S. P., Iyer, S. S., Bhagavan, S. M., Beladakere-Ramaswamy, S., & Zaheer, A. (2017).

144 Fairweather, D., Bruno, K. A., Darakjian, A. A., Bruce, B. K., Gehin, J. M., Kotha, A., Jain, A., Peng, Z., Hodge, D. O., Rozen, T. D., Munipalli, B., Rivera, F. A., Malavet, P. A., & Knight, D. R. T. (2023). High overlap in patients diagnosed with hypermobile Ehlers-Danlos Syndrome or Hypermobile Spectrum Disorders with fibromyalgia and 40 self-reported symptoms and comorbidities. *Frontiers in Medicine*, *10*, 1096180. https://doi.org/10.3389/fmed.2023.1096180 .

145 Dhaliwal, J. S., Rosani, A., & Saadabadi, A. (2023, August 28). Diazepam. *StatPearls*. https://www.ncbi.nlm.nih.gov/books/NBK537022/ .

146 Gannage, J. (2022, February 2).

147 Shin, H. S., Bae, M. J., Choi, D. W., & Shon, D. H. (2014). Skullcap (*Scutellaria baicalensis*) extract and its active compound, wogonin, inhibit ovalbumin-induced Th2-mediated response. *Molecules (Basel, Switzerland)*, *19*(2), 2536-2545. https://doi.org/10.3390/molecules19022536.

148 Science Daily. (2018, April 25). Drinking baking soda could be an inexpensive, safe way to combat autoimmune disease. *ScienceDaily*. www.sciencedaily.com/releases/2018/04/180425093745.htm .

149 Fu, S., Ni, S., Wang, D., Fu, M., & Hong, T. (2019). Berberine suppresses mast cell-mediated allergic responses via regulating FcεRI-mediated and MAPK signaling. *International Immunopharmacology*, *71*, 1-6. https://doi.org/10.1016/j.intimp.2019.02.041 .

150 Akkol, E. K., Yalçin, F. N., Kaya, D., Caliş, I., Yesilada, E., & Ersöz, T. (2008). In vivo anti-inflammatory and antinociceptive actions of some *Lamium* species. *Journal of Ethnopharmacology*, *118*(1), 166-172. https://doi.org/10.1016/j.jep.2008.04.001

151 Greaves, M.W., Yamamoto, S., & Mahzoon, B. (1976). The mast cell: Interrelationships between histamine and prostaglandins. *Clinical and Experimental Dermatology*, *1*, 327-329. https://doi.org/10.1111/j.1365-2230.1976.tb01438.x .

152 Greaves, M.W., Yamamoto, S., & Mahzoon, B. (1976).

153 Greaves, M.W., Yamamoto, S., & Mahzoon, B. (1976).

154 Salehi, B., Mishra, A. P., Nigam, M., Sener, B., Kilic, M., Sharifi-Rad, M., Fokou, P. V. T., Martins, N., & Sharifi-Rad, J. (2018). Resveratrol: A double-edged sword in health benefits. *Biomedicines*, *6*(3), 91. https://doi.org/10.3390/biomedicines6030091 .

155 Carnahan, J. (2018, March 12). Mold is a major trigger of mast cell activation syndrome. *Dr. Jill.* https://www.jillcarnahan.com/2018/03/12/mold-is-a-major-trigger-of-mast-activation-cell-syndrome/ .

156 Miller, C. S. (1996). Chemical sensitivity: Symptom, syndrome or mechanism for disease? *Toxicology, 111*(1-3), 69-86. https://doi.org/10.1016/0300-483X(96)03393-8 .

157 Haanes, J. V., Nordin, S., Hillert, L., Witthöft, M., van Kamp, I., van Thriel, C., & Van den Bergh, O. (2020). "Symptoms associated with environmental factors" (SAEF) - Towards a paradigm shift regarding "idiopathic environmental intolerance" and related phenomena. *Journal of Psychosomatic Research, 131,* 109955. Advance online publication. https://doi.org/10.1016/j.jpsychores.2020.109955 .

158 Palmer, R. F., Dempsey, T. T., & Afrin, L. B. (2023). Chemical intolerance and mast cell activation: A suspicious synchronicity. *Journal of Xenobiotics*, *13*(4), 704–718. https://doi.org/10.3390/jox13040045 .

159 Carnahan, J. (2017, November 13). Safe and effective detox binders that actually work. *Dr. Jill.* https://www.jillcarnahan.com/2017/11/13/safe-effective-detox-binders/ .

160 Bagasra, O., Golkar, Z., Garcia, M., Rice, L. N., & Pace, D. G. (2013). Role of perfumes in pathogenesis of autism. *Medical Hhypotheses*, *80*(6), 795-803. https://doi.org/10.1016/j.mehy.2013.03.014 .

161 Palmer, R. F., Dempsey, T. T., & Afrin, L. B. (2023).

[162] Palmer, R. F., Dempsey, T. T., & Afrin, L. B. (2023).

163 Sandström, M., Lyskov, E., Berglund, A., Medvedev, S., & Mild, K. H. (1997). Neurophysiological effects of flickering light in patients with perceived electrical hypersensitivity. *Journal of Occupational and Environmental Medicine*, *39*(1), 15-22. https://doi.org/10.1097/00043764-199701000-00006 .

164 Belyaev, I., Dean, A., Eger, H., Hubmann, G., Jandrisovits, R., Kern, M., Kundi, M/, Moshammer, H., Lercher, P., Müller, K., Oberfeld, G., Ohnsorge, P., Pelzmann, P., Scheingraber, C., & Thill, R. (2016). EUROPAEM EMF guideline 2016 for the prevention, diagnosis and treatment of EMF-related health problems and illnesses. *Reviews on Environmental Health*, *31*(3), 363-397. https://doi.org/10.1515/reveh-2016-0011 .

165 Palmieri, B., Corazzari, V., Vadala', M., Vallelunga, A., Morales-Medina, J. C., & Iannitti, T. (2021). The role of sensory and olfactory pathways in multiple chemical sensitivity. *Reviews on Environmental Health*, *36*(3), 319-326. https://doi.org/10.1515/reveh-2020-0058 .

166 Haehner A., Hummel, T., Heinritz, W., Krueger, S., Meinhardt, M., Whitcroft, K. L., Sabatowski, R., & Gossrau, G.. (2018, June 23). Mutation in Nav1.7 causes high olfactory sensitivity. https://doi.org/10.1002/ejp.1272.

167 Andersson, L., Claeson, A. S., Nyberg, L., & Nordin, S. (2017). Short-term olfactory sensitization involves brain networks relevant for pain, and indicates chemical intolerance. *International Journal of Hygiene and Environmental Health, 220*(2), Part B, 503-509, https://doi.org/10.1016/j.ijheh.2017.02.002.

168 Sandström, M., Lyskov, E., Berglund, A., Medvedev, S., & Mild, K. H. (1997). Neurophysiological effects of flickering light in patients with perceived electrical hypersensitivity. *Journal of Occupational and Environmental Medicine*, *39*(1), 15-22. https://doi.org/10.1097/00043764-199701000-00006 .

169 Sandström, M., Lyskov, E., Berglund, A., Medvedev, S., & Mild, K. H. (1997).

170 Sobel, N., Prabhakaran, V., Hartley, C. A., Desmond, J. E., Glover, G. H., Sullivan, E. V., & Gabrieli, J. D. (1999). Blind smell: brain activation induced by an undetected air-borne chemical. *Brain : A Journal of Neurology*, *122 (Pt 2)*, 209-217. https://doi.org/10.1093/brain/122.2.209 .

171 Meggs, W. J., & Cleveland, C. H., Jr (1993). Rhinolaryngoscopic examination of patients with the multiple chemical sensitivity syndrome. *Archives of Environmental Health*, *48*(1), 14-18. https://doi.org/10.1080/00039896.1993.9938388 .

172 Hillert, L., Musabasic, V., Berglund, H., Ciumas, C., & Savic, I. (2007). Odor processing in multiple chemical sensitivity. *Human Brain Mapping*, *28*(3), 172-182. https://doi.org/10.1002/hbm.20266 .

173 Courseault, J., Kingry, C., Morrison, V., Edstrom, C., Morrell, K., Jaubert, L., Elia, V., & Bix, G. (2023). Folate-dependent hypermobility syndrome: A proposed mechanism and diagnosis. *Heliyon*, *9*(4), e15387. https://doi.org/10.1016/j.heliyon.2023.e15387 .

174 Gibson, P. R., Elms, A. N., & Ruding, L. A. (2003). Perceived treatment efficacy for conventional and alternative therapies reported by persons with multiple chemical sensitivity. *Environmental Health Perspectives, 111*(12), 1498—1504. https://doi.org/10.1289/ehp.5936 .

175 Anderson, P. (2023, December 8). *Multiple chemical sensitivity: What is it & how to treat it* [Video]. Dr. Paul Anderson (YouTube). https://www.youtube.com/watch?v=4Sedxm3Nq00&list=PL3Tsd5WqoummfmUrdXHzA3tS8oRCxShtG&index=19 .

176 Belyaev, I., Dean, A., Eger, H., Hubmann, G., Jandrisovits, R., Kern, M., Kundi, M., Moshammer, H., Lercher, P., Müller, K., Oberfeld, G., Ohnsorge, P., Pelzmann, P., Scheingraber, C., & Thill, R. (2016). EUROPAEM EMF guideline 2016 for the prevention, diagnosis and treatment of EMF-related health problems and illnesses. *Reviews on Environmental Health, 31(*3), 363-397. https://doi.org/10.1515/reveh-2016-0011 .

177 Sandström, M., Lyskov, E., Berglund, A., Medvedev, S., & Mild, K. H. (1997).

178 Segura, C. (2021, June 24). How to stop fragrance & smoke coming in from neighbors. *My Chemical-Free House*. https://www.mychemicalfreehouse.net/2021/06/how-to-stop-fragrance-smoke-coming-in-from-neighbours.html .

179 This is a lovely compilation of the energies for each day of the week; be sure to click through to the exercises for the day as well as the subsequent days: Devi, S. (2012, November 5). Monday: Colour of the day and other energies by Rudolf Steiner. *Well Wishers Group*. https://wellwishersgroup.wordpress.com/2012/09/24/monday-right-word-exercises-for-the-days-of-the-week-by-rudolf-steiner/ .

180 Gibson, P. R., Elms, A. N., & Ruding, L. A. (2003).

181 Immel, J. How to improve digestion with ayurveda's easy to digest foods. *Joyful Belly*. https://www.joyfulbelly.com/Ayurveda/herbal-action/Easy .

182 Maz. (2018, January 17). Warm salads for optimal wellness & digestive health. *Balanced*. https://balancedacupuncture.com.au/2018/01/17/warm-salads-optimal-wellness-digestive-health/ .

183 Carmody, R. N., & Wrangham, R. W. (2009). Cooking and the human commitment to a high-quality diet. *Cold Spring Harbor Symposia on Quantitative Biology, 74*, 427-434. https://doi.org/10.1101/sqb.2009.74.019 .

184 Many MCAS food lists suggest that you should eat these foods, but my Ayurveda practitioner disagreed and was right. I and numerous people I know with hyperactive immune systems such as in Allergy/MCAS/MCS have done significantly better when we stopped eating onions, garlic, and peppers.

185 Seneviratne, S. L., Maitland, A., & Afrin. L. (2017, March 6). Mast cell disorders in Ehlers-Danlos Syndrome. *American Journal of Medical Genetics*. https://doi.org/10.1002/ajmg.c.31555 .

186 Schnedl, W. J., Schenk, M., Lackner, S., Enko, D., Mangge, H., & Forster, F. (2019). Diamine oxidase supplementation improves symptoms in patients with histamine intolerance. *Food Science and Biotechnology, 28*(6), 1779-1784. https://doi.org/10.1007/s10068-019-00627-3.

187 Afrin, P. (2023, March 31). *5 best holistic treatments for MCAS (mast cell activation syndrome)* [Video]. Dr. Paul Afrin (YouTube). https://www.youtube.com/watch?v=_q6_2wDX1i8 .

188 Carnahan, J. (2018, March 12). Mold is a major trigger of mast cell activation syndrome. *Dr. Jill.* https://www.jillcarnahan.com/2018/03/12/mold-is-a-major-trigger-of-mast-activation-cell-syndrome/ .

189 G., M. (2023, December 13). Should I use a DAO supplement? (diamine oxidase). Low Histamine Eats. https://lowhistamineeats.com/dao-supplement/ .

190 Nemati, D., Hinrichs, R., Johnson, A., Lauche, R., & Munk, N. (2024). Massage therapy as a self-management strategy for musculoskeletal pain and chronic conditions: A systematic review of feasibility and scope. *Journal of Integrative and Complementary Medicine, 30*(4), 319-335. https://doi.org/10.1089/jicm.2023.0271 .

191 Tapping or thumping the thymus is a technique of Traditional Chinese Medicine. It is described on this patient sheet from Seattle Children's Hospital, "The Three Thumps." https://www.seattlechildrens.org/globalassets/documents/for-patients-and-families/pfe/pe2256.pdf .

192 International Sports Sciences Association. (2023, March 25). Magnesium for muscle recovery: How it works and how to use it. https://www.issaonline.com/blog/post/magnesium-for-muscle-recovery-how-it-works-how-to-use-it .

193 Hartanto, A., Majeed, N. M., Lua, V. Y. Q., Wong, J., & Chen, N. R. Y. (2022). Dispositional gratitude, health-related factors, and lipid profiles in midlife: A biomarker study. *Scientific Reports, 12*(1), 6034. https://doi.org/10.1038/s41598-022-09960-w .

194 Cunha, L. F., Pellanda, L. C., & Reppold, C. T. (2019). Positive psychology and gratitude interventions: A randomized clinical trial. *Frontiers in Psychology, 10*, 584. https://doi.org/10.3389/fpsyg.2019.00584 .

195 Kubzansky, L. D., Huffman, J. C., Boehm, J. K., Hernandez, R., Kim, E. S., Koga, H. K., Feig, E. H., Lloyd-Jones, D. M., Seligman, M. E. P., & Labarthe, D. R. (2018). Positive psychological well-being and cardiovascular disease: JACC health promotion series. *Journal of the American College of Cardiology, 72*(12), 1382-1396. https://doi.org/10.1016/j.jacc.2018.07.042 .

196 Tindle, H. A., Chang, Y. F., Kuller, L. H., Manson, J. E., Robinson, J. G., Rosal, M. C., Siegle, G. J., & Matthews, K. A. (2009). Optimism, cynical hostility, and incident coronary heart disease and mortality in the Women's Health Initiative. *Circulation, 120*(8), 656-662. https://doi.org/10.1161/CIRCULATIONAHA.108.827642 .

197 Franco, L. S., Shanahan, D. F., & Fuller, R. A. (2017). A Review of the benefits of nature experiences: More than meets the eye. *International Journal of Environmental Research and Public Health, 14*(8), 864. https://doi.org/10.3390/ijerph14080864 .

198 Grilli, G., & Sacchelli, S. (2020). Health benefits derived from forest: A review. *International Journal of Environmental Research and Public Health, 17*(17), 6125. https://doi.org/10.3390/ijerph17176125 .

199 Addas, A. (2023). Impact of forestry on environment and human health: An evidence-based investigation. *Frontiers in Public Health, 11*, 1260519. https://doi.org/10.3389/fpubh.2023.1260519 .

200 Sivarajah, S., Smith, S. M., & Thomas, S. C. (2018). Tree cover and species composition effects on academic performance of primary school students. *PloS One, 13*(2), e0193254. https://doi.org/10.1371/journal.pone.0193254 .

201 Sharkey, L. & Lamoreux, K. (2021, April 8). What does it mean to be touch starved? https://www.healthline.com/health/touch-starved#long-term-solutions .

202 Floyd, K. (2014). Relational and health correlates of affection deprivation. *Western Journal of Communication, 78*(4), 383-403. https://doi.org/10.1080/10570314.2014.927071 .

203 van Raalte, L. J. & Floyd, K. (2021). Daily hugging predicts lower levels of two proinflammatory cytokines. *Western Journal of Communication, 85*(4), 487-506. https://doi..org/10.1080/10570314.2020.1850851 .

204 Lindqvist, P. G., Epstein, E., Nielsen, K., Landin-Olsson, M., Ingvar, C., & Olsson, H. (2016). Avoidance of sun exposure as a risk factor for major causes of death: A competing risk analysis of the melanoma in Southern Sweden cohort. *Journal of Internal Medicine, 280*(4), 375-387. https://doi.org/10.1111/joim.12496 .

205 Sandström, M., Lyskov, E., Berglund, A., Medvedev, S., & Mild, K. H. (1997). Neurophysiological effects of flickering light in patients with perceived electrical hypersensitivity. *Journal of Occupational and Environmental Medicine, 39*(1), 15-22. https://doi.org/10.1097/00043764-199701000-00006 .

206 Marais, S. D. (2022, November 10). The importance of play for adults. *Psych Central.* https://psychcentral.com/blog/the-importance-of-play-for-adults .

207 Vocally. (2021, April 28). https://vocally.nl/singing-and-the-vagus-nerve/ .

208 Ellis, R. J., & Thayer, J. F. (2010). Music and autonomic nervous system (dys)function. *Music Perception, 27*(4), 317-326. https://doi.org/10.1525/mp.2010.27.4.317 .

209 Ellis, R. J., & Thayer, J. F. (2010).

210 This statement is based on my observations while treating clients at my holistic healing center, Vibrant Life, over the course of over 10 years, where I saw clients with a very wide variety of ailments who all benefited from improved health and happiness after trading their fast-paced lifestyle for a slower one. It is also backed up by this article, among others: Mateus, J. (2023, May 13). The hidden risks of rushing: Impact on health and well-being. *Joana Mateus Biokinetics.* https://jmbiokineticist.co.za/f/the-hidden-risks-of-rushing-impact-on-health-and-well-being .

211 Salamanca, A., Almodóvar, P., Jarama, I., González-Hedström, D., Prodanov, M., & Inarejos-García, A. M. (2021). Anti-influenza virus activity of the elenolic acid rich olive leaf (*Olea europaea* L.) extract Isenolic®. *Antiviral Chemistry & Chemotherapy, 29*, 20402066211063391. https://doi.org/10.1177/20402066211063391 .

212 Toulabi, T., Delfan, B., Rashidipour, M., Yarahmadi, S., Ravanshad, F., Javanbakht, A., & Almasian, M. (2022). The efficacy of olive leaf extract on healing herpes simplex virus labialis: A randomized double-blind study. *Explore (New York, N.Y.), 18*(3), 287—292. https://doi.org/10.1016/j.explore.2021.01.003 .

213 Georgiou, N., Kakava, M. G., Routsi, E. A., Petsas, E., Stavridis, N., Freris, C., Zoupanou, N., Moschovou, K., Kiriakidi, S., & Mavromoustakos, T. (2023). Quercetin: A potential polydynamic drug. *Molecules (Basel, Switzerland)*, *28*(24), 8141. https://doi.org/10.3390/molecules28248141 .

214 Horwitz, R. J. (2018). Chapter 30 - The allergic patient. In Rakel, D. (Ed.), *Integrative Medicine* (Fourth Edition). Elsevier, 300-309.e2, https://doi.org/10.1016/B978-0-323-35868-2.00030-X .

215 Ding, Y., Che, D., Li, C., Cao, J., Wang, J., Ma, P., Zhao, T., An, H., & Zhang, T. (2019). Quercetin inhibits Mrgprx2-induced pseudo-allergic reaction via PLCγ-IP3R related Ca2+ fluctuations. *International Immunopharmacology*, *66*, 185-197. https://doi.org/10.1016/j.intimp.2018.11.025 .

216 Fu, S., Ni, S., Wang, D., Fu, M., & Hong, T. (2019). Berberine suppresses mast cell-mediated allergic responses via regulating FcεRI-mediated and MAPK signaling. *International Immunopharmacology*, *71*, 16. https://doi.org/10.1016/j.intimp.2019.02.041 .

217 Lesjak, M., Hoque, R., Balesaria, S., Skinner, V., Debnam, E. S., Srai, S. K., & Sharp, P. A. (2014). Quercetin inhibits intestinal iron absorption and ferroportin transporter expression in vivo and in vitro. *PloS* One, *9*(7), e102900. https://doi.org/10.1371/journal.pone.0102900 .

218 Modern Neuropathy. (2019, April 18). 6 powerhouse herbs for nerve damage regeneration. https://modernneuropathy.com/6-powerhouse-herbs-for-nerve-damage/ .

219 Akkol, E. K., Yalçin, F. N., Kaya, D., Caliş, I., Yesilada, E., & Ersöz, T. (2008). In vivo anti-inflammatory and antinociceptive actions of some *Lamium* species. *Journal of Ethnopharmacology*, *118*(1), 166-172. https://doi.org/10.1016/j.jep.2008.04.001 .

220 Bush, Z., Gildea, J., Roberts, D., & Matavelli, L. (2019). The effects of ION* gut health dietary supplement on markers of intestinal permeability and immune system function in healthy subjects: A double-blind, placebo-controlled clinical trial. ION* Biome. https://cdn.shopify.com/s/files/1/0354/2789/t/51/assets/IONBiome_Science_Paper_White_Paper_DigitalFile.pdf .

221 Marengo, K. (2020, April 24). What is fulvic acid, and does it have benefits? *Healthline*. https://www.healthline.com/nutrition/fulvic-acid .

222 Winkler, J., & Ghosh, S. (2018). Therapeutic potential of fulvic acid in chronic inflammatory diseases and diabetes. *Journal of Diabetes Research*, 5391014. https://doi.org/10.1155/2018/5391014 .

223 Hou, P. W., Hsu, H. C., Lin, Y. W., Tang, N. Y., Cheng, C. Y., & Hsieh, C. L. (2015). The history, mechanism, and clinical application of auricular therapy in traditional chinese medicine. evidence-based complementary and alternative medicine. *eCAM*, 495684. https://doi.org/10.1155/2015/495684 .

224 Bernal, M., Huecker, M., Shreffler, J., Mittel, O., Mittel, J., & Soliman, N. (2021). Successful treatment for alpha gal mammal product allergy using auricular acupuncture: A case series. *Medical Acupuncture*, *33*(5), 343-348. https://doi.org/10.1089/acu.2021.0010 .

225 Klimas, L. (2015, April 26). Mast cell mediators: Prostaglandin D2 (PGD2). *Mast Attack*. https://www.mastattack.org/2015/04/mast-cell-mediators-prostaglandin-d2-pgd2/ .

226 St. John's Hospital Dermatological Society: Symposium on the Mast Cell (1976). The mast cell: Interrelationships between histamine and prostaglandins. *Clinical and Experimental Dermatology*, *1*, 327.

227 Butterfield, J. H., & Weiler, C. R. (2008, November 1). Prevention of mast cell activation disorder-associated clinical sequelae of excessive prostaglandin D2 production. *Intionalterna Archives of Allergy Immunology*, *147*(4), 338-343. https://doi.org/10.1159/000144042 .

228 Zhang, S., Grabauskas, G., Wu, X., Joo, M. K., Heldsinger, A., Song, I., Owyang, C., & Yu, S. (2013). Role of prostaglandin D2 in mast cell activation-induced sensitization of esophageal vagal afferents. *American Journal Of Physiolog,. Gastrointestinal And Liver Physiology*, *304*(10), G908-G916. https://doi.org/10.1152/ajpgi.00448.2012 .

229 You and Your Hormones. (2017, July). Prostaglandins. https://www.yourhormones.info/hormones/prostaglandins/ .

230 Habashy, J. (2020, September 16). Mastocystosis treatment and management. *Medscape*. https://emedicine.medscape.com/article/1057932-treatment#d6?form=fpf .

231 Salehi, B., Mishra, A. P., Nigam, M., Sener, B., Kilic, M., Sharifi-Rad, M., Fokou, P. V. T., Martins, N., & Sharifi-Rad, J. (2018). Resveratrol: A double-edged sword in health benefits. *Biomedicines*, *6*(3), 91. https://doi.org/10.3390/biomedicines6030091 .

232 Chai, S. C., Davis, K., Zhang, Z., Zha, L., & Kirschner, K. F. (2019). Effects of tart cherry juice on biomarkers of inflammation and oxidative stress in older adults. *Nutrients*, *11*(2), 228. https://doi.org/10.3390/nu11020228 .

233 Kim, D. W., Jung, D. H., Sung, J., Min, I. S., & Lee, S. J. (2021). Tart cherry extract containing chlorogenic acid, quercetin, and kaempferol inhibits the mitochondrial apoptotic cell death elicited by airborne pm10 in human epidermal keratinocytes. *Antioxidants (Basel, Switzerland)*, *10*(3), 443. https://doi.org/10.3390/antiox10030443 .

234 Johnston, C. S., Martin, L. J., & Cai, X. (1992). Antihistamine effect of supplemental ascorbic acid and neutrophil chemotaxis. *Journal of the American College of Nutrition*, *11*(2), 172—176.

235 Clemetson, C. A. (1980). Histamine and ascorbic acid in human blood. *The Journal of Nutrition*, *110*(4), 662-668. https://doi.org/10.1093/jn/110.4.662 .

236 Carr, A. C., & Maggini, S. (2017). Vitamin C and immune function. *Nutrients*, *9*(11), 1211. https://doi.org/10.3390/nu9111211 .

237 Błach, J., Nowacki, W., Mazur A., et al. (2007). Magnesium in skin allergy. *Advances in Hygiene and Experimental Medicine*, *61*, 548-554. https://pubmed.ncbi.nlm.nih.gov/17928798/ .

238 Bornhöft, G., Wolf, U., von Ammon, K., Righetti, M., Maxion-Bergemann, S., Baumgartner, S., Thurneysen, A. E., & Matthiessen, P. F. (2006). Effectiveness, safety and cost-effectiveness of homeopathy in general practice — Summarized health technology assessment. *Forschende Komplementarmedizin (2006)*, *13 Suppl 2*, 19-29. https://doi.org/10.1159/000093586 .

239 Yu, S., Peng, W., Qiu, F., & Zhang, G. (2022). Research progress of astragaloside IV in the treatment of atopic diseases. *Biomedicine & Pharmacotherapy*, *156*, 113989. https://doi.org/10.1016/j.biopha.2022.113989 .

240 Qi, Y., Gao, F., Hou, L., & Wan, C. (2017). Anti-inflammatory and immunostimulatory activities of astragalosides. *The American Journal of Chinese Medicine*, *45*(6), 1157—1167. https://doi.org/10.1142/S0192415X1750063X .

241 Esmaeil, N., Anaraki, S. B., Gharagozloo, M., & Moayedi, B. (2017). Silymarin impacts on immune system as an immunomodulator: One key for many locks. *International Immunopharmacology*, *50*, 194-201. https://doi.org/10.1016/j.intimp.2017.06.030 .

242 Matsui, E. C., & Matsui, W. (2009). Higher serum folate levels are associated with a lower risk of atopy and wheeze. *The Journal of Allergy and Clinical Immunology*, *123*(6), 1253-9.e2. https://doi.org/10.1016/j.jaci.2009.03.007 .

243 Chesini, D., & Caminati, M. (2022). Vitamin B12 and atopic dermatitis: Any therapeutic relevance for oral supplementation? *Journal of Dietary Supplements*, *19*(2), 238—242. https://doi.org/10.1080/19390211.2020.1860180 .

244 Real Food RN. What are cell salts and how are they used? https://realfoodrn.com/what-are-cell-salts-how-are-they-used/ .

245 Schnedl, W. J., Schenk, M., Lackner, S., Enko, D., Mangge, H., & Forster, F. (2019). Diamine oxidase supplementation improves symptoms in patients with histamine intolerance. *Food Science and Biotechnology*, *28*(6), 1779-1784. https://doi.org/10.1007/s10068-019-00627-3.

246 Afrin, P. (2023, March 31). *5 best holistic treatments for MCAS (mast cell activation syndrome)* [Video]. Dr. Paul Afrin (YouTube). https://www.youtube.com/watch?v=_q6_2wDX1i8 .

247 Carnahan, J. (2018, March 12). Mold is a major trigger of mast cell activation syndrome. *Dr. Jill.* https://www.jillcarnahan.com/2018/03/12/mold-is-a-major-trigger-of-mast-activation-cell-syndrome/ .

248 G., M. (2023, December 13). Should I use a DAO supplement? (diamine oxidase). Low Histamine Eats. https://lowhistamineeats.com/dao-supplement/ .

249 Grinshpun, S. A., Mainelis, G., Trunov, M., Adhikari, A. Reponen, T., & Willeke, K. (2005). Evaluation of ionic air purifiers for reducing aerosol exposure in confined indoor spaces. https://weinproducts.com/news/entry/evaluation-of-ionic-air-purifiers-for-reducing-aerosol-exposure-in-confined-indoor-spaces .

250 Kim, K. H., Szulejko, J. E., Kumar, P., Kwon, E. E., Adelodun, A. A., & Reddy, P. A. K. (2017). Air ionization as a control technology for off-gas emissions of volatile organic compounds. *Environmental Pollution (Barking, Essex : 1987)*, *225*, 729-743. https://doi.org/10.1016/j.envpol.2017.03.026 .

251 Walker, A. (2017, November 17). Checklist for the newly diagnosed: 20 tips for MCAS. *Mast Cells United.* https://mastcellsunited.com/2017/11/17/checklist-for-the-newly-diagnosed-20-tips-for-mcas/ .

252 Oğuz, O., Manole, F., Bayar Muluk, N., & Cingi, C. (2023). Facial mask for prevention of allergic rhinitis symptoms. *Frontiers in Allergy*, *4*, 1265394. https://doi.org/10.3389/falgy.2023.1265394 .

253 Lin, T. K., Zhong, L., & Santiago, J. L. (2017). Anti-inflammatory and skin barrier repair effects of topical application of some plant oils. *International Journal of Molecular Sciences*, *19*(1), 70. https://doi.org/10.3390/ijms19010070 .

254 Veritasnaut. (2019, June 15). *Medium.* https://medium.com/@veritasnaut/sunglasses-are-killing-you-dbadb93f935d .

255 Vital Veda. (2020, December 22). Why wearing sunglasses is not healthy. https://vitalveda.com.au/learn/emotional-health/sunglasses/ .

256 Friedman, D.I., & De Ver Dye, T. (2009), Migraine and the environment. *Headache: The Journal of Head and Face Pain, 49,* 941-952. https://doi.org/10.1111/j.1526-4610.2009.01443.x .

257 Main, A., Dowson, A., & Gross, M. (1997), Photophobia and phonophobia in migraineurs between attacks. *Headache: The Journal of Head and Face Pain, 37,* 492-495. https://doi.org/10.1046/j.1526-4610.1997.3708492.x .

258 Helmut. (2022, March 19). My favorite earplugs for noise sensitivity and sensory overload. *NoisyWorld.* https://noisyworld.org/earplugs-for-noise-sensitivity-sensory-overload/.

259 Duyan, M., & Vural, N. (2022). The utilization of activated charcoal in the management of anaphylaxis: A case series. *Cureus, 14*(11), e31949. https://doi.org/10.7759/cureus.31949 .

260 Błach, J., Nowacki, W., Mazur A., et al. (2007). Magnesium in skin allergy. *Advances in Hygiene and Experimental Medicine, 61,* 548-554.

261 Souza, A. C. R., Vasconcelos, A. R., Dias, D. D., Komoni, G., & Name, J. J. (2023). The integral role of magnesium in muscle integrity and aging: A comprehensive review. *Nutrients, 15*(24), 5127. https://doi.org/10.3390/nu15245127 .

262 Zhang, J., Zhang, B., Zhang, J., Lin, W., & Zhang, S. (2021). Magnesium promotes the regeneration of the peripheral nerve. *Frontiers in Cell and Developmental Biology, 9,* 717854. https://doi.org/10.3389/fcell.2021.717854 .

263 Carnahan, J. (2018, March 12). Mold is a Major Trigger of Mast Cell Activation Syndrome. *Dr. Jill.* https://www.jillcarnahan.com/2018/03/12/mold-is-a-major-trigger-of-mast-activation-cell-syndrome/ .

264 Carnahan, J. (2018, March 12).

265 Johnston, C. S., Martin, L. J., & Cai, X. (1992). Antihistamine effect of supplemental ascorbic acid and neutrophil chemotaxis. *Journal of the American College of Nutrition, 11*(2), 172—176.

266 Johnston, C. S., Martin, L. J., & Cai, X. (1992).

267 Clemetson, C. A. (1980). Histamine and ascorbic acid in human blood. *The Journal of Nutrition, 110*(4), 662—668. https://doi.org/10.1093/jn/110.4.662 .

268 Carr, A. C., & Maggini, S. (2017). Vitamin C and immune function. *Nutrients, 9*(11), 1211. https://doi.org/10.3390/nu9111211 .

269 Li, Q., Tang, X., Huang, L., Wang, T., Huang, Y., & Jiang, S. (2024). Anti-allergic effect of vitamin C through inhibiting degranulation and regulating TH 1/TH 2 cell polarization. *Journal of the Science of Food and Agriculture,* 10.1002/jsfa.13419. Advance online publication. https://doi.org/10.1002/jsfa.13419.

270 Roschek, B., Jr, Fink, R. C., McMichael, M., & Alberte, R. S. (2009). Nettle extract (*Urtica dioica*) affects key receptors and enzymes associated with allergic rhinitis. *Phytotherapy research: PTR,* 23(7), 920-926. https://doi.org/10.1002/ptr.2763 .

271 Abenavoli, L., Izzo, A. A., Milić, N., Cicala, C., Santini, A., & Capasso, R. (2018). Milk thistle (*Silybum marianum*): A concise overview on its chemistry, pharmacological, and nutraceutical uses in liver diseases. *Phytotherapy Research: PTR, 32*(11), 2202-2213. https://doi.org/10.1002/ptr.6171 .

272 Huskisson, E., Maggini, S., & Ruf, M. (2007). The role of vitamins and minerals in energy metabolism and well-being. *The Journal of International Medical Research, 35*(3), 277-289. https://doi.org/10.1177/147323000703500301 .

273 Garland, E. M., Gamboa, A., Nwazue, V. C., Celedonio, J. E., Paranjape, S. Y., Black, B. K., Okamoto, L. E., Shibao, C. A., Biaggioni, I., Robertson, D., Diedrich, A., Dupont, W. D., & Raj, S. R. (2021). Effect of high dietary sodium intake in patients with postural tachycardia syndrome. *Journal of the American College of Cardiology, 77*(17), 2174-2184. https://doi.org/10.1016/j.jacc.2021.03.005 .

274 For myself and many of my friends who have Multiple Chemical Sensitivity, as well as among many of the people in many of the social media groups about Multiple Chemical Sensitivity, there is agreement that eating high-fat-containing foods soon after being exposed to a trigger will reduce the severity of the reaction. It is well known that most toxins are fat-soluble, so the prevailing conjecture is that the fat in the digestive system binds the offending toxins so that they can be flushed from the system. I have not found a study to describe the actual mechanism at play, but for whatever reason, when I have been triggered by a chemical, I do feel much better after having eaten something containing fat.

275 ScienceDaily. (2018, April 25). Drinking baking soda could be an inexpensive, safe way to combat autoimmune disease. *ScienceDaily.* www.sciencedaily.com/releases/2018/04/180425093745.htm.

276 Chai, S. C., Davis, K., Zhang, Z., Zha, L., & Kirschner, K. F. (2019). Effects of tart cherry juice on biomarkers of inflammation and oxidative stress in older adults. *Nutrients*, *11*(2), 228. https://doi.org/10.3390/nu11020228 .

277 Bøhn, S. K., Myhrstad, M. C. W., Thoresen, M., Erlund, I., Vasstrand, A. K., Marciuch, A., Carlsen, M. H., Bastani, N. E., Engedal, K., Flekkøy, K. M., & Blomhoff, R. (2021). Bilberry/red grape juice decreases plasma biomarkers of inflammation and tissue damage in aged men with subjective memory impairment -a randomized clinical trial. *BMC nutrition*, *7*(1), 75. https://doi.org/10.1186/s40795-021-00482-8 .

278 Martins, N. C., Dorneles, G. P., Blembeel, A. S., Marinho, J. P., Proença, I. C. T., da Cunha Goulart, M. J. V., Moller, G. B., Marques, E. P., Pochmann, D., Salvador, M., Elsner, V., Peres, A., Dani, C., & Ribeiro, J. L. (2020). Effects of grape juice consumption on oxidative stress and inflammation in male volleyball players: A randomized, double-blind, placebo-controlled clinical trial. https://doi.org/10.1016/j.ctim.2020.102570 .

279 Salehi, B., Mishra, A. P., Nigam, M., Sener, B., Kilic, M., Sharifi-Rad, M., Fokou, P. V. T., Martins, N., & Sharifi-Rad, J. (2018). Resveratrol: A double-edged sword in health benefits. *Biomedicines*, *6*(3), 91. https://doi.org/10.3390/biomedicines6030091 .

280 Abed, H., Ball, P. A., & Wang, L. X. (2012). Diagnosis and management of postural orthostatic tachycardia syndrome: A brief review. *Journal of Geriatric Cardiology : JGC*, *9*(1), 61—67. https://doi.org/10.3724/SP.J.1263.2012.00061 .

281 Lopresti, A. L. (2020). The effects of psychological and environmental stress on micronutrient concentrations in the body: A review of the evidence. *Advances in Nutrition (Bethesda, Md.)*, *11*(1), 103-112. https://doi.org/10.1093/advances/nmz082 .

282 Alka Seltzer Gold essentially contains baking soda, which was discussed above, and potassium bicarbonate and citric acid. Some people report getting better results from this product than baking soda alone for diminishing allergy reactions.

283 Laurino, C., & Palmieri, B. (2015). Zeolite: "The magic stone"; Main nutritional, environmental, experimental and clinical fields of application. *Nutricion Hospitalaria*, *32*(2), 573-581. https://doi.org/10.3305/nh.2015.32.2.8914 .

284 Kraljević Pavelić, S., Simović Medica, J., Gumbarević, D., Filošević, A., Pržulj, N., & Pavelić, K. (2018). Critical review on zeolite clinoptilolite safety and medical applications *in vivo*. *Frontiers in Pharmacology*, *9*, 1350. https://doi.org/10.3389/fphar.2018.01350 .

285 Coseva. The safest, most effective method of toxin removal : Advanced TRS user guide. ttps://www.thrivedirecthealthcare.com/uploads/1/0/7/7/107723313/coseva_atrs_product_guide.pdf .

286 Pu, S. Y., Huang, Y. L., Pu, C. M., Kang, Y. N., Hoang, K. D., Chen, K. H., & Chen, C. (2023). Effects of oral collagen for skin anti-aging: A systematic review and meta-analysis. *Nutrients*, *15*(9), 2080. https://doi.org/10.3390/nu15092080 .

287 Butterfield, J. H., & Weiler, C. R. (2008). Prevention of mast cell activation disorder-associated clinical sequelae of excessive prostaglandin D(2) production. *International Archives Of Allergy And Immunology*, *147*(4), 338-343. https://doi.org/10.1159/000144042

288 Zhang, J., Zhang, B., Zhang, J., Lin, W., & Zhang, S. (2021). Magnesium promotes the regeneration of the peripheral nerve. *Frontiers in Cell and Developmental Biology*, *9*, 717854. https://doi.org/10.3389/fcell.2021.717854 .

289 Harkin, C. Natural medicine phase 1 & 2 liver detox & cleanse. *Cara Health*. https://www.carahealth.com/health-articles/digestive-liver-detox-nutrition-weight-loss/phase-1-2-liver-detoxification .

290 Venkat, S. R. (2022, October 4). What is dysmetria? *Web*MD. https://www.webmd.com/brain/what-s-dysmetria .

291 Yan, J., & Dussor, G. (2014). Ion channels and Migraine. *Headache*, *54*(4), 619-639. https://doi.org/10.1111/head.12323 .

292 Hauser, R. (2023, April 10). *Essential tremor coming from the neck? The connection to cervical dysstructure* [Video]. Caring Medical and Hauser Neck Center (YouTube). https://www.youtube.com/watch?v=nbSr2ORGXkg .

293 Pan, M. K., & Kuo, S. H. (2022). Essential tremor: Clinical perspectives and pathophysiology. *Journal of the Neurological Sciences*, *435*, 120198. https://doi.org/10.1016/j.jns.2022.120198 .

294 Pan, M. K., & Kuo, S. H. (2022).

295 Manorenj, S., Shravani, C., & Jawalker, S. (2019). Clinical characteristics of essential tremor in South India: A hospital-based cohort study. *Journal of Neurosciences in Rural Practice, 10*(2), 245-249. https://doi.org/10.4103/jnrp.jnrp_348_18 .

296 Hauser, R. (2023, April 10).

297 Pan, M. K., & Kuo, S. H. (2022).

298 Hauser, R. (2023, April 10).

299 Amlang, C. J., Diaz, D. T., & Louis, E. D. (2020, March 24). Essential tremor as a "waste basket" diagnosis: Diagnosing essential tremor remains a challenge. *Front. Neurol*, 11. https://doi.org/10.3389/fneur.2020.00172 .

300 Hamonet, C., Ducret, L., Marié-Tanay, C., & Brock, I. (2016). Dystonia in the joint hypermobility syndrome (a.k.a. Ehlers-Danlos Syndrome, Hypermobility Type). *SOJ Neurol 3*(1), 1-3. https://doi.org/10.15226/2374-6858/3/1/00123 .

301 Wang, T. J., Stecco, A., & Dashtipour, K. (2021). the effect of low dose onabotulinumtoxina on cervical dystonia in Hypermobile Ehlers-Danlos Syndrome. *Tremor and Other Hyperkinetic Movements (New York, N.Y.), 11*, 42. https://doi.org/10.5334/tohm.647 .

302 Hamonet, C., Schatz, P. M., Bezire, P., Ducret, L., Brissot, & R. (2018). Cognitive and psychopathological aspects of Ehlers-Danlos Syndrome — Experience in a specialized medical consultation. *Research Advances in Brain Disorders and Therapy*. DOI: 10.29011/ RABDT-104. 100004. https://www.gavinpublishers.com/assets/articles_pdf/1525934180article_pdf97661175.pdf .

303 Hauser, R., Woldin, B., Evans, B., Hutcheson, B., Matias, D., & Rawlings, B. (2021). Intermittent cerebral ischemia as a cause of dystonic storms in hypermobile Ehlers-Danlos syndrome with upper cervical
instability, and prolotherapy as a successful treatment: 4 case series. *Open Journal of Clinical & Medical Case Reports, 7*(7).

304 Shakkottai, V. G. (2014). Physiologic changes associated with cerebellar dystonia. *Cerebellum (London, England), 13*(5), 637-644. https://doi.org/10.1007/s12311-014-0572-5 .

305 Cloud, L. J., & Jinnah, H. A. (2010). Treatment strategies for dystonia. *Expert Opinion on Pharmacotherapy, 11*(1), 5–15. https://doi.org/10.1517/14656560903426171 .

306 Hamonet C, Schatz PM, Bezire P, Ducret L, & Brissot R (2018) Cognitive and psychopathological aspects of Ehlers-Danlos Syndrome - Experience in a specialized medical consultation. *Research Advances in Brain Disorders and Therapy.* RABDT-104. https://doi.org/10.29011/ RABDT-104. 100004 .

307 Hamonet, C., Schatz, P. M., Bezire, P., Ducret, L., & Brissot, R. (2018). Cognitive and psychopathological aspects of Ehlers-Danlos Syndrome — Experience in a specialized medical consultation. *Res Adv Brain Disord Ther:* RABDT-104. DOI: 10.29011/ RABDT-104. 100004 .

308 Singhal, A. B., Maas, M. B., Goldstein, J. N., Mills, B. B., Chen, D. W., Ayata, C., Kacmarek, R. M., & Topcuoglu, M. A. (2017). High-flow oxygen therapy for treatment of acute migraine: A randomized crossover trial. *Cephalalgia: An International Journal of Headache, 37*(8), 730-736. https://doi.org/10.1177/0333102416651453 .

309 Bennett, M. H., French, C., Schnabel, A., Wasiak, J., Kranke, P., & Weibel, S. (2015). Normobaric and hyperbaric oxygen therapy for the treatment and prevention of migraine and cluster headache. *The Cochrane Database of Systematic Reviews, 2015*(12), CD005219. https://doi.org/10.1002/14651858.CD005219.pub3 .

310 Thwaites, P.A., Gibson, P.R., Burgell, R.E. (2022, September). Hypermobile Ehlers-Danlos Syndrome and disorders of the gastrointestinal tract: What the gastroenterologist needs to know. *Journal of Gastroenterology and Hepatology, 37*(9), 1693-1709. https://doi:.org/10.1111/jgh.15927 .

311 Mila, E. ((2022, January 23). The ultimate list of coconut derivatives in skincare. *Sensitive Skin Oasis*. https://sensitiveskinoasis.com/coconut-derivatives-in-skin-care/ .

312 This is a common topic of conversation in social media groups. Every time it is brought up, at least one person replies that all of their symptoms were alleviated by switching to a certain diet, but many different diets have been credited, with no discernible pattern emerging.

313 Kong, W., Xie, Y., Zhong, J., & Cao, C. (2022). Ultra-processed foods and allergic symptoms among children and adults in the United States: A population-based analysis of NHANES 2005-2006. *Frontiers in Public Health, 10*, 1038141. https://doi.org/10.3389/fpubh.2022.1038141 .

314 Costa de Miranda, R., Rauber, F., & Levy, R. B. (2021). Impact of ultra-processed food consumption on metabolic health. *Current Opinion in Lipidology, 32*(1), 24-37. https://doi.org/10.1097/MOL.0000000000000728 .

315 Mie, A., Andersen, H. R., Gunnarsson, S., Kahl, J., Kesse-Guyot, E., Rembiałkowska, E., Quaglio, G., & Grandjean, P. (2017). Human health implications of organic food and organic agriculture: a comprehensive review. *Environmental health : A global access science source*, *16*(1), 111. https://doi.org/10.1186/s12940-017-0315-4 .

316 Biodynamic Demeter Alliance. What is biodynamics? https://www.biodynamics.com/what-is-biodynamics.

317 Ramírez Carnero, A., Lestido-Cardama, A., Vazquez Loureiro, P., Barbosa-Pereira, L., Rodríguez Bernaldo de Quirós, A., & Sendón, R. (2021). Presence of perfluoroalkyl and polyfluoroalkyl substances (PFAS) in food contact materials (FCM) and its migration to food. *Foods (Basel, Switzerland)*, *10*(7), 1443. https://doi.org/10.3390/foods10071443 .

318 Ramírez Carnero, A., Lestido-Cardama, A., Vazquez Loureiro, P., Barbosa-Pereira, L., Rodríguez Bernaldo de Quirós, A., & Sendón, R. (2021).

319 Esquerre, N., Basso, L., Dubuquoy, C., Djouina, M., Chappard, D., Blanpied, C., Desreumaux, P., Vergnolle, N., Vignal, C., & Body-Malapel, M. (2019). Aluminum ingestion promotes colorectal hypersensitivity in rodents. *Cellular and Molecular Gastroenterology and Hepatology*, *7*(1), 185-196. https://doi.org/10.1016/j.jcmgh.2018.09.012 .

320 Fujiwara, Y., Machida, A., Watanabe, Y., Shiba, M., Tominaga, K., Watanabe, T., Ocrapani, N., Higuchi, K., & Arakawa, T. (2005). Association between dinner-to-bed time and gastro-esophageal reflux disease. *The American Journal of Gastroenterology*, *100*(12), 2633-2636. https://doi.org/10.1111/j.1572-0241.2005.00354.x .

321 Takasu, N., Furuoka, S., Inatsugi, N., Rutkowska, D., & Tokura, H. (2000). The effects of skin pressure by clothing on whole gut transit time and amount of feces. *Journal of Physiological Anthropology and Applied Human Science*, *19*(3), 151-156. https://doi.org/10.2114/jpa.19.151 .

322 Hirano, Y., & Onozuka, M. (2014). *Brain and nerve = Shinkei kenkyu no shinpo*, *66*(1), 25-32.

323 Carmody, R. N., & Wrangham, R. W. (2009). Cooking and the human commitment to a high-quality diet. *Cold Spring Harbor Symposia on Quantitative Biology*, *74*, 427-434. https://doi.org/10.1101/sqb.2009.74.019 .

324 Miller, K., & Gleim, S. (2023, September 13). Common heartburn triggers. *WebMD*. https://www.webmd.com/heartburn-gerd/triggers .

325 Crum, A. J., Corbin, W. R., Brownell, K. D., & Salovey, P. (2011). Mind over milkshakes: Mindsets, not just nutrients, determine ghrelin response. *Health Psychology : Official Journal of the Division of Health Psychology, American Psychological Association*, *30*(4), 424-431. https://doi.org/10.1037/a0023467 .

326 Hagerty, B. B. (2009, May 20). Prayer may reshape your brain...and your reality. *NPR: All Things Considered*. https://www.npr.org/2009/05/20/104310443/prayer-may-reshape-your-brain-and-your-reality .

327 Fujiwara, Y., Machida, A., Watanabe, Y., Shiba, M., Tominaga, K., Watanabe, T., Ocrapani, N., Higuchi, K., & Arakawa, T. (2005). Association between dinner-to-bed time and gastro-esophageal reflux disease. *The American Journal of Gastroenterology*, *100*(12), 2633-2636. https://doi.org/10.1111/j.1572-0241.2005.00354.x .

328 Ajbani, K., Chansky, M. E., & Baumann, B. M. (2011). Homespun remedy, homespun toxicity: Baking soda ingestion for dyspepsia. *The Journal of Emergency Medicine*, *40*(4), e71-e74. https://doi.org/10.1016/j.jemermed.2007.04.027 .

329 Medical College of Georgia at Augusta University. (2018, April 25). Drinking baking soda could be an inexpensive, safe way to combat autoimmune disease. *ScienceDaily*. www.sciencedaily.com/releases/2018/04/180425093745.htm .

330 Grgic, J., Pedisic, Z., Saunders, B., Artioli, G. G., Schoenfeld, B. J., McKenna, M. J., Bishop, D. J., Kreider, R. B., Stout, J. R., Kalman, D. S., Arent, S. M., VanDusseldorp, T. A., Lopez, H. L., Ziegenfuss, T. N., Burke, L. M., Antonio, J., & Campbell, B. I. (2021). International Society of Sports Nutrition position stand: Sodium bicarbonate and exercise performance. *Journal of the International Society of Sports Nutrition*, *18*(1), 61. https://doi.org/10.1186/s12970-021-00458-w .

331 Angus, K., Asgharifar, S., & Gleberzon, B. (2015). What effect does chiropractic treatment have on gastrointestinal (GI) disorders: A narrative review of the literature. *The Journal of the Canadian Chiropractic Association*, *59*(2), 122-133.

332 Bush, Z., Gildea, J., Roberts, D., & Matavelli, L. (2019). The effects of ION* gut health dietary supplement on markers of intestinal permeability and immune system function in healthy subjects: A double-blind, placebo-controlled clinical trial. ION* Biome.

https://cdn.shopify.com/s/files/1/0354/2789/t/51/assets/IONBiome_Science_Paper_White_Paper_DigitalFile.pdf .

333 Marengo, K. (2020, April 24). What is fulvic acid, and does it have benefits? *Healthline*. https://www.healthline.com/nutrition/fulvic-acid .

334 Winkler, J., & Ghosh, S. (2018). Therapeutic potential of fulvic acid in chronic inflammatory diseases and diabetes. *Journal of Diabetes Research*, 5391014. https://doi.org/10.1155/2018/5391014 .

335 Huynh, D. T. K., Shamash, K., Burch, M., Phillips, E., Cunneen, S., Van Allan, R. J., & Shouhed, D. (2019). Median arcuate ligament syndrome and its associated conditions. *The American Surgeon*, *85*(10), 1162-1165.

336 Smereczyński, A., Kołaczyk, K., & Kiedrowicz, R. (2021). New perspective on median arcuate ligament syndrome: Case reports. *Journal of Ultrasonography*, *21*(86), e234-e236. https://doi.org/10.15557/JoU.2021.0037 .

337 Becker, E., Mohammed, T., & Wysocki, J. (2021, October). Often overlooked diagnosis: Median arcuate ligament syndrome as a mimicker of Crohn's disease. *ACG Case Reports Journal, 8*(10):p e00675. https://doi.org/10.14309/crj.0000000000000675 .

338 Smereczyński, A., Kołaczyk, K., & Kiedrowicz, R. (2021).

339 Asanad, S., Bayomi, M., Brown, D., Buzzard, J., Lai, E., Ling, C., Miglani, T., Mohammed, T., Tsai, J., Uddin, O., & Singman, E. (2022). Ehlers-Danlos Syndromes and their manifestations in the visual system. *Frontiers in Medicine*, *9*, 996458. https://doi.org/10.3389/fmed.2022.996458 .

340 Han, X., Liu, C., Chen, Y., & He, M. (2022). Myopia prediction: A systematic review. *Eye (London, England)*, *36*(5), 921-929. https://doi.org/10.1038/s41433-021-01805-6 .

341 Wang, J., Li, Y., Musch, D. C., Wei, N., Qi, X., Ding, G., Li, X., Li, J., Song, L., Zhang, Y., Ning, Y., Zeng, X., Hua, N., Li, S., & Qian, X. (2021). Progression of myopia in school-aged children after COVID-19 home confinement. *JAMA Ophthalmology*, *139*(3), 293-300. https://doi.org/10.1001/jamaophthalmol.2020.6239 .

342 Danilenko, K. V., & Samoilova, E. A. (2007). Stimulatory effect of morning bright light on reproductive hormones and ovulation: Results of a controlled crossover trial. *PloS Clinical Trials*, *2*(2), e7. https://doi.org/10.1371/journal.pctr.0020007 .

343 Maffetone, P. (2015, April 29). Sunlight: Good for the eyes as well as the brain. *MAF*. https://philmaffetone.com/sun-and-brain/ .

344 Vital Veda. (2020, December 22). Why wearing sunglasses is not healthy. https://vitalveda.com.au/learn/emotional-health/sunglasses/ .

345 Veritasnaut. (2019, June 15). Sunglasses are killing you. *Medium*. https://medium.com/@veritasnaut/sunglasses-are-killing-you-dbadb93f935d .

346 Pearce, G., Bell, L., Pezaro, S., & Reinhold, E. (2023). Childbearing with Hypermobile Ehlers-Danlos Syndrome and Hypermobility Spectrum Disorders: A large international survey of outcomes and complications. *International Journal of Environmental Research and Public Health*, *20*(20), 6957. https://doi.org/10.3390/ijerph20206957 .

347 Smoley, B. A., & Robinson, C. M. (2012). Natural family planning. *American Family Physician*, *86*(10), 924-928.

348 Caliogna, L., Guerrieri, V., Annunziata, S., Bina, V., Brancato, A. M., Castelli, A., Jannelli, E., Ivone, A., Grassi, F. A., Mosconi, M., et al. (2021). Biomarkers for Ehlers-Danlos Syndromes: There is a role? *International Journal of Molecular Sciences*, *22*(18), 10149. https://doi.org/10.3390/ijms221810149 .

349 Sharma, R., Biedenharn, K. R., Fedor, J. M., & Agarwal, A. (2013). Lifestyle factors and reproductive health: taking control of your fertility. *Reproductive Biology And Endocrinology : RB&E*, *11*, 66. https://doi.org/10.1186/1477-7827-11-66 .

350 Angus, K., Asgharifar, S., & Gleberzon, B. (2015). What effect does chiropractic treatment have on gastrointestinal (GI) disorders: A narrative review of the literature. *The Journal of the Canadian Chiropractic Association*, *59*(2), 122-133.

351 Xu, J. Y., Zhao, A. L., Xin, P., Geng, J. Z., Wang, B. J., & Xia, T. (2022). Acupuncture for female infertility: Discussion on action mechanism and application. *Evidence-Based Complementary* and *Alternative Medicine: eCAM*, 3854117. https://doi.org/10.1155/2022/3854117 .

352 Zheng, X., Yu, S., Liu, L., Yang, H., Wang, F., Yang, H., Lv, X., & Yang, J. (2022). The dose-related efficacy of acupuncture on endometrial receptivity in infertile women: A systematic review and meta-analysis. *Frontiers in Public Health*, *10*, 858587. https://doi.org/10.3389/fpubh.2022.858587 .

353 Novy, M, Eschenbach, D, *et al*, (2008). Infections as a cause of infertility. *Global Library of Women's Medicine. (ISSN: 1756-2228).* DOI 10.3843/GLOWM.10328. https://www.glowm.com/section-view/heading/Infections%20as%20a%20Cause%20of%20Infertility/item/327# .

354 Rooney, K. L., & Domar, A. D. (2018). The relationship between stress and infertility. *Dialogues in Clinical Neuroscience, 20*(1), 41-47. https://doi.org/10.31887/DCNS.2018.20.1/klrooney .

355 MacDonald, D., & Arvigo, R. (2017, November 21). Can this ancient Mayan massage technique increase fertility? *Massage Magazine.* https://www.massagemag.com/mayan-fertility-massage-technique-87497/ .

356 Pearce, G., Bell, L., Pezaro, S., & Reinhold, E. (2023).

357 Mysels, D. J., & Sullivan, M. A. (2010). The relationship between opioid and sugar intake: Review of evidence and clinical applications. *Journal of Opioid Management, 6*(6), 445-452. https://doi.org/10.5055/jom.2010.0043 .

358 Mphande, A. N., Killowe, C., Phalira, S., Jones, H. W., & Harrison, W. J. (2007). Effects of honey and sugar dressings on wound healing. *Journal of Wound Care, 16*(7), 317-319. https://doi.org/10.12968/jowc.2007.16.7.27053

359 Yamamoto, T., Sako, N., & Maeda, S. (2000). Effects of taste stimulation on beta-endorphin levels in rat cerebrospinal fluid and plasma. *Physiology & Behavior, 69*(3), 345-350. https://doi.org/10.1016/s0031-9384(99)00252-8 .

360 Ahmed, S. H., Guillem, K., & Vandaele, Y. (2013). Sugar addiction: Pushing the drug-sugar analogy to the limit. *Current Opinion in Clinical Nutrition and Metabolic Care, 16*(4), 434-439. https://doi.org/10.1097/MCO.0b013e328361c8b8 .

361 Bray, G. A. (2016, July 1). Is sugar addictive? *Diabetes, 65*(7), 1797-1799. https://doi.org/10.2337/dbi16-0022 .

362 Goran, M. I., Plows, J. F., & Ventura, E. E. (2019). Effects of consuming sugars and alternative sweeteners during pregnancy on maternal and child health: Evidence for a secondhand sugar effect. *The Proceedings of the Nutrition Society, 78*(3), 262-271. https://doi.org/10.1017/S002966511800263X .

363 Campbell, B. The role of histamine in pregnancy. *Dr. Becky Campbell Functional Medicine.* https://drbeckycampbell.com/histamine-intolerance-and-pregnancy/ .

364 Tagauov, Y. D., Abu-Elsaoud, A. M., Abdrassulova, Z. T., Tuleukhanov, S. T., Salybekova, N. N., Tulindinova, G., & Al-Abkal, F. (2023). Improvement of blood parameters of male rats exposed to different injection doses of liquid chlorophyll. *Cureus, 15*(3), e36044. https://doi.org/10.7759/cureus.36044 .

365 This treatment was taught to me by a friend who learned it when getting chemotherapy for cancer many years ago. I have talked online with other women who also had the experience of fountain sodas helping their HG.

366 Neri, W. (2024, May 30). Why do so many people turn to Coca-Cola during a migraine attack? *Migraine Again.* https://www.migraineagain.com/coca-cola-during-migraine-attack/ .

367 Mysels, D. J., & Sullivan, M. A. (2010). The relationship between opioid and sugar intake: Review of evidence and clinical applications. *Journal of Opioid Management, 6*(6), 445-452. https://doi.org/10.5055/jom.2010.0043 .

368 Butler, N. (2023, October 5). How does chewing gum affect your digestive system? *Healthnews.* https://healthnews.com/nutrition/healthy-eating/how-does-chewing-gum-affect-your-digestive-system/ .

369 Dodds, M. W. J., Haddou, M. B., & Day, J. E. L. (2023). The effect of gum chewing on xerostomia and salivary flow rate in elderly and medically compromised subjects: A systematic review and meta-analysis. *BMC Oral Health 23*, 406. https://doi.org/10.1186/s12903-023-03084-x .

370 Koren, G., & Pairaideau, N. (2006). Compliance with prenatal vitamins: Patients with morning sickness sometimes find it difficult. *Canadian Family Physician Medecin de Famille Canadien, 52*(11), 1392-1393.

371 Iftikhar, N. (2020, September 25). Side effects of prenatal vitamins: What they are and how to treat them. *Healthline.* https://www.healthline.com/health/pregnancy/prenatal-vitamins-side-effects#takeaway .

372 O'Donnell, A., McParlin, C., Robson, S. C., et al. (2016, October). Treatments for hyperemesis gravidarum and nausea and vomiting in pregnancy: A systematic review and economic assessment. *Southampton (UK): NIHR Journals Library. (Health Technology Assessment, No. 20.74.) Scientific summary.* https://www.ncbi.nlm.nih.gov/books/NBK390535/ .

373 O'Donnell, A., McParlin, C., Robson, S. C., et al. (2016, October).

374 Van den Heuvel, E., Goossens, M., Vanderhaegen, H., Sun, H. X., & Buntinx, F. (2016). Effect of acustimulation on nausea and vomiting and on hyperemesis in pregnancy: A systematic review of Western and Chinese literature. *BMC Complementary and Alternative Medicine, 16*, 13. https://doi.org/10.1186/s12906-016-0985-4 .

375 Xu, T., Lun, W., & He, Y. (2024). Subchorionic hematoma: Research status and pathogenesis (Review). *Medicine international*, *4*(2), 10. https://doi.org/10.3892/mi.2024.134 .

376 Redmond, A. & Siddle, H. (2016, January 5). Footcare in Hypermobile Ehlers-Dalos Syndrome. *Ehlers-Danlos Support UK.* https://www.ehlers-danlos.org/information/footcare-in-hypermobile-ehlers-danlos-syndrome/ .

377 Trojian, T., & Tucker, A. K. (2019). Plantar fasciitis. *American Family Physician*, *99*(12), 744-750.

378 Kim, C. (2022, August 5). Plantar fasciitis and knee hypermobility. *Dr. Cathy A. Kim.* https://drcathykim.com/2022/08/plantar-fasciitis-and-knee-hypermobility/ .

379 Menz, H. B., & Morris, M. E. (2005). Footwear characteristics and foot problems in older people. *Gerontology*, *51*(5), 346-351. https://doi.org/10.1159/000086373 .

380 Silfverskiöld J. P. (1991). Common foot problems. Relieving the pain of bunions, keratoses, corns, and calluses. *Postgraduate Medicine*, *89*(5), 183-188. https://doi.org/10.1080/00325481.1991.11700901 .

381 Edimo, C. O., Wajsberg, J. R., Wong, S., Nahmias, Z. P., & Riley, B. A. (2021). The dermatological aspects of hEDS in women. *International Journal of Women's Dermatology*, *7*(3), 285-289. https://doi.org/10.1016/j.ijwd.2021.01.020 .

382 Hara, S., Kitano, M., & Kudo, S. (2023). The effects of short foot exercises to treat flat foot deformity: A systematic review. *Journal of Back and Musculoskeletal Rehabilitation*, *36*(1), 21-33. https://doi.org/10.3233/BMR-210374 .

383 Goodyear-Smith, F., & Arroll, B. (2006). Growing pains. *BMJ (Clinical research ed.)*, *333*(7566), 456-457. https://doi.org/10.1136/bmj.38950.463877.80 .

384 Uziel, Y., & Hashkes, P. J. (2007). Growing pains in children. *Pediatric Rheumatology Online Journal*, *5*, 5. https://doi.org/10.1186/1546-0096-5-5 .

385 Goodyear-Smith, F., & Arroll, B. (2006).

386 Mathews, L. (2011). Pain in children: Neglected, unaddressed and mismanaged. *Indian Journal of Palliative Care*, *17*(Suppl), S70-S73. https://doi.org/10.4103/0973-1075.76247 .

387 Wang, Z. R., & Ni, G. X. (2021). Is it time to put traditional cold therapy in rehabilitation of soft-tissue injuries out to pasture? *World Journal of Clinical Cases*, *9*(17), 4116-4122. https://doi.org/10.12998/wjcc.v9.i17.4116 .

388 Nakano, J., Yamabayashi, C., Scott, A., & Reid, W. D. (2012). The effect of heat applied with stretch to increase range of motion: A systematic review. *Physical Therapy in Sport, 13*, 3, 180-188. https://doi.org/10.1016/j.ptsp.2011.11.003 .

389 Staiger C. (2012). Comfrey: A clinical overview. *Phytotherapy research : PTR, 26*(10), 1441-1448. https://doi.org/10.1002/ptr.4612 .

390 Zhang, J., Zhang, B., Zhang, J., Lin, W., & Zhang, S. (2021). Magnesium promotes the regeneration of the peripheral nerve. *Frontiers in Cell and Developmental Biology, 9*, 717854. https://doi.org/10.3389/fcell.2021.717854 .

391 Staiger C. (2012).

392 Walthall, J., Anand, P., & Rehman, U. H. (2023, February 26). Dupuytren contracture. In: *StatPearls*. https://www.ncbi.nlm.nih.gov/books/NBK526074/ .

393 Nakano, J., Yamabayashi, C., Scott, A., & Reid, W. D. (2012). The effect of heat applied with stretch to increase range of motion: A systematic review. *Physical Therapy in Sport, 13*, 3, 180-188. https://doi.org/10.1016/j.ptsp.2011.11.003 .

394 Staiger C. (2012).

395 Brund, R. B. K., Rasmussen, S. Nielsen, R. O., Kersting, U. G., Laessoe, U., & Voigt, M. (2017, May 24). The association between eccentric hip abduction strength and hip and knee angular movements in recreational male runners: An explorative study. *Scandinavian Journal of Medicine and Science in Sports*, *28*(2). https://doi.org/10.1111/sms.12923 .

396 Gavin Daly. Knee pain — Are my feet to blame? *Posture Podiatry.* https://posturepodiatry.com.au/ .

397 Morales-Brown, P. (2023, July 26). What's to know about crepitus of the knee. *Medical News Today.* https://www.medicalnewstoday.com/articles/310547#causes-of-crepitus .

398 McCoy, K. (2018, September 3). Crepitus symptoms, natural remedies, and how to prevent. *Dr. Axe*. https://draxe.com/health/crepitus/ .

399 Cleveland Clinic. (2023, August 22). Lymph. https://my.clevelandclinic.org/health/body/25209-lymph .

400 Medline Plus. (2022, July 25). Lymph system. https://medlineplus.gov/ency/article/002247.htm .

401 Skobe, M., & Detmar, M. (2000). Structure, function, and molecular control of the skin lymphatic system. *Journal of Investigative Dermatology Symposium Proceedings, 5*(1), 14-19. ISSN 1087-0024. https://doi.org/10.1046/j.1087-0024.2000.00001.x .

402 Venugopal, A. M., Stewart, R. H., Laine, G. A., Dongaonkar, R. M., & Quick, C. M. (2007). Lymphangion coordination minimally affects mean flow in lymphatic vessels. *American Journal of Physiology: Heart and Circulatory Physiology, 293*(2), H1183-H1189. https://doi.org/10.1152/ajpheart.01340.2006 .

403 Hardy, D. (2022, October). What is lymphoedema? *The Lymphoedema Support Network*. https://www.lymphoedema.org/information/what-is-lymphoedema/ .

404 National Heart, Lung, and Blood Institute. (2022, May 18). What is metabolic syndrome? https://www.nhlbi.nih.gov/health/metabolic-syndrome .

405 Guillermo, O., et al. (2020, July). The lymphatic vasculature in the 21st century: Novel functional roles in homeostasis and disease. *Cell, 182.* https://doi.org/10.1016/j.cell.2020.06.039.

406 Scallan, J. P., Zawieja, S. D., Castorena-Gonzalez, J. A., & Davis, M. J. (2016, August 2). Lymphatic pumping: Mechanics, mechanisms and malfunction. *Journal of Physiology*, 15;594(20), 5749-5768. https://doi.org/10.1113/JP272088.

407 LibreTexts. Lymphatic vessel structure. https://med.libretexts.org/Bookshelves/Anatomy_and_Physiology/Anatomy_and_Physiology_(Boundless)/19:_Lymphatic_System/19.2:_Lymphatic_Vessels/19.2A:_Lymphatic_Vessel_Structure .

408 Seymour, T. (2017, July 27). How to perform a lymphatic drainage massage. *Medical News Today.* https://www.medicalnewstoday.com/articles/318628#Outlook .

409 Yuan, S. L. K., Matsutani. L. A., & Marques, A. P. (2015). Effectiveness of different styles of massage therapy in fibromyalgia: A systematic review and meta-analysis. *Manual Therapy, 20*(2) 257-264. ISSN 1356-689X. https://doi.org/10.1016/j.math.2014.09.003 .

410 Wang, M., Tutt, J. O., Dorricott, N. O., Parker, K. L., Russo, A. F., & Sowers, L. P. (2022). Involvement of the cerebellum in migraine. *Frontiers in Systems Neuroscience, 16*. https://www.frontiersin.org/articles/10.3389/fnsys.2022.984406 . DOI=10.3389/fnsys.2022.984406.

411 American Migraine Foundation. (2018, January 18). The timeline of a migraine attack. https://americanMigrainefoundation.org/resource-library/timeline-migraine-attack/ .

412 Karsan, N., Bose, P., Newman, J., & Goadsby, P. J. (2021). Are some patient-perceived migraine triggers simply early manifestations of the attack?. *Journal of Neurology, 268*(5), 1885-1893. https://doi.org/10.1007/s00415-020-10344-1 .

413 American Migraine Foundation. (2018, January 18).

414 Gazit, Y., Jacob, G., & Grahame, R. (2016). Ehlers-Danlos Syndrome-Hypermobility Type: A much neglected multisystemic disorder. *Rambam Maimonides Medical Journal, 7*(4), e0034. https://doi.org/10.5041/RMMJ.10261 .

415 Yan, J., & Dussor, G. (2014). Ion channels and migraine. *Headache, 54*(4), 619-639. https://doi.org/10.1111/head.12323 .

416 Temple, K. M. (2020, August 26).The alcoholic beverage: An elixir, and yet a poison? *RHI Hub*. https://www.ruralhealthinfo.org/rural-monitor/alcohol-elixir-poison .

417 Wachholtz, A. B., Malone, C. D., & Pargament, K. I. (2017). Effect of different meditation types on migraine headache medication use. *Behavioral Medicine (Washington, D.C.), 43*(1), 1-8. https://doi.org/10.1080/08964289.2015.1024601 .

418 Karsan, N., Bose, P., Newman, J., & Goadsby, P. J. (2021).

419 Lum, B. (2024). Functional medicine treatment of histamine intolerance. *Functional Helathcare Institute*. https://www.drbrianlum.com/histamine-intolerance .

420 Harkin, C. Natural medicine phase 1 & 2 liver detox & cleanse. *Cara Health*. https://www.carahealth.com/health-articles/digestive-liver-detox-nutrition-weight-loss/phase-1-2-liver-detoxification .

421 Morris, T., Stables, M., Hobbs, A., de Souza, P., Colville-Nash, P., Warner, T., Newson, J., Bellingan, G., & Gilroy, D. W. (2009, August 1). Effects of low-dose aspirin on acute inflammatory

responses in humans. *Journal of Immunology (Baltimore, Md. : 1950), 183*(3), 2089-2096. https://doi.org/10.4049/jimmunol.0900477 .

422 Medical College of Georgia at Augusta University. (2018, April 25). Drinking baking soda could be an inexpensive, safe way to combat autoimmune disease. *ScienceDaily*. https://www.sciencedaily.com/releases/2018/04/180425093745.htm .

423 Grgic, J., Pedisic, Z., Saunders, B., Artioli, G. G., Schoenfeld, B. J., McKenna, M. J., Bishop, D. J., Kreider, R. B., Stout, J. R., Kalman, D. S., Arent, S. M., VanDusseldorp, T. A., Lopez, H. L., Ziegenfuss, T. N., Burke, L. M., Antonio, J., & Campbell, B. I. (2021). International Society of Sports Nutrition position stand: Sodium bicarbonate and exercise performance. *Journal of the International Society of Sports Nutrition, 18*(1), 61. https://doi.org/10.1186/s12970-021-00458-w .

424 Singhal, A. B., Maas, M. B., Goldstein, J. N., Mills, B. B., Chen, D. W., Ayata, C., Kacmarek, R. M., & Topcuoglu, M. A. (2017). High-flow oxygen therapy for treatment of acute migraine: A randomized crossover trial. *Cephalalgia : An International Journal of Headache, 37*(8), 730-736. https://doi.org/10.1177/0333102416651453 .

425 Bennett, M. H., French, C., Schnabel, A., Wasiak, J., Kranke, P., & Weibel, S. (2015). Normobaric and hyperbaric oxygen therapy for the treatment and prevention of migraine and cluster headache. *The Cochrane Database of Systematic Reviews*, 2015(12), CD005219. https://doi.org/10.1002/14651858.CD005219.pub3 .

426 Shaik, M. M., & Gan, S. H. (2015). Vitamin supplementation as possible prophylactic treatment against migraine with aura and menstrual migraine. *BioMed Research International*, 469529. https://doi.org/10.1155/2015/469529 .

427 Rainero, I., Vacca, A., Roveta, F., Govone, F., Gai, A., & Rubino, E. (2019). Targeting MTHFR for the treatment of migraines. *Expert Opinion on Therapeutic Targets, 23*(1), 29-37. https://doi.org/10.1080/14728222.2019.1549544 .

428 Altura, B. T., & Altura, B. M. (1984). Interactions of Mg and K on cerebral vessels — Aspects in view of stroke. Review of present status and new findings. *Magnesium, 3*(4-6), 195-211.

429 Hirano, Y., & Onozuka, M. (2014). *Brain and nerve = Shinkei kenkyu no shinpo, 66*(1), 25-32.

430 Todd, C. (2019, June 4). Here's what actually happens in your body when you eat fat. *Self.* https://www.self.com/story/what-fat-does-in-your-body .

431 Chaibi, A., Tuchin, P. J., & Russell, M. B. (2011). Manual therapies for migraine: A systematic review. *The Journal of Headache and Pain, 12*(2), 127-133. https://doi.org/10.1007/s10194-011-0296-6 .

432 Lopresti, A. L., Smith, S. J., & Drummond, P. D. (2020). Herbal treatments for migraine: A systematic review of randomised-controlled studies. *Phytotherapy Research : PTR, 34*(10), 2493-2517. https://doi.org/10.1002/ptr.6701 .

433 Faridzadeh, A., Salimi, Y., Ghasemirad, H., Kargar, M., Rashtchian, A., Mahmoudvand, G., Karimi, M. A., Zerangian, N., Jahani, N., Masoudi, A., Sadeghian Dastjerdi, B., Salavatizadeh, M., Sadeghsalehi, H., & Deravi, N. (2022). Neuroprotective potential of aromatic herbs: Rosemary, sage, and lavender. *Frontiers in Neuroscience, 16*, 909833. https://doi.org/10.3389/fnins.2022.909833 .

434 Zhang, C. S., Lyu, S., Zhang, A. L., Guo, X., Sun, J., Lu, C., Luo, X., & Xue, C. C. (2022). Natural products for migraine: Data-mining analyses of Chinese Medicine classical literature. *Frontiers in Pharmacology, 13*, 995559. https://doi.org/10.3389/fphar.2022.995559 .

435 Sujan, M. U., Rao, M. R., Kisan, R., Abhishekh, H. A., Nalini, A., Raju, T. R., & Sathyaprabha, T. N. (2016). Influence of hydrotherapy on clinical and cardiac autonomic function in migraine patients. *Journal of Neurosciences in Rural Practice, 7*(1), 109-113. https://doi.org/10.4103/0976-3147.165389 .

436 Mysels, D. J., & Sullivan, M. A. (2010). The relationship between opioid and sugar intake: Review of evidence and clinical applications. *Journal of Opioid Management, 6*(6), 445-452. https://doi.org/10.5055/jom.2010.0043 .

437 Nowaczewska, M., Wiciński, M., & Kaźmierczak, W. (2020). The ambiguous role of caffeine in migraine headache: From trigger to treatment. *Nutrients, 12*(8), 2259. https://doi.org/10.3390/nu12082259 .

438 Echeverri, D., Montes, F. R., Cabrera, M., Galán, A., & Prieto, A. (2010). Caffeine's vascular mechanisms of action. *International Journal of Vascular Medicine, 2010*, 834060. https://doi.org/10.1155/2010/834060 .

439 Rouge. (2023, May 3). Red light therapy for headaches and migraines: Relief for relentless pain. https://rouge.care/blogs/rouge-red-light-therapy-blog/red-light-therapy-for-headaches-and-Migraines-relief-for-relentless-pain .

440 Bigal, M. E., & Hargreaves, R. J. (2013). Why does sleep stop migraine? *Current Pain and Headache Reports*, *17*(10), 369. https://doi.org/10.1007/s11916-013-0369-0 .

441 Although I cannot currently find the original source for this statement, I do remember that it has been confirmed numerous times in social media group conversations.

442 Nguyen, C,T., & Basso, M. (2022, October 24). Epley maneuver. *StatPearls.* https://www.ncbi.nlm.nih.gov/books/NBK563287/ .

443 Cunningham, S. (2023, December 6). The power of peppermint. UC Health. https://www.uchealth.org/today/the-power-of-peppermint/ .

444 Mysels, D. J., & Sullivan, M. A. (2010). The relationship between opioid and sugar intake: Review of evidence and clinical applications. *Journal of Opioid Management*, *6*(6), 445-452. https://doi.org/10.5055/jom.2010.0043 .

445 Lepperdinger, U., Zschocke, J., & Kapferer-Seebacher, I. (2021). Oral manifestations of Ehlers-Danlos Syndromes. *American Journal of Medical Genetics. Part C, Seminars in Medical Genetics*, *187*(4), 520-526. https://doi.org/10.1002/ajmg.c.31941 .

446 Marsh, P. D. (2006). Dental plaque as a biofilm and a microbial community — implications for health and disease. *BMC Oral Health*, *6 Suppl 1*(Suppl 1), S14. https://doi.org/10.1186/1472-6831-6-S1-S14 .

447 Tinkle, B., Castori, M., Berglund, B., Cohen, H., Grahame, R., Kazkaz, H., & Levy, H. (2017). Hypermobile Ehlers-Danlos Syndrome (a.k.a. Ehlers-Danlos Syndrome Type III and Ehlers-Danlos Syndrome Hypermobility Type): Clinical description and natural history. *American Journal of Medical Genetics. Part C, Seminars in Medical Genetics*, *175*(1), 48-69. https://doi.org/10.1002/ajmg.c.31538 .

448 Wang, C., Wang, L., Wang, X., & Cao, Z. (2022). Beneficial effects of melatonin on periodontitis management: Far more than oral cavity. *International Journal of Molecular Sciences*, *23*(23), 14541. https://doi.org/10.3390/ijms232314541 .

449 Nagel, R. (2011). *Cure Tooth Decay: Remineralize Cavities and Repair Your Teeth Naturally with Good Food.* Golden Child Publishing, Los Angeles, CA. https://amzn.to/3NWMKuW .

450 Nagel, R. (2011).

451 Abou Neel, E. A., Aljabo, A., Strange, A., Ibrahim, S., Coathup, M., Young, A. M., Bozec, L., & Mudera, V. (2016). Demineralization-remineralization dynamics in teeth and bone. *International Journal of Nanomedicine*, *11*, 4743-4763. https://doi.org/10.2147/IJN.S107624 .

452 Akamai. The not so good ingredients found in natural toothpastes. https://www.akamaibasics.com/blogs/learn-more/the-facts-on-ingredients-in-natural-toothpastes .

453 Fluoride Action Network. Health effects. https://fluoridealert.org/issues/health/ .

454 Attin, T., & Hornecker, E. (2005). Tooth brushing and oral health: How frequently and when should tooth brushing be performed? *Oral Health & Preventive Dentistry*, *3*(3), 135-140.

455 Nagel, R. (2011).

456 Danser, M. M., Gomez, S. M., & Van der Weijden, G. A. (2005, November 24). Tongue coating and tongue brushing: A literature review. *International Journal of Dental Hygiene.* https://doi.org/10.1034/j.1601-5037.2003.00034.x .

457 Barnes, C. M., Russell, C. M., Reinhardt, R. A., Payne, J. B., & Lyle, D. M. (2005). Comparison of irrigation to floss as an adjunct to tooth brushing: Effect on bleeding, gingivitis, and supragingival plaque. *The Journal of Clinical Dentistry*, *16*(3), 71-77.

458 Shanbhag, V. K. L. (2017). Oil pulling for maintaining oral hygiene — A review. *Journal of Traditional and Complementary Medicine*, *7*(1), 106-109. ISSN 2225-4110. https://doi.org/10.1016/j.jtcme.2016.05.004 .

459 Asokan, S. A., Rathan, J. A., Muthu, M. S. B., Rathna, Prabhu V. C., Emmadi, P. D., Raghuraman, D., & Chamundeswari, E. (2008, Jan-Mar). Effect of oil pulling on *Streptococcus mutans* count in plaque and saliva using Dentocult SM Strip mutans test: A randomized, controlled, triple-blind study. *Journal of Indian Society of Pedodontics and Preventive Dentistry*, *26*(1), 12-17. https://doi.org/10.4103/0970-4388.40315 .

460 Brookes, Z., Teoh, L., Cieplik, F., & Kumar, P. (2023). Mouthwash effects on the oral microbiome: Are they good, bad, or balanced? *International Dental Journal*, *73 Suppl 2*(Suppl 2), S74-S81. https://doi.org/10.1016/j.identj.2023.08.010 .

461 Ask the Doctors. (2022, August 22). Brushing your tongue could have adverse health effects. *UCLA Health*. https://www.uclahealth.org/news/brushing-your-tongue-could-have-adverse-health-effects .

462 Rathore, M., Singh, A., & Pant, V. A. (2012). The dental amalgam toxicity fear: A myth or actuality. *Toxicology International, 19*(2), 81-88. https://doi.org/10.4103/0971-6580.97191 .

463 Cuthbert, S.C., & Goodheart, G.J. (2007). On the reliability and validity of manual muscle testing: A literature review . *Chiropractic and Manual Therapies, 15*, 4. https://doi.org/10.1186/1746-1340-15-4 .

464 Tinkle, B., Castori, M., Berglund, B., Cohen, H., Grahame, R., Kazkaz, H., & Levy, H. (2017). Hypermobile Ehlers-Danlos Syndrome (a.k.a. Ehlers-Danlos Syndrome Type III and Ehlers-Danlos Syndrome Hypermobility Type): Clinical description and natural history. *American Journal of Medical Genetics. Part C, Seminars in Medical Genetics, 175*(1), 48-69. https://doi.org/10.1002/ajmg.c.31538 .

465 International Association of Facial Growth Guidance. Orthotropics evidence. https://orthotropics.com/ .

466 Mew J. (2007). Facial changes in identical twins treated by different orthodontic techniques. *World Journal of Orthodontics, 8*(2), 174-188.

467 Lee, U. K., Graves, L. L., & Friedlander, A. H. (2019). Mewing: Social media's alternative to orthognathic surgery? *Journal of Oral and Maxillofacial Surgery: Official Journal of the American Association of Oral and Maxillofacial Surgeons, 77*(9), 1743-1744. https://doi.org/10.1016/j.joms.2019.03.024 .

468 Singh, D., Medina, L. E., & Hang, W. M. (2009). Soft tissue facial changes using Biobloc Appliances: Geometric morphometrics. *International Journal of orthodontics (Milwaukee, Wis.), 20*(2), 29-34.

469 Cottrell, M. (2023, September 25). Straight teeth without braces: How craniosacral therapy can bring the mouth and teeth into alignment. https://www.craniosacralgr.com/post/straight-teeth-without-braces-how-craniosacral-therapy-can-bring-the-mouth-and-teeth-into-alignment .

470 Craniosacral Fascial Therapy. CFT supports myofunctional therapy. https://www.craniosacralfascialtherapy.com/myofunctional-therapy .

471 Alghadir, A. H., Zafar, H., & Iqbal, Z. A. (2015). Effect of tongue position on postural stability during quiet standing in healthy young males. *Somatosensory & Motor Research, 32*(3), 183-186. https://doi.org/10.3109/08990220.2015.1043120 .

472 di Vico, R., Ardigò, L. P., Salernitano, G., Chamari, K., & Padulo, J. (2014). The acute effect of the tongue position in the mouth on knee isokinetic test performance: a highly surprising pilot study. *Muscles, Ligaments and Tendons Journal, 3*(4), 318-323.

473 Devasya, A., & Sarpangala, M. (2017). Familial ankyloglossia -A rare report of three cases in a family. *Journal of Clinical and Diagnostic Research : JCDR, 11*(2), ZJ03–ZJ04. https://doi.org/10.7860/JCDR/2017/24035.9308 .

474 Cirino, E. (2021, February 11). Identifying and treating tongue-tie in adults. *Healthline.* https://www.healthline.com/health/dental-and-oral-health/tongue-tie-in-adults#9 .

475 Mills, N., Pransky, S. M., Geddes, D. T., & Mirjalili, S. A. (2019). What is a tongue tie? Defining the anatomy of the in-situ lingual frenulum. *Clinical Anatomy (New York, N.Y.), 32*(6), 749-761. https://doi.org/10.1002/ca.23343 .

476 Correa, E. J., O'Connor-Reina, C., Rodríguez-Alcalá, L., Benjumea, F., Casado-Morente, J. C., Baptista, P. M., Casale, M., Moffa, A., & Plaza, G. (2022). Does frenotomy modify upper airway collapse in adult patients? Case report and systematic review. *Journal of Clinical Medicine, 12*(1), 201. https://doi.org/10.3390/jcm12010201 .

477 Kahn, S., Ehrlich, P., Feldman, M., Sapolsky, R., & Wong, S. (2020, September). The jaw epidemic: Recognition, origins, cures, and prevention. *BioScience*, 70(9), 759-771. https://doi.org/10.1093/biosci/biaa073

478 North American Association of Facial Orthotropics. (2019, July 24). Live a healthier life by taping your mouth shut. https://orthotropics-na.org/live-a-healthier-life-by-taping-your-mouth-shut/ .

479 Kahn, S., Ehrlich, P., Feldman, M., Sapolsky, R., Wong, S. (2020, September).

480 Carboni, L. (2022). Active folate versus folic acid: The role of 5-MTHF (methylfolate) in human health. *Integrative Medicine (Encinitas, Calif.), 21*(3), 36-41. https://www.ncbi.nlm.nih.gov/pmc/articles/PMC9380836/ .

481 Wang, T. J., & Stecco, A. (2021). Fascial thickness and stiffness in hypermobile Ehlers-Danlos Syndrome. *American Journal of Medical Genetics. Part C, Seminars in Medical Genetics, 187*(4), 446-452. https://doi.org/10.1002/ajmg.c.31948 .

482 Liew, S. C., & Gupta, E. D. (2015). Methylenetetrahydrofolate reductase (MTHFR) C677T polymorphism: Epidemiology, metabolism and the associated diseases. *European Journal of Medical Genetics, 58*(1), 1-10. https://doi.org/10.1016/j.ejmg.2014.10.004 .

483 Gualtieri, P., AlWadart, M., De Santis, G. L., Alwadart, N., Della Morte, D., Clarke, C., Best, T., Salimei, C., Bigioni, G., Cianci, R., De Lorenzo, A., & Di Renzo, L. (2023). The role of MTHFR polymorphisms in the risk of lipedema. *European Review for Medical and Pharmacological Sciences, 27*(4), 1625-1632. https://doi.org/10.26355/eurrev_202302_31407 .

484 Sturm, K. (2023, May). Folate-dependent hypermobility: Researchers at Tulane's EDS clinic look into new possible mechanism for hypermobile EDS. *EDS Awareness*. https://www.chronicpainpartners.com/folate-dependent-hypermobility-researchers-at-tulanes-eds-clinic-look-into-new-possible-mechanism-for-hypermobile-eds/ .

485 Hodges, R. E., & Minich, D. M. (2015). Modulation of metabolic detoxification pathways using foods and food-derived components: A scientific review with clinical application. *Journal of Nutrition and Metabolism, 2015*, 760689. https://doi.org/10.1155/2015/760689 .

486 Courseault, J., Kingry, C., Morrison, V., Edstrom, C., Morrell, K., Jaubert, L., Elia, V., & Bix, G. (2023). Folate-dependent hypermobility syndrome: A proposed mechanism and diagnosis. *Heliyon, 9*(4), e15387. https://doi.org/10.1016/j.heliyon.2023.e15387 .

487 Lohkamp, L. N., Marathe, N., & Fehlings, M. G. (2022). Craniocervical instability in Ehlers-Danlos Syndrome — A systematic review of diagnostic and surgical treatment criteria. *Global Spine Journal, 12*(8), 1862-1871. https://doi.org/10.1177/21925682211068520 .

488 Henderson Sr., F. C., Austin, C., Benzel, C., Bolognese, P., Ellenbogen, R., Francomano, C. A., Ireton, C., Klinge, P., Koby, M., Long, D., Patel, S., Singman, E. L., & Voermans, N. C., adapted by Guscott, B. Neurological and spinal manifestations of the Ehlers-Danlos Syndromes (for non-experts). *The Ehlers-Danlos Society.* https://www.ehlers-danlos.com/2017-eds-classification-non-experts/neurological-spinal-manifestations-ehlers-danlos-syndromes/ .

489 Larsen, K. (2017, September 10). Atlas joint instability: Causes, consequences and solutions. *MSK Neurology*. https://mskneurology.com/atlas-joint-instability-causes-consequences-solutions/ .

490 Depta, B. (2016, March 1). *How understanding the tensegrity model can help you prevent injuries and train better* [Video]. Barbara Depta (YouTube). https://www.youtube.com/watch?v=DNyY5DUP1RU .

491 Hargrove, T. (2010, January 17). Why slow movement builds coordination. *Better Movement.* https://www.bettermovement.org/blog/2010/why-practice-slow-movement .

492 Häkkinen, A., Kautiainen, H., Hannonen, P., & Ylinen, J. (2008). Strength Training and stretching versus stretching only in the treatment of patients with chronic neck pain: A randomized one-year follow-up study. *Clinical Rehabilitation, 22*(7), 592-600. https://doi.org/10.1177/0269215507087486

493 Hauser, R. (2023, April 10). *Essential tremor coming from the neck? The connection to cervical dysstructure* [Video]. Caring Medical and Hauser Neck Neck (YouTube). https://www.youtube.com/watch?v=nbSr2ORGXkg .

494 Nakano, J., Yamabayashi, C., Scott, A., & Reid, W. D. (2012). The effect of heat applied with stretch to increase range of motion: A systematic review. *Physical Therapy in Sport, 13*(3), 180-188. https://doi.org/10.1016/j.ptsp.2011.11.003 .

495 Haleem, Z., Philip, J., & Muhammad, S. (2021). Erythema ab igne: A rare presentation of toasted skin syndrome with the use of a space heater. *Cureus, 13*(2), e13401. https://doi.org/10.7759/cureus.13401.

496 Aria, A. B., Chen, L., & Silapunt, S. (2018). Erythema ab igne from heating pad use: A report of three clinical cases and a differential diagnosis. *Cureus, 10*(5), e2635. https://doi.org/10.7759/cureus.2635.

497 Childress, M. A., & Becker, B. A. (2016). Nonoperative management of cervical radiculopathy. *American Family Physician, 93*(9), 746-754.

498 Ylinen, J., Kautiainen, H., Wirén, K., & Häkkinen, A. (2007). Stretching exercises vs manual therapy in treatment of chronic neck pain: A randomized, controlled cross-over trial. *Journal of Rehabilitation Medicine, 39*(2), 126-132. https://doi.org/10.2340/16501977-0015.

499 Zhang, J., Zhang, B., Zhang, J., Lin, W., & Zhang, S. (2021). Magnesium promotes the regeneration of the peripheral nerve. *Frontiers in Cell and Developmental Biology, 9*, 717854. https://doi.org/10.3389/fcell.2021.717854 .

500 Staiger C. (2012). Comfrey: A clinical overview. *Phytotherapy Research : PTR, 26*(10), 1441-1448. https://doi.org/10.1002/ptr.4612 .

501 Glaser, D. L., & Kaplan, F. S. (1997). Osteoporosis: Definition and clinical presentation. *Spine, 22*(24 Suppl), 12S-16S. https://doi.org/10.1097/00007632-199712151-00003.

502 Eller-Vainicher, C., Bassotti, A., Imeraj, A., Cairoli, E., Ulivieri, F. M., Cortini, F., Dubini, M., Marinelli, B., Spada, A., & Chiodini, I. (2016). Bone involvement in adult patients affected with Ehlers-Danlos Syndrome. *Osteoporosis International: A Journal Established as Result Of Cooperation Between the European Foundation for Osteoporosis and the National Osteoporosis Foundation of the USA*, *27*(8), 2525-2531. https://doi.org/10.1007/s00198-016-3562-2 .

503 Tucker, L. A., Strong, J. E., LeCheminant, J. D., & Bailey, B. W. (2015). Effect of two jumping programs on hip bone mineral density in premenopausal women: A randomized controlled trial. *American Journal of Health Promotion: AJHP*, *29*(3), 158-164. https://doi.org/10.4278/ajhp.130430-QUAN-200 .

504 Holubiac, I. Ș., Leuciuc, F. V., Crăciun, D. M., & Dobrescu, T. (2022). Effect of Strength Training protocol on bone mineral density for postmenopausal women with osteopenia/osteoporosis assessed by Dual-Energy X-ray Absorptiometry (DEXA). *Sensors (Basel, Switzerland)*, *22*(5), 1904. https://doi.org/10.3390/s22051904 .

505 Hinton, P. S., Nigh, P., & Thyfault, J. (2015). Effectiveness of resistance training or jumping-exercise to increase bone mineral density in men with low bone mass: A 12-month randomized, clinical trial. *Bone*, *79*, 203-212. https://doi.org/10.1016/j.bone.2015.06.008 .

506 Watson, S. L., Weeks, B. K., Weis, L. J., Harding, A. T., Horan, S. A., & Beck, B. R. (2018), High-intensity resistance and impact training improves bone mineral density and physical function in postmenopausal women with osteopenia and osteoporosis: The LIFTMOR randomized controlled trial. *The Journal of Bone and Mineral Research*, *33*, 211-220. https://doi.org/10.1002/jbmr.3284 .

507 Tucker, L. A., Strong, J. E., LeCheminant, J. D., & Bailey, B. W. (2015). Effect of two jumping programs on hip bone mineral density in premenopausal women: A randomized controlled trial. *American Journal of Health Promotion: AJHP*, *29*(3), 158-164. https://doi.org/10.4278/ajhp.130430-QUAN-200 .

508 Holubiac, I. Ș., Leuciuc, F. V., Crăciun, D. M., & Dobrescu, T. (2022). Effect of Strength Training protocol on bone mineral density for postmenopausal women with osteopenia/osteoporosis assessed by dual-energy X-ray absorptiometry (DEXA). *Sensors (Basel, Switzerland)*, *22*(5), 1904. https://doi.org/10.3390/s22051904 .

509 König, D., Oesser, S., Scharla, S., Zdzieblik, D., & Gollhofer, A. (2018). Specific collagen peptides improve bone mineral density and bone markers in postmenopausal women — A randomized controlled study. *Nutrients*, *10*(1), 97. https://doi.org/10.3390/nu10010097 .

510 König, D., Oesser, S., Scharla, S., Zdzieblik, D., & Gollhofer, A. (2018).

511 Föger-Samwald, U., Dovjak, P., Azizi-Semrad, U., Kerschan-Schindl, K., & Pietschmann, P. (2020). Osteoporosis: Pathophysiology and therapeutic options. *EXCLI Journal*, *19*, 1017-1037. https://doi.org/10.17179/excli2020-2591 .

512 Schaafsma, A., de Vries, P. J. F., & Saris, W. H. M. (2001) Delay of natural bone loss by higher intakes of specific minerals and vitamins. Critical Reviews in Food Science and Nutrition, 41(3), 225-249, https://doi.org/10.1080/20014091091805 .

513 Lee, H. J., Kim, C. O., & Lee, D. C. (2021). Association between daily sunlight exposure and fractures in older Korean adults with osteoporosis: A nationwide population-based cross-sectional study. Yonsei Medical Journal, 62(7), 593-599. https://doi.org/10.3349/ymj.2021.62.7.593 .

514 Föger-Samwald, U., Dovjak, P., Azizi-Semrad, U., Kerschan-Schindl, K., & Pietschmann, P. (2020).

515 Föger-Samwald, U., Dovjak, P., Azizi-Semrad, U., Kerschan-Schindl, K., & Pietschmann, P. (2020).

516 Gazit, Y., Jacob, G., & Grahame, R. (2016). Ehlers-Danlos Syndrome-Hypermobility Type: A much neglected multisystemic disorder. Rambam Maimonides Medical Journal, 7(4), e0034. https://doi.org/10.5041/RMMJ.10261 .

517 Patel, M., & Khullar, V. (2021). Urogynaecology and Ehlers-Danlos Syndrome. American Journal of Medical Genetics: Part C, Seminars in Medical Genetics, 187(4), 579-585. https://doi.org/10.1002/ajmg.c.31959 .

518 Grimes, W. R., & Stratton, M. (2023, June 26). Pelvic floor dysfunction. StatPearls. https://www.ncbi.nlm.nih.gov/books/NBK559246/ .

519 Kenway, M. (2021, July 9). 7 Rectocele REPAIR Rules | Complete Physiotherapy Guide to RECTOCOELE RECOVERY [Video]. Michele Kenway, YouTube. https://www.youtube.com/watch?v=k99g5uUHcck&t=9s .

520 Carley, M. E., & Schaffer, J. (2000). Urinary incontinence and pelvic organ prolapse in women with Marfan or Ehlers Danlos syndrome. American journal of obstetrics and gynecology, 182(5), 1021–1023. https://doi.org/10.1067/mob.2000.105410 .

521 McIntosh, L. J., Stanitski, D. F., Mallett, V. T., Frahm, J. D., Richardson, D. A., & Evans, M. I. (1996). Ehlers-Danlos syndrome: relationship between joint hypermobility, urinary incontinence, and pelvic floor prolapse. Gynecologic and obstetric investigation, 41(2), 135–139. https://doi.org/10.1159/000292060 .

522 Gilliam, E., Hoffman, J. D., & Yeh, G. (2020). Urogenital and pelvic complications in the Ehlers-Danlos syndromes and associated hypermobility spectrum disorders: A scoping review. Clinical genetics, 97(1), 168–178. https://doi.org/10.1111/cge.13624 .

523 Cleveland Clinic. (2022, August 22). Pelvic organ prolapse. https://my.clevelandclinic.org/health/diseases/24046-pelvic-organ-prolapse .

524 Barrell, K. & Smith, A. G. (2019). Peripheral neuropathy. Medical Clinics of North America, 103(2), 383-397. ISSN 0025-7125, ISBN 9780323654715. https://doi.org/10.1016/j.mcna.2018.10.006 .

525 Menorca, R. M., Fussell, T. S., & Elfar, J. C. (2013). Nerve physiology: Mechanisms of injury and recovery. Hand Clinics, 29(3), 317-330. https://doi.org/10.1016/j.hcl.2013.04.002 .

526 Anavara Health and Wellness Facilitators. Axonotmesis. https://anavara.com/treatment/axonotmesis/.

527 Hakim, A. (2004, October 22). Hypermobile Ehlers-Danlos Syndrome. In Adam, M. P., Feldman, J., Mirzaa, G. M., et al. (Eds.), GeneReviews®. Seattle (WA): University of Washington, Seattle; 1993-2024. https://www.ncbi.nlm.nih.gov/books/NBK1279/ .

528 Chaney, B. & Nadi, M. (2023, September 4). Axonotmesis. StatPearls. https://www.ncbi.nlm.nih.gov/books/NBK562304/ .

529 Tohidi, V. How nerves heal after trauma. Orlando Health. https://www.orlandohealth.com/content-hub/how-nerves-recover-after-trauma /

530 Grisold, W., & Carozzi, V. A. (2021). Toxicity in peripheral nerves: An overview. Toxics, 9(9), 218. https://doi.org/10.3390/toxics9090218 .

531 Grisold, W., & Carozzi, V. A. (2021).

532 B10Numb3r5. Length of neuron from base of spine to big toe-longest cell in human body. https://bionumbers.hms.harvard.edu/bionumber.aspx?id=104901 .

533 Shem, K., Wong, J., & Dirlikov, B. (2020). Effective self-stretching of carpal ligament for the treatment of carpal tunnel syndrome: A double-blinded randomized controlled study. *Journal of Hand Therapy: Official Journal of the American Society of Hand Therapists, 33*(3), 272-280. https://doi.org/10.1016/j.jht.2019.12.002 .

534 Hauser, R. & Steilen-Matias, D. R. Brachioradial pruritus — Neuropathic itch. *Caring Medical Florida*. https://caringmedical.com/prolotherapy-news/brachioradial-pruritis-neuropathic-itch-hysterical-itching/ .

535 Pinto, A. C., Wachholz, P. A., Masuda, P. Y., & Martelli, A. C. (2016). Clinical, epidemiological and therapeutic profile of patients with brachioradial pruritus in a reference service in dermatology. *Anais Brasileiros de Dermatologia, 91*(4), 549-51. https://doi.org/10.1590/abd1806-4841.201644767 .

536 Burstein, R., Blake, P., Schain, A., & Perry, C. (2017). Extracranial origin of headache. *Current Opinion in Neurology, 30*(3), 263-271. https://doi.org/10.1097/WCO.0000000000000437 .

537 Pan, W., Peng, J., & Elmofty, D. (2021). Occipital neuralgia. *Current Pain and Headache Reports, 25*(9), 61. https://doi.org/10.1007/s11916-021-00972-1 .

538 Henssen, D. J. H. A., Derks, B., van Doorn, M., Verhoogt, N., Van Cappellen van Walsum, A. M., Staats, P., & Vissers, K. (2019). Vagus nerve stimulation for primary headache disorders: An anatomical review to explain a clinical phenomenon. *Cephalalgia : An International Journal of Headache, 39*(9), 1180-1194. https://doi.org/10.1177/0333102419833076 .

539 Huff, T., Weisbrod, L. J. & Daly, D. T. (2022, November 9). Neuroanatomy, cranial nerve 5 (trigeminal). *StatPearls*. https://www.ncbi.nlm.nih.gov/books/NBK482283/ .

540 Oaklander, A. L. (2011). Neuropathic itch. *Seminars in Cutaneous Medicine And Surgery, 30*(2), 87-92. https://doi.org/10.1016/j.sder.2011.04.006 .

541 Yu, M. & Wang, S. M. (2022, October 31). Anatomy, head and neck, occipital nerves. *StatPearls*. https://www.ncbi.nlm.nih.gov/books/NBK542213/ .

542 Anavara Health and Wellness Facilitators. Axonotmesis. https://anavara.com/treatment/axonotmesis/

543 Chaney, B. & Nadi, M. (2023, September 4). Axonotmesis. *StatPearls*. https://www.ncbi.nlm.nih.gov/books/NBK562304/ .

544 Precision Physical Therapy. (2024, April 30). To stretch or not to stretch?: Muscle vs. nerve pain, identifying the difference. https://www.precisionstl.com/blog/2021/4-30-nervepain.

545 Thomas, E., Bellafiore, M., Petrigna, L., Paoli, A., Palma, A., & Bianco, A. (2021). Peripheral nerve responses to muscle stretching: A systematic review. *Journal of Sports Science & Medicine*, *20*(2), 258-267. https://doi.org/10.52082/jssm.2021.258 .

546 Genetic Disease Investigators, LLC. (2016, January). Correcting the missing piece in chronic fatigue syndrome — Part 1. *Discovery Genetic Disease Investigators*. https://vagusnervesupport.com/wp-content/uploads/2017/11/Chronic-Disease-Digest-Text-Correcting-the-Missing-Piece-in-Chronic-Fatigue-Syndrome.pdf .

547 Cronkleton, E. (2023, August 23). 6 best supplements for neuropathy. *Healthline*. https://www.healthline.com/health/neuropathy-supplements#b-vitamins .

548 Geller, M., Oliveira, L., Nigri, R., Mezitis, S. G. E., Ribeiro, M. G., de Souza da Fonseca, A., Guimarães, O. R., Kaufman. R., & Wajnsztajn, F. (2017). B vitamins for neuropathy and neuropathic pain. *Vitamins and Minerals, 6(*2). https://www.omicsonline.org/open-access/b-vitamins-for-neuropathy-and-neuropathic-pain-2376-1318-1000161.php?aid=90896 .

549 Geller M, et al. (2017).

550 Ajmera, R. (2024, March 18). 15 foods high in folate (folic acid). *Healthline*. https://www.healthline.com/nutrition/foods-high-in-folate-folic-acid#1.-Legumes .

551 Tohidi, V. How nerves heal after trauma. *Orlando Health*. https://www.orlandohealth.com/content-hub/how-nerves-recover-after-trauma /

552 Zhang, J., Zhang, B., Zhang, J., Lin, W., & Zhang, S. (2021). Magnesium promotes the regeneration of the peripheral nerve. *Frontiers in Cell and Developmental Biology, 9*, 717854. https://doi.org/10.3389/fcell.2021.717854 .

553 Forouzanfar, F. & Hosseinzadeh, H. (2018). Medicinal herbs in the treatment of neuropathic pain: A review. *Iranian Journal of Basic Medical Sciences*, *21*(4), 347-358. https://doi.org/10.22038/IJBMS.2018.24026.6021 .

554 Modern Neuropathy. (2019, April 18). 6 powerhouse herbs for nerve damage regeneration. https://modernneuropathy.com/6-powerhouse-herbs-for-nerve-damage/ .

555 Jeon, Y., Kim, C.-E., Jung, D., Kwak, K., Park, S., Lim, D., Kim, S., Baek, W. (2013). Curcumin could prevent the development of chronic neuropathic pain in rats with peripheral nerve injury. *Current Therapeutic Research, 74*, 1-4. ISSN 0011-393X. https://doi.org/10.1016/j.curtheres.2012.10.001 .

556 Jeon, Y., Kim, C.-E., Jung, D., Kwak, K., Park, S., Lim, D., Kim, S., Baek, W. (2013).

557 Babu A, et al. (2014). *Effect of curcumin in mice model of vincristine-induced neuropathy*. https://www.tandfonline.com/doi/full/10.3109/13880209.2014.943247 .

558 Cameron, N. E., Cotter, M. A., Dines, K. C., Robertson, S., & Cox, D. (1993). The effects of evening primrose oil on nerve function and capillarization in streptozotocin-diabetic rats: Modulation by the cyclo-oxygenase inhibitor flurbiprofen. *British Journal of Pharmacology*, *109*(4), 972-979. https://doi.org/10.1111/j.1476-5381.1993.tb13716.x .

559 Ramli, D., Aziz, I. Mohamad, M., Abdulahi, D., & Sanusi, J. (2017, May 23). The changes in rats with sciatic nerve crush injury supplemented with evening primrose oil: Behavioural, morphologic, and morphometric analysis. *Hindawi*. https://doi.org/10.1155/2017/3476407 .

560 Precision Physical Therapy. (2024, April 30). To stretch or not to stretch?: Muscle vs. nerve - pain, identifying the difference. https://www.precisionstl.com/blog/2021/4-30-nervepain .

561 Oaklander, A. L. (2011). Neuropathic itch. *Seminars in Cutaneous Medicine And Surgery, 30*(2), 87-92. https://doi.org/10.1016/j.sder.2011.04.006 .

562 Cameron, N. E., Cotter, M. A., Dines, K. C., Robertson, S., & Cox, D. (1993). The effects of evening primrose oil on nerve function and capillarization in streptozotocin-diabetic rats: Modulation by the cyclo-oxygenase inhibitor flurbiprofen. *British Journal of Pharmacology*, *109*(4), 972-979. https://doi.org/10.1111/j.1476-5381.1993.tb13716.x .

563 Ramli, D., Aziz, I. Mohamad, M., Abdulahi, D., & Sanusi, J. (2017, May 23). The changes in rats with sciatic nerve crush injury supplemented with evening primrose oil: Behavioural, morphologic, and morphometric analysis. *Hindawi*. https://doi.org/10.1155/2017/3476407 .

564 Pavlov, V. A., Wang, H., Czura, C. J., Friedman, S. G., & Tracey, K. J. (2003). The cholinergic anti-inflammatory pathway: A missing link in neuroimmunomodulation. *Molecular Medicine (Cambridge, Mass.)*, *9*(5-8), 125-134.

565 Genetic Disease Investigators, LLC. (2016, January). Correcting the missing piece in chronic fatigue syndrome — Part 1. *Discovery Genetic Disease Investigators.* https://vagusnervesupport.com/wp-content/uploads/2017/11/Chronic-Disease-Digest-Text-Correcting-the-Missing-Piece-in-Chronic-Fatigue-Syndrome.pdf .

566 Wang, Z. R., & Ni, G. X. (2021). Is it time to put traditional cold therapy in rehabilitation of soft-tissue injuries out to pasture? *World Journal of Clinical Cases, 9*(17), 4116-4122. https://doi.org/10.12998/wjcc.v9.i17.4116 .

567 Nakano, J., Yamabayashi, C., Scott, A., & Reid, W. D. (2012). The effect of heat applied with stretch to increase range of motion: A systematic review. *Physical Therapy in Sport,* 13(3), 180-188. https://doi.org/10.1016/j.ptsp.2011.11.003 .

568 Salehi, B., Mishra, A. P., Nigam, M., Sener, B., Kilic, M., Sharifi-Rad, M., Fokou, P. V. T., Martins, N., & Sharifi-Rad, J. (2018). Resveratrol: A double-edged sword in health benefits. *Biomedicines, 6*(3), 91. https://doi.org/10.3390/biomedicines6030091

569 Candelario-Jalil, E., de Oliveira, A.C.P., Gräf, S. *et al.* (2007). Resveratrol potently reduces prostaglandin E2production and free radical formation in lipopolysaccharide-activated primary rat microglia. *J Neuroinflammation 4*, 25. https://doi.org/10.1186/1742-2094-4-25 .

570 Modern Neuropathy. (2019, April 18). 6 powerhouse herbs for nerve damage regeneration. https://modernneuropathy.com/6-powerhouse-herbs-for-nerve-damage/ .

571 Jeon, Y., Kim, C.-E., Jung, D., Kwak, K., Park, S., Lim, D., Kim, S., Baek, W. (2013). Curcumin could prevent the development of chronic neuropathic pain in rats with peripheral nerve injury. *Current Therapeutic Research, 74*, 1-4. ISSN 0011-393X. https://doi.org/10.1016/j.curtheres.2012.10.001 .

572 Jeon, Y., Kim, C.-E., Jung, D., Kwak, K., Park, S., Lim, D., Kim, S., Baek, W. (2013).

573 Babu A, et al. (2014). *Effect of curcumin in mice model of vincristine-induced neuropathy.* https://www.tandfonline.com/doi/full/10.3109/13880209.2014.943247 .

574 Chaney, B. & Nadi, M. (2023, September 4). Axonotmesis. *StatPearls.* https://www.ncbi.nlm.nih.gov/books/NBK562304/ .

575 Grisold, W., & Carozzi, V. A. (2021). Toxicity in peripheral nerves: An overview. *Toxics, 9*(9), 218. https://doi.org/10.3390/toxics9090218 .

576 Standing Up to POTS. Ehlers-Danlos Syndrome: Common POTS comorbidity. https://www.standinguptopots.org/EDS .

577 Nwazue, V. C., & Raj, S. R. (2013). Confounders of vasovagal syncope: Orthostatic hypotension. *Cardiology Clinics, 31*(1), 89-100. https://doi.org/10.1016/j.ccl.2012.09.003 .

578 Fu, Q., VanGundy, T. B., Shibata, S., Auchus, R. J., Williams, G. H., & Levine, B. D. (2010). Menstrual cycle affects renal-adrenal and hemodynamic responses during prolonged standing in the postural orthostatic tachycardia syndrome. Hypertension (Dallas, Tex.: 1979), 56(1), 82-90. https://doi.org/10.1161/HYPERTENSIONAHA.110.151787 .

579 Weitzel, L. (2019, July 9). *Heads UP - Episode 22: POTS and migraine disease* [Video]. National Headache Foundation (YouTube). https://www.youtube.com/watch?v=Lf_3rD7BtR4 .

580 Olshansky, B., Cannom, D., Fedorowski, A., Stewart, J., Gibbons, C., Sutton, R., Shen, W. K., Muldowney, J., Chung, T. H., Feigofsky, S., Nayak, H., Calkins, H., & Benditt, D. G. (2020). Postural orthostatic tachycardia syndrome (POTS): A critical assessment. *Progress in Cardiovascular Diseases, 63*(3), 263-270. https://doi.org/10.1016/j.pcad.2020.03.010 .

581 Szmuilowicz, E. D., Adler, G. K., Williams, J. S., Green, D. E., Yao, T. M., Hopkins, P. N., & Seely, E. W. (2006). Relationship between aldosterone and progesterone in the human menstrual cycle. *The Journal of Clinical Endocrinology and Metabolism, 91*(10), 3981-3987. https://doi.org/10.1210/jc.2006-1154 .

582 Fu, Q., VanGundy, T. B., Shibata, S., Auchus, R. J., Williams, G. H., & Levine, B. D. (2010). Menstrual cycle affects renal-adrenal and hemodynamic responses during prolonged standing in the postural orthostatic tachycardia syndrome. *Hypertension (Dallas, Tex.: 1979), 56*(1), 82-90. https://doi.org/10.1161/HYPERTENSIONAHA.110.151787 .

583 Katayama, K., & Saito, M. (2019). Muscle sympathetic nerve activity during exercise. *The Journal of Physiological Sciences : JPS, 69*(4), 589-598. https://doi.org/10.1007/s12576-019-00669-6 .

584 Johns Hopkins Medicine. Postural Orthostatic Tachycardia Syndrome (POTS). https://www.hopkinsmedicine.org/health/conditions-and-diseases/postural-orthostatic-tachycardia-syndrome-pots .

585 Fu, Q., VanGundy, T. B., Shibata, S., Auchus, R. J., Williams, G. H., & Levine, B. D. (2010).

586 Hall, J., Bourne, K. M., Sheldon, R. S., Vernino, S., Raj, V., Ng, J., Okamoto, L. E., Arnold, A. C., Bryarly, M., Phillips, L., Paranjape, S. Y., & Raj, S. R. (2021). A comparison of health-related quality of life in autonomic disorders: Postural tachycardia syndrome versus vasovagal syncope. *Clinical Autonomic Research : Official Journal of the Clinical Autonomic Research Society*, *31*(3), 433-441. https://doi.org/10.1007/s10286-021-00781-x .

587 Nwazue, V. C. & Raj, S. R. (2013). Confounders of vasovagal syncope: Orthostatic hypotension. *Cardiology Clinics*, *31*(1), 89-100. https://doi.org/10.1016/j.ccl.2012.09.003 .

588 Katayama, K., & Saito, M. (2019). Muscle sympathetic nerve activity during exercise. *The Journal of Physiological Sciences : JPS*, *69*(4), 589-598. https://doi.org/10.1007/s12576-019-00669-6 .

589 Katayama, K., & Saito, M. (2019).

590 Standing Up To POTS. Managing POTS symptoms: Lifestyle modifications that can decrease symptom load. https://www.standinguptopots.org/livingwithpots/pots-tricks .

591 I noticed that cimbing stairs or hills was once of my worst triggers for POTS, especially if I was climbing the stairs while holding a full laundry basket. Going slowly, keeping my posture straight, and not carrying heavy things has solved the problem for me. I have seen other people comment about difficulty with stairs and hills, but I have not found an article that addresses this problem. There may be other triggers that you experience that are not addressed here, so pay attention to what brings your symptoms on, remembering that it can take up to 10 minutes for the symptoms to become noticeable.

592Katayama, K., & Saito, M. (2019).

593 Katayama, K., & Saito, M. (2019).

594 Standing Up To POTS. Managing POTS symptoms: Lifestyle modifications that can decrease symptom load.

595 Johns Hopkins Medicine. Postural orthostatic tachycardia syndrome (POTS). https://www.hopkinsmedicine.org/health/conditions-and-diseases/postural-orthostatic-tachycardia-syndrome-pots

596 Katayama, K., & Saito, M. (2019).

597 Katayama, K., & Saito, M. (2019).

598 Tiwari, R., Kumar, R., Malik, S., Raj, T., & Kumar, P. (2021). Analysis of heart rate variability and implication of different factors on heart rate variability. *Current Cardiology Reviews*, *17*(5), e160721189770. https://doi.org/10.2174/1573403X16999201231203854 .

599 Katayama, K., & Saito, M. (2019).

600 Chaitow, L. & DeLany, J. (2011). Chapter 14 - The leg and foot. In Chaitow, L. & DeLany, J. (Eds.), *Clinical Application of Neuromuscular Techniques, Volume 2 (Second Edition),* Churchill Livingstone, 503-577. https://doi.org/10.1016/B978-0-443-06815-7.00014-0 .

601 Herman, H. (2017, November 21). Knee hyperextension: It's all in your mind! *Ellie Herman Pilates.* https://www.elliehermanpilates.com/ellies-blog/2017/11/20/how-to-help-hyperextension-its-all-in-your-mind .

602 Katayama, K., & Saito, M. (2019).

603 Katayama, K., & Saito, M. (2019).

604 Abed, H., Ball, P. A., & Wang, L. X. (2012). Diagnosis and management of postural orthostatic tachycardia syndrome: A brief review. *Journal of Geriatric Cardiology : JGC,* *9*(1), 61-67. https://doi.org/10.3724/SP.J.1263.2012.00061 .

605 Shepherd, J. T., Rusch, N. J., & Vanhoutte, P. M. (1983). Effect of cold on the blood vessel wall. *General Pharmacology*, *14*(1), 61-64. https://doi.org/10.1016/0306-3623(83)90064-2.

606 Johns Hopkins Medicine. Postural orthostatic tachycardia syndrome (POTS). https://www.hopkinsmedicine.org/health/conditions-and-diseases/postural-orthostatic-tachycardia-syndrome-pots

607 Cleveland Clinic. (2022, June 9). Valsalva maneuver. https://my.clevelandclinic.org/health/treatments/23209-valsalva-maneuver .

608 Foster, A. Hypermobility rib subluxation: A practical guide. *The Fibro Guy.* https://www.thefibroguy.com/blog/hypermobility-rib-subluxation/ .

609 Costochondritis.com. (2019, November 28). Costochondritis and Elhers-Danlos Syndrome. https://Costochondritis.com/Costochondritis-and-ehlers-danlos-syndrome/ .

610 Slipping Rib Syndrome.org. (2024). What are the symptoms of slipping rib syndrome? https://www.slippingribsyndrome.org/symptoms-of-srs .

611 Ayloo, A., Cvengros, T. & Marella, S. (2013). Evaluation and treatment of musculoskeletal chest pain. *Primary Care, 40*(4), 863-viii. https://doi.org/10.1016/j.pop.2013.08.007 .

612 Hamilton, A. Slipping rib syndrome: A pain in the upper back. *Sports Performance Bulletin.* https://www.sportsperformancebulletin.com/injuries-health/endurance-injuries-and-health/slipping-rib-syndrome-a-pain-in-the-upper-back .

613 van den Hoorn, W., Bruijn, S. M., Meijer, O. G., Hodges, P. W., & van Dieën, J. H. (2012). Mechanical coupling between transverse plane pelvis and thorax rotations during gait is higher in people with low back pain. *Journal of Biomechanics, 45*(2), 342-347. https://doi.org/10.1016/j.jbiomech.2011.10.024 .

614 Nakano, J., Yamabayashi, C., Scott, A., & Reid, W. D. (2012). The effect of heat applied with stretch to increase range of motion: A systematic review. *Physical Therapy in Sport, 13*(3), 180-188. https://doi.org/10.1016/j.ptsp.2011.11.003 .

615 Higuera, V. (2019, September 23). Heating pads for back pain: Benefits and best practices. *Healthline.* https://www.healthline.com/health/heating-pad-for-back-pain .

616 Bervoets, D. C., Luijsterburg, P. A., Alessie, J. J., Buijs, M. J., & Verhagen, A. P. (2015). Massage therapy has short-term benefits for people with common musculoskeletal disorders compared to no treatment: A systematic review. *Journal of Physiotherapy, 61*(3), 106-116. https://doi.org/10.1016/j.jphys.2015.05.018 .

617 English, N., & McLean, S. (2023, August 7). The 7 best serratus exercises for chiseled abs and shoulder stability. Bar Bend. https://barbend.com/serratus-exercises/ .

618 Staiger, C. (2012). Comfrey: A clinical overview. *Phytotherapy Research : PTR, 26*(10), 1441-1448. https://doi.org/10.1002/ptr.4612 .

619 Yen, J. L., Lin, S. P., Chen, M. R., & Niu, D. M. (2006). Clinical features of Ehlers-Danlos Syndrome. *Journal of the Formosan Medical Association, Taiwan yi zhi, 105*(6), 475-480. https://doi.org/10.1016/S0929-6646(09)60187-X .

620 Myers, A. Are swimming pools sabotaging your thyroid? *Amy Myers MD.* https://www.amymyersmd.com/article/swimming-pools-thyroid .

621 Lin, T. K., Zhong, L., & Santiago, J. L. (2017). Anti-inflammatory and skin barrier repair effects of topical application of some plant oils. *International Journal of Molecular Sciences, 19*(1), 70. https://doi.org/10.3390/ijms19010070 .

622 Edimo, C. O., Wajsberg, J. R., Wong, S., Nahmias, Z. P., & Riley, B. A. (2021). The dermatological aspects of hEDS in women. *International Journal of Women's Dermatology, 7*(3), 285-289. https://doi.org/10.1016/j.ijwd.2021.01.020 .

623 Caporuscio, J. (2020, April 30). Can you use epson salts for acne? *Medical News Today.* https://www.medicalnewstoday.com/articles/epsom-salt-for-acne .

624 Edimo, C. O., Wajsberg, J. R., Wong, S., Nahmias, Z. P., & Riley, B. A. (2021).

625 Murad, H. Eat Your Watermelon! *Howard Murad MD.* https://drhowardmurad.com/eat-your-watermelon/ .

626 Broida, S. E., Sweeney, A. P., Gottschalk, M. B., & Wagner, E. R. (2021). Management of shoulder instability in hypermobility-type Ehlers-Danlos Syndrome, *JSES Reviews, Reports, and Techniques, 1*(3), 155-164, ISSN 2666-6391. https://doi.org/10.1016/j.xrrt.2021.03.002 .

627 Stanford Medecine. Scapular dyskinesis. https://stanfordhealthcare.org/medical-conditions/bones-joints-and-muscles/scapular-dyskinesis.html .

628 Wang, Z. R., & Ni, G. X. (2021). Is it time to put traditional cold therapy in rehabilitation of soft-tissue injuries out to pasture? *World Journal of Clinical Cases, 9*(17), 4116-4122. https://doi.org/10.12998/wjcc.v9.i17.4116 .

629 Nakano, J., Yamabayashi, C., Scott, A., & Reid, W. D. (2012). The effect of heat applied with stretch to increase range of motion: A systematic review. *Physical Therapy in Sport, 13*(3), 180-188. https://doi.org/10.1016/j.ptsp.2011.11.003 .

630 Although it is documented that hEDS causes weakness in mucous membranes, I actually was not able to find documentation of hEDS patients having more frequent or more severe sinusitis conditions. My family does not suffer from this problem, though I have known hypermobile people who have persistent, chronic sinus infections.

631 Cunningham, S. (2023, December 6). The power of peppermint. *UC Health.* https://www.uchealth.org/today/the-power-of-peppermint/ .

632 Laccourreye, O., Werner, A., Giroud, J.-P., Couloigner, V., Bonfils, P., & Bondon-Guitton, E. (2015). Benefits, limits and danger of ephedrine and pseudoephedrine as nasal decongestants. *European Annals of Otorhinolaryngology, Head and Neck Diseases, 132*(1), 31-34. ISSN 1879-7296. https://doi.org/10.1016/j.anorl.2014.11.001 .

633 National Center for Complementary and Integrative Health. (2020, July). Ephedra. https://www.nccih.nih.gov/health/ephedra .

634 National Center for Complementary and Integrative Health. (2020, July).

635 Panther, E. J., Reintgen, C. D., Cueto, R. J., Hao, K. A., Chim, H., & King, J. J. (2022). Thoracic outlet syndrome: A review. *Journal of Shoulder and Elbow Surgery, 31*(11), e545-e561. https://doi.org/10.1016/j.jse.2022.06.026 .

636 Larsen, K., Galluccio, F. C., & Chand, S. K. (2019, February 27). Does thoracic outlet syndrome cause cerebrovascular hyperperfusion? Diagnostic markers for occult craniovascular congestion. *Anaesthesia, Pain & Intensive Care.* https://www.academia.edu/43278645/Does_thoracic_outlet_syndrome_cause_cerebrovascular_hyperperfusion_Diagnostic_markers_for_occult_craniovascular_congestion .

637 Lim, C., Kavousi, Y., Lum, Y. W., & Christo, P. J. (2021). Evaluation and management of neurogenic thoracic outlet syndrome with an overview of surgical approaches: A comprehensive review. *Journal of Pain Research, 14*, 3085-3095. https://doi.org/10.2147/JPR.S282578 .

638 The TMJ Association. What is TMJ? https://tmj.org/living-with-tmj/basics/ .

639 Yap, A. U., Qiu, L. Y., Natu, V. P., & Wong, M. C. (2020). Functional, physical and psychosocial impact of temporomandibular Disorders in adolescents and young adults. *Medicina Oral, Patologia Oral y Cirugia Bucal, 25*(2), e188–e194. https://doi.org/10.4317/medoral.23298 .

640 Diep, D., Fau, V., Wdowik, S., Bienvenu, B., Bénateau, H., & Veyssière, A. (2016). Dysfonction de l'appareil manducateur et syndrome d'Ehlers-Danlos de type hypermobile : Etude cas-témoin [Temporomandibular disorders and Ehlers-Danlos Syndrome, hypermobility type: A case-control study]. *Revue de Stomatologie, de Chirurgie Maxillo-Faciale et de Chirurgie Orale, 117*(4), 228-233. https://doi.org/10.1016/j.revsto.2016.07.009 .

641 Goldstein, L. & Makofsky, H. (2009). Deep cervical muscle dysfunction and head/neck/face pain — Part 1. *Practical Pain Management, 9*(1).

642 Tabrizi, R., Shourmaej, Y., Pourdanesh, F., Shafiei, S., & Moslemi, H. (2024). Does lifestyle modification (physical exercise and listening to music) improve symptoms in patients with a temporomandibular disorder? A randomized clinical trial. *National Journal of Maxillofacial Surgery, 15*(1), 55-58. https://doi.org/10.4103/njms.njms_23_23 ,

643 Halverson, C. M. E., Cao, S., Perkins, S. M., & Francomano, C. A. (2003). Comorbidity, misdiagnoses, and the diagnostic odyssey in patients with Hypermobile Ehlers-Danlos Syndrome. *Genetics in Medicine Open 1*(1). https://doi.org/10.1016/j.gimo.2023.100812 .

644 Fibromyalgia Care Society of America. What is fibromyalgia? https://www.fibro.org/what-is-fibromyalgia .

645 Fairweather, D., Bruno, K. A., Darakjian, A. A., Bruce, B. K., Gehin, J. M., Kotha, A., Jain, A., Peng, Z., Hodge, D. O., Rozen, T. D., Munipalli, B., Rivera, F. A., Malavet, P. A., & Knight, D. R. T. (2023). High overlap in patients diagnosed with Hypermobile Ehlers-Danlos Syndrome or Hypermobile Spectrum Disorders with fibromyalgia and 40 self-reported symptoms and comorbidities. *Frontiers in Medicine, 10*, 1096180. https://doi.org/10.3389/fmed.2023.1096180 .

646 Eccles, J. A., Thompson, B., Themelis, K., Amato, M. L., Stocks, R., Pound, A., Jones, A. M., Cipinova, Z., Shah-Goodwin, L., Timeyin, J., Thompson, C. R., Batty, T., Harrison, N. A., Critchley, H. D., & Davies, K. A. (2021). Beyond bones: The relevance of variants of connective tissue (hypermobility) to fibromyalgia, ME/CFS and controversies surrounding diagnostic classification: an observational study. *Clinical Medicine (London, England), 21*(1), 53-58. https://doi.org/10.7861/clinmed.2020-0743 .

647 Action for ME. What is ME? https://www.actionforme.org.uk/get-information/what-is-me/what-does-me-feel-like/ .

648 Wells, D. (2023, May 26). Blood test for fibromyalgia: What you need to know. *Healthline.* https://www.healthline.com/health/fibromyalgia/blood-test .

649 Bulbena, A., Baeza-Velasco, C., Bulbena-Cabre, A., Pailhez, G., Critchley, H., Chopra, P., Mallorquı-Bague, N., Frank, C., & Porges, S. (2017). Psychiatric and psychological aspects in the Ehlers-Danlos Syndromes. *American Journal of Medical Genetics Part C Seminar on Medical Genetics, 175C*, 237-245. https://doi.org/10.1002/ajmg.c.31544 .

650 Bulbena-Cabré, A., Baeza-Velasco, C., Rosado-Figuerola, S., & Bulbena, A. (2021, November 9). Updates on the psychological and psychiatric aspects of the Ehlers-Danlos Syndromes and Hypermobility Spectrum Disorders. *American Journal of Medical Genetics*. https://doi.org/10.1002/ajmg.c.31955 .

651 Bulbena A, Baeza-Velasco C, Bulbena-Cabre A, Pailhez G, Critchley H, Chopra P, Mallorqui-Bague N, Frank C, Porges S. (2017).

652 Bulbena-Cabré, A., Baeza-Velasco, C., Rosado-Figuerola, S., & Bulbena, A. (2021, November 9).

653 Bulbena, A. (2022) *Anxiety: A quick immersion.* Tibidabo Publishing, Inc.

654 Bulbena, A., Baeza-Velasco, C., Bulbena-Cabre, A., Pailhez, G., Critchley, H., Chopra, P., Mallorqui-Bague, N., Frank, C., & Porges, S. (2017).

655 Casanova, E. L., Baeza-Velasco, C., Buchanan, C. B., & Casanova, M. F. (2020). The Relationship between autism and Ehlers-Danlos Syndromes/Hypermobility Spectrum Disorders. *Journal of Personalized Medicine, 10*(4), 260. https://doi.org/10.3390/jpm10040260 .

656 Bulbena-Cabré, A., Baeza-Velasco, C., Rosado-Figuerola, S., & Bulbena, A. (2021, November 9).

657 Bulbena-Cabré, A., Baeza-Velasco, C., Rosado-Figuerola, S., & Bulbena, A. (2021, November 9).

658 Espiridion, E. D., Daniel, A., & Van Allen, J. R. (2018). recurrent depression and borderline personality disorder in a patient with Ehlers-Danlos Syndrome. *Cureus, 10*(12), e3760. https://doi.org/10.7759/cureus.3760 .

659 Bulbena-Cabré, A., Baeza-Velasco, C., Rosado-Figuerola, S., & Bulbena, A. (2021, November 9).

660 National Institute of Neurological Disorders and Stroke. Multiple sclerosis. https://www.ninds.nih.gov/health-information/disorders/multiple-sclerosis .

661 Vilisaar, J., Harikrishnan, S., Suri, M., & Constantinescu, C. S. (2008). Ehlers-Danlos Syndrome and multiple sclerosis: A possible association. *Multiple Sclerosis (Houndmills, Basingstoke, England), 14*(4), 567-570. https://doi.org/10.1177/1352458507083187

662 Kidd, B. L., Moore, K., Walters, M. T., Smith, J. L., & Cawley, M. I. (1989). Immunohistological features of synovitis in ankylosing spondylitis: A comparison with rheumatoid arthritis. *Annals of the Rheumatic Diseases, 48*(2), 92-98. https://doi.org/10.1136/ard.48.2.92 .

663 Smith, M. D. (2011). The normal synovium. *The Open Rheumatology Journal, 5*, 100-106. https://doi.org/10.2174/1874312901105010100 .

664 Arthritis Foundation. Rheumatoid arthritis: Causes, symptoms, treatments and more. https://www.arthritis.org/diseases/rheumatoid-arthritis .

665 National Institute of Arthritis and Musculoskeletal and Skin Diseases. Rheumatoid arthritis: Diagnosis, treatment, and steps to take. https://www.niams.nih.gov/health-topics/rheumatoid-arthritis/diagnosis-treatment-and-steps-to-take .

666 Arthritis Foundation. Ankylosing spondylitis & nonradiographic axial spondyloarthritis. https://www.arthritis.org/diseases/ankylosing-spondylitis .

667 Arthritis Foundation. Rheumatoid arthritis: Causes, symptoms, treatments and more.

668 Rheumatoid Arthritis Foundation. Rheumatoid arthritis FAQ. https://www.helpfightra.org/rheumatoid-arthritis-faqs/ .

669 Makol, A. K., Chakravorty, Heller, M. B., & Riley, B. (2021). The association between Hypermobility Ehlers-Danlos Syndrome and other rheumatologic diseases. *EMJ.* https://doi.org/10.33590/emj/21-00078R2 .

670 Baeza-Velasco, C., Cohen, D., Hamonet, C., Vlamynck, E., Diaz, L., Cravero, C., Cappe, E., & Guinchat, V. (2018). Autism, joint hypermobility-related disorders and pain. *Frontiers in Psychiatry, 9*, 656. https://doi.org/10.3389/fpsyt.2018.00656 .

671 Casanova, E. L., Baeza-Velasco, C., Buchanan, C. B., & Casanova, M. F. (2020). The relationship between autism and Ehlers-Danlos Syndromes/Hypermobility Spectrum Disorders. *Journal of Personalized Medicine, 10*(4), 260. https://doi.org/10.3390/jpm10040260

672 Bulbena-Cabré, A., Baeza-Velasco, C., Rosado-Figuerola, S., & Bulbena, A. (2021, November 9). Updates on the psychological and psychiatric aspects of the Ehlers-Danlos Syndromes and Hypermobility Spectrum Disorders. *American Journal of Medical Genetics*. https://doi.org/10.1002/ajmg.c.31955 .

673 Zhang, P., Omanska, A., Ander, B. P., Gandal, M. J., Stamova, B., & Schumann, C. M. (2023). Neuron-specific transcriptomic signatures indicate neuroinflammation and altered neuronal activity in ASD temporal cortex. *Proceedings of the National Academy of Sciences, e2206758120*(120), 10. https://doi.org/10.1073/pnas.2206758120 .

674 Moore J. W. (2016). What is the sense of agency and why does it matter? *Frontiers in Psychology*, *7*, 1272. https://doi.org/10.3389/fpsyg.2016.01272 .

675 The Pulse. 5 surprising benefits of abhyanga. https://mapi.com/blogs/articles/5-surprising-benefits-of-abhyanga .

676 Basler, A. J. (2011). Pilot study investigating the effects of Ayurvedic Abhyanga massage on subjective stress experience. *Journal of Alternative and Complementary Medicine, (New York, N.Y.)*, *17*(5), 435-440. https://doi.org/10.1089/acm.2010.0281 .

677 Cohen, G. L., & Shermal, D. K. (2014). The psychology of change: Self-affirmation and social psychological intervention. *The Annual Review of Psychology*, *65*, 333-71. https://doi.org/10.1146/annurev-psych-010213-115137 . https://ed.stanford.edu/sites/default/files/annurev-psych-psychology_of_change_final_e2.pdf.

678 Cohen, G. L. & Shermal, D. K. (2014).

679 Moore J. W. (2016). what is the sense of agency and why does it matter? *Frontiers in Psychology*, *7*, 1272. https://doi.org/10.3389/fpsyg.2016.01272 .

680 Liu, L. Y., Chen, X. D., Wu, B. Y., & Jiang, Q. (2010). Influence of aloe polysaccharide on proliferation and hyaluronic acid and hydroxyproline secretion of human fibroblasts in vitro. *Journal of Chinese Integrative Medicine*, *8*(3), 256-262. https://doi.org/10.3736/jcim20100310 . https://pubmed.ncbi.nlm.nih.gov/20226148/ .

681 Chen, X. D., Wu, B. Y., Jiang, Q., Wang, S. B., Huang, L. Y., & Wang, Z. C. (2005). Influence of polysaccharide from aloe vera on the proliferation of the human epithelial cells cultured in vitro. *Journal Of Burns*, *21*(6), 430-433.

682 Natsch, A. (2015). What makes us smell: The biochemistry of body odour and the design of new deodorant ingredients. *Chimia*, *69*(7-8), 414-420. https://doi.org/10.2533/chimia.2015.414 .

683 Baker, L. B. (2019). Physiology of sweat gland function: The roles of sweating and sweat composition in human health. *Temperature (Austin, Tex.)*, *6*(3), 211-259. https://doi.org/10.1080/23328940.2019.1632145 .

684 Pineau, A., Fauconneau, B., Sappino, A.-P., Deloncle, R., & Guillard, O. (2014). If exposure to aluminium in antiperspirants presents health risks, its content should be reduced. *Journal of Trace Elements in Medicine and Biology*, *28*(2), 147-150, ISSN 0946-672X, https://doi.org/10.1016/j.jtemb.2013.12.002 .

685 Meier, L., Stange, R., Michalsen, A., & Uehleke, B. (2012). Clay jojoba oil facial mask for lesioned skin and mild acne — Results of a prospective, observational pilot study. *Forschende Komplementarmedizin (2006)*, *19*(2), 75-79. https://doi.org/10.1159/000338076 .

686 McDonald, B. C., *et al. (2018).* Volatile chemical products emerging as largest petrochemical source of urban organic emissions. *Science*, 359,760-764. https://doil.org/10.1126/science.aaq0524 .

687 Persellin, K. (2023, July 25). What is fragrance? *Environmental Working Group.* https://www.ewg.org/news-insights/news/2023/07/what-fragrance .

688 United States Congress House Committee on Science and Technology. (1989). Neurotoxins, at home and the workplace: Report to the committee on science and technology, *U.S. House of Representatives, Ninety-ninth Congress, second session. Washington: U.S. G.P.O.* https://catalog.libraries.psu.edu/catalog/10031231 .

689 Grisold, W., & Carozzi, V. A. (2021). Toxicity in peripheral nerves: An overview. *Toxics*, *9*(9), 218. https://doi.org/10.3390/toxics9090218 .

690 Ahn, C., & Jeung, E. B. (2023). Endocrine-disrupting chemicals and disease endpoints. *International Journal of Molecular Sciences*, *24*(6). 5342. https://doi.org/10.3390/ijms24065342 .

691 Ravichandran, J., Karthikeyan, B. S., Jost, J., & Samal, A. (2022). An atlas of fragrance chemicals in children's products. *Science of The Total Environment*, *818*, 151682, ISSN 0048-9697. https://doi.org/10.1016/j.scitotenv.2021.151682 .

692 Bagasra, O., Golkar, Z., Garcia, M., Rice, L. N., & Pace, D. G. (2013). Role of perfumes in pathogenesis of autism. *Medical Hypotheses*, *80*(6), 795-803. https://doi.org/10.1016/j.mehy.2013.03.014.

693 Bagasra, O., Golkar, Z., Garcia, M., Rice, L. N., & Pace, D. G. (2013).

694 Steinemann, A. (2016). Fragranced consumer products: Exposures and effects from emissions. *Air Quality, Atmosphere, & Health*, *9*(8), 861-866. https://doi.org/10.1007/s11869-016-0442-z.

695 Pizzorno, L. (2015). Nothing boring about boron. *Integrative Medicine (Encinitas, Calif.)*, *14*(4), 35-48.

696 Stüttgen, G., Siebel, T., & Aggerbeck, B. (1982). Absorption of boric acid through human skin depending on the type of vehicle. *Archives of Dermatological Research*, *272*(1-2), 21-29. https://doi.org/10.1007/BF00510389 .

697 Matei, A. (2023, November 2). Thread carefully: Your gym clothes could be leaching toxic chemicals. *The Guardian*. https://www.theguardian.com/wellness/2023/nov/02/workout-clothes-sweat-chemicals-cancer .

698 Chevalier, G., Sinatra, S. T., Oschman, J. L., Sokal, K., & Sokal, P. (2012). Earthing: Health implications of reconnecting the human body to the Earth's surface electrons. *Journal of Environmental and Public Health*, 291541. https://doi.org/10.1155/2012/291541 .

699 Oschman, J. L., Chevalier, G., & Brown, R. (2015). The effects of grounding (earthing) on inflammation, the immune response, wound healing, and prevention and treatment of chronic inflammatory and autoimmune diseases. *Journal of Inflammation Research*, *8*, 83-96. https://doi.org/10.2147/JIR.S69656 .

700 Sinatra, S. T., Sinatra, D. S., Sinatra, S. W., & Chevalier, G. (2023). Grounding - The universal anti-inflammatory remedy. *Biomedical Journal*, *46*(1), 11-16. https://doi.org/10.1016/j.bj.2022.12.002 .

701 Park, H. J., Jeong, W., Yu, H. J., Ye, M., Hong, Y., Kim, M., Kim, J. Y., & Shim, I. (2022). The effect of earthing mat on stress-induced anxiety-like behavior and neuroendocrine changes in the rat. *Biomedicines*, *11*(1), 57. https://doi.org/10.3390/biomedicines11010057 .

702 Chevalier, G., Sinatra, S. T., Oschman, J. L., Sokal, K., & Sokal, P. (2012). Earthing: Health implications of reconnecting the human body to the Earth's surface electrons. *Journal of Environmental and Public Health*, *2012*, 291541. https://doi.org/10.1155/2012/291541 .

703 Oschman, J. L., Chevalier, G., & Brown, R. (2015). The effects of grounding (earthing) on inflammation, the immune response, wound healing, and prevention and treatment of chronic inflammatory and autoimmune diseases. *Journal of Inflammation Research*, *8*, 83-96. https://doi.org/10.2147/JIR.S69656 .

704 Tindle, H. A., Chang, Y. F., Kuller, L. H., Manson, J. E., Robinson, J. G., Rosal, M. C., Siegle, G. J., & Matthews, K. A. (2009). Optimism, cynical hostility, and incident coronary heart disease and mortality in the Women's Health Initiative. *Circulation*, *120*(8), 656-662. https://doi.org/10.1161/CIRCULATIONAHA.108.827642 .

705 Adorni, R., Zanatta, F., D'Addario, M., Atella, F., Costantino, E., Iaderosa, C., Petarle, G., & Steca, P. (2021). Health-related lifestyle profiles in healthy adults: Associations with sociodemographic indicators, dispositional optimism, and sense of coherence. *Nutrients*, *13*(11), 3778. https://doi.org/10.3390/nu13113778 .

706 Adorni, R., Zanatta, F., D'Addario, M., Atella, F., Costantino, E., Iaderosa, C., Petarle, G., & Steca, P. (2021).

707 Anthony, E. G., Kritz-Silverstein, D., & Barrett-Connor, E. (2016). Optimism and mortality in older men and women: The Rancho Bernardo study. *Journal of Aging Research*, 5185104. https://doi.org/10.1155/2016/5185104 .

708 Association for Psychological Science. (2012, July 30). Grin and bear it: Smiling facilitates stress recovery. *ScienceDaily*. www.sciencedaily.com/releases/2012/07/120730150113.htm .

709 Yim, J. (2016). Therapeutic benefits of laughter in mental health: A theoretical review. *The Tohoku Journal of Experimental Medicine*, *239*(3), 243-249. https://doi.org/10.1620/tjem.239.243 .

710 Takayanagi, K. (2007). Laughter education and the psycho-physical effects: introduction of smile-sun method. *Japan-Hospitals: The Journal of the Japan Hospital Association*, (26), 31-35.

711 Neumann, I. D.. (2004, April). Oxytocin: The neuropeptide of love reveals some of its secrets. *Elsevier*, *5*(4), 231-233. https://doi.org/10.1016/j.cmet.2007.03.008 .

712 Ozerkan K. N. (2001). The effects of smiling or crying facial expressions on grip strength, measured with a hand dynamometer and the bi-digital O-ring test. *Acupuncture & Electro-Therapeutics Research*, *26*(3), 171-186. https://pubmed.ncbi.nlm.nih.gov/11761446/ .

713 I do not know if this was the specific article my PT was referring to; there are many showing similar results: Brown, D. K., Barton, J. L., & Gladwell, V. F. (2013). Viewing nature scenes positively affects recovery of autonomic function following acute-mental stress. *Environmental Science & Technology*, *47*(11), 5562-5569. https://doi.org/10.1021/es305019p .

714 *Time*. 'Forest Bathing' is great for your health: Here's how to do it. https://time.com/5259602/japanese-forest-bathing/ .

715 Li, Q., Ochiai, H., Ochiai, T., Takayama, N., Kumeda, S., Miura, T., Aoyagi, Y., & Imai, M. (2022). Effects of forest bathing (shinrin-yoku) on serotonin in serum, depressive symptoms and subjective

sleep quality in middle-aged males. *Environmental Health and Preventive Medicine, 27*, 44. https://doi.org/10.1265/ehpm.22-00136 .

716 Mao, G. X., Lan, X. G., Cao, Y. B., Chen, Z. M., He, Z. H., Lv, Y. D., Wang, Y. Z., Hu, X. L., Wang, G. F., & Yan, J. (2012). Effects of short-term forest bathing on human health in a broad-leaved evergreen forest in Zhejiang Province, China. *Biomedical and Environmental Sciences: BES, 25*(3), 317-324. https://doi.org/10.3967/0895-3988.2012.03.010 .

717 Tomasso, L. P., Yin, J., Cedeño Laurent, J. G., Chen, J. T., Catalano, P. J., & Spengler, J. D. (2021). The relationship between nature deprivation and individual wellbeing across urban gradients under COVID-19. *International Journal Of Environmental Research and Public Health, 18*(4), 1511. https://doi.org/10.3390/ijerph18041511 .

718 Lindqvist, P. G., Epstein, E., Nielsen, K., Landin-Olsson, M., Ingvar, C., & Olsson, H. (2016). Avoidance of sun exposure as a risk factor for major causes of death: A competing risk analysis of the melanoma in Southern Sweden cohort. *Journal of Internal Medicine, 280*(4), 375-387. https://doi.org/10.1111/joim.12496 .

719 Eleanor, R. (2021). Sound and soundscape in restorative natural environments: A narrative literature review. *Frontiers in Psychology*, 12. https://doi.org/10.3389/fpsyg.2021.570563 .

720 Franco, L.S., Shanahan, D.F., & Fuller, R.A. (2017). A review of the benefits of nature experiences: More than meets the eye. *International Journal of Environmental Research and Public Health, 14*, 864. https://doi.org/10.3390/ijerph14080864 .

721 Han, X., Liu, C., Chen, Y., & He, M. (2022). Myopia prediction: A systematic review. *Eye (London, England), 36*(5), 921-929. https://doi.org/10.1038/s41433-021-01805-6 .

722 Rose, K. A., Morgan, I. G., Ip, J., Kifley, A., Huynh, S., Smith, W., & Mitchell, P. (2008a). Outdoor activity reduces the prevalence of myopia in children. *Ophthalmology, 115*(8), 1279-1285. https://pubmed.ncbi.nlm.nih.gov/18294691/ .

723 Xiong, S., Sankaridurg, P., Naduvilath, T., Zang, J., Zou, H., Zhu, J., Lv, M., He, X. and Xu, X. (2017). Time spent in outdoor activities in relation to myopia prevention and control: A meta-analysis and systematic review. *Acta Opthalmologica, 95*(6), 551-566. https://www.ncbi.nlm.nih.gov/pmc/articles/PMC5599950/ .

724 Williams, K. M., Bentham, G. C. G., & Young, I. S. (2017). Association between myopia, ultraviolet B radiation exposure, serum vitamin D concentrations, and genetic polymorphisms in vitamin D metabolic pathways in a multicountry European study. *JAMA Opthalmology, 135*(1), 47-53. https://pubmed.ncbi.nlm.nih.gov/27918775/ .

725 I have not been able to find this study during the process of writing this book, so you will have to trust my memory on this one.

726 Hunting, E. R., England, S. J., & Robert, D. (2021, July 15). Tree canopies influence ground level atmospheric electrical and biogeochemical variability. *Frontiers in Earth Sciences, Section on Atmospheric Science, 9.* https://doi.org/10.3389/feart.2021.671870 .

727 Marsh, J. (2023, February 24). 4 phytoncides benefits: how trees improve our health. *Environment.* https://environment.co/phytoncides-benefits/ .

728 Shanahan, D., Bush, R., Gaston, K., *et al.* (2016). Health benefits from nature experiences depend on dose. *Scientific Reports, 6*, 28551. https://doi.org/10.1038/srep28551 .

729 Jarvis, S. (2019, July 9). The health beefits of seawater. *Patient.* https://patient.info/news-and-features/the-health-benefits-of-seawater .

730 Marris, E. (2014, May 25). Let kids run wild in the woods. *Slate.* https://slate.com/technology/2014/05/kid-play-zones-in-parks-leave-no-trace-inhibits-fun-and-bonding-with-nature.html .

731 Finch, K. (2014). Nature play: Nurturing children and strengthening conservation through connections to the land. *Pennsylvania Land Trust Association.* https://library.weconservepa.org/guides/135-nature-play .

732 Null, M., Arbor, T. C., & Agarwal, M. (2023, March 6). Anatomy, lymphatic system. *StatPearls.* PMID: 30020619. https://pubmed.ncbi.nlm.nih.gov/30020619/ .

733 Seattle Children's. (2022, February). The three thumps. https://www.seattlechildrens.org/globalassets/documents/for-patients-and-families/pfe/pe2256.pdf .

734 Null, M., Arbor, T. C., & Agarwal, M. (2023, March 6).

735 Seattle Children's. (2022, February).

736 This happened to a friend of mine.

737 Bornhöft, G., Wolf, U., von Ammon, K., Righetti, M., Maxion-Bergemann, S., Baumgartner, S., Thurneysen, A. E., & Matthiessen, P. F. (2006). Effectiveness, safety and cost-effectiveness of homeopathy in general practice — Summarized health technology assessment. *Forschende Komplementarmedizin (2006), 13 Suppl 2*, 19-29. https://doi.org/10.1159/000093586 .

738 LibreTexts. Lymphatic vessel structure. https://med.libretexts.org/Bookshelves/Anatomy_and_Physiology/Anatomy_and_Physiology_(Boundless)/19:_Lymphatic_System/19.2:_Lymphatic_Vessels/19.2A:_Lymphatic_Vessel_Structure .

739 Yuan, S. L. K., Matsutani. L. A., & Marques, A. P. (2015). Effectiveness of different styles of massage therapy in fibromyalgia: A systematic review and meta-analysis. *Manual Therapy, 20*(2), 2015, 257-264. ISSN 1356-689X. https://doi.org/10.1016/j.math.2014.09.003 .

740 Bordoni, B., Mahabadi, N., & Varacallo, M. (2023, July 17). Anatomy, fascia. *StatPearls*. PMID: 29630284.

741 Wang, T. J., & Stecco, A. (2021). Fascial thickness and stiffness in hypermobile Ehlers-Danlos Syndrome. *American Journal of Medical Genetics. Part C, Seminars in Medical Genetics, 187*(4), 446-452. https://doi.org/10.1002/ajmg.c.31948 .

742 Shem, K., Wong, J., & Dirlikov, B. (2020). Effective self-stretching of carpal ligament for the treatment of carpal tunnel syndrome: A double-blinded randomized controlled study. *Journal of Hand Therapy: Official Journal of the American Society of Hand Therapists, 33*(3), 272-280. https://doi.org/10.1016/j.jht.2019.12.002 .

743 Tsai, S. R. & Hamblin, M. R. (2017). Biological effects and medical applications of infrared radiation. *Journal of Photochemistry and Photobiology. B, Biology, 170*, 197-207. https://doi.org/10.1016/j.jphotobiol.2017.04.014 .

744 Zhu, Q., Cao, X., Zhang, Y., Zhou, Y., Zhang, J., Zhang, X., Zhu, Y., & Xue, L. (2023). Repeated low-level red-light therapy for controlling onset and progression of myopia-a review. *International Journal of Medical Sciences, 20*(10), 1363-1376. https://doi.org/10.7150/ijms.85746 .

745 Heiskanen, V., Pfiffner, M., & Partonen, T. (2020). Sunlight and health: Shifting the focus from vitamin D3 to photobiomodulation by red and near-infrared light. *Ageing Research Reviews, 61*, 101089. https://doi.org/10.1016/j.arr.2020.101089 .

746 Li, W. H., Seo, I., Kim, B., Fassih, A., Southall, M. D., & Parsa, R. (2021). Low-level red plus near infrared lights combination induces expressions of collagen and elastin in human skin in vitro. *International Journal of Cosmetic Science, 43*(3), 311-320. https://doi.org/10.1111/ics.12698 .

747 Lin, T. K., Zhong, L., & Santiago, J. L. (2017). Anti-Inflammatory and skin barrier repair effects of topical application of some plant oils. *International Journal of Molecular Sciences, 19*(1), 70. https://doi.org/10.3390/ijms19010070 .

748 Meier, L., Stange, R., Michalsen, A., & Uehleke, B. (2012). Clay jojoba oil facial mask for lesioned skin and mild acne — Results of a prospective, observational pilot study. *Forschende Komplementarmedizin (2006), 19*(2), 75-79. https://doi.org/10.1159/000338076 .

749 This is not the report that I distinctly remember reading some years ago, but like many others, it shows that prayer makes a difference: Byrd, R. C. (1988). Positive therapeutic effects of intercessory prayer in a coronary care unit population. *Southern Medical Journal, 81*(7), 826-829. https://doi.org/10.1097/00007611-198807000-00005 .

750 Wachholtz, A. B., Malone, C. D., & Pargament, K. I. (2017). Effect of different meditation types on migraine headache medication use. *Behavioral Medicine (Washington, D.C.), 43*(1), 1-8. https://doi.org/10.1080/08964289.2015.1024601 .

751 Koseki, T., Kakizaki, F., Hayashi, S., Nishida, N., & Itoh, M. (2019). Effect of forward head posture on thoracic shape and respiratory function. *Journal of Physical Therapy Science, 31*(1), 63-68. https://doi.org/10.1589/jpts.31.63 .

752 Physiopedia. Forward Head Posture. https://www.physio-pedia.com/Forward_Head_Posture .

753 Alghadir, A. H., Zafar, H., & Iqbal, Z. A. (2015). Effect of tongue position on postural stability during quiet standing in healthy young males. *Somatosensory & Motor Research, 32*(3), 183-186. https://doi.org/10.3109/08990220.2015.1043120 .

754 Page, P. (2012). Current concepts in muscle stretching for exercise and rehabilitation. *International Journal of Sports Physical Therapy, 7*(1), 109-119. https://www.ncbi.nlm.nih.gov/pmc/articles/PMC3273886/ .

755 Bass, E. (2012). Tendinopathy: Why the difference between tendinitis and tendinosis matters. *International Journal of Therapeutic Massage & Bodywork, 5*(1), 14-17. https://doi.org/10.3822/ijtmb.v5i1.153 .

756 Hargrove, T. (2010, January 17). Why slow movement builds coordination. *Better Movement.* https://www.bettermovement.org/blog/2010/why-practice-slow-movement .

757 Great Ape Grips. (2023, August 17). The history of the rice bucket workout: A tale of forearm and grip Strength Training. https://www.greatapegrips.com/blogs/news/the-history-of-the-rice-bucket-workout-a-tale-of-forearm-and-grip-strength-training .

758 VAHVA Fitness. (2018, February 4). Ancient Shaolin secret for powerful forearms. https://vahvafitness.com/shaolin-secret-forearms/ .

759 Zamil, D. H., Khan, R. M., Braun, T. L., & Nawas, Z. Y. (2022). Dermatological uses of rice products: Trend or true? *Journal of cosmetic dermatology*, *21*(11), 6056-6060. https://doi.org/10.1111/jocd.15099 .

760 Luo, Y., Chen, X., Qi, S., You, X., & Huang, X. (2018). Well-being and anticipation for future positive events: evidences from an fMRI study. *Frontiers in Psychology*, *8*, 2199. https://doi.org/10.3389/fpsyg.2017.02199 .

761 Malm, C., Jakobsson, J., & Isaksson, A. (2019). Physical activity and sports-real health benefits: A review with insight into the public health of Sweden. *Sports (Basel, Switzerland)*, *7*(5), 127. https://doi.org/10.3390/sports7050127 .

762 Ozerkan, K. N. (2001). The effects of smiling or crying facial expressions on grip strength, measured with a hand dynamometer and the bi-digital O-ring test. *Acupuncture & Electro-Therapeutics Research*, *26*(3), 171-186. https://pubmed.ncbi.nlm.nih.gov/11761446/ .

763 Tindle, H. A., Chang, Y. F., Kuller, L. H., Manson, J. E., Robinson, J. G., Rosal, M. C., Siegle, G. J., & Matthews, K. A. (2009). Optimism, cynical hostility, and incident coronary heart disease and mortality in the Women's Health Initiative. *Circulation*, *120*(8), 656-662. https://doi.org/10.1161/CIRCULATIONAHA.108.827642 .

764 Lindqvist, P. G., Epstein, E., Nielsen, K., Landin-Olsson, M., Ingvar, C., & Olsson, H. (2016). Avoidance of sun exposure as a risk factor for major causes of death: A competing risk analysis of the melanoma in Southern Sweden cohort. *Journal of Internal Medicine*, *280*(4), 375-387. https://doi.org/10.1111/joim.12496 .

765 Ozerkan, K. N. (2001). The effects of smiling or crying facial expressions on grip strength, measured with a hand dynamometer and the bi-digital O-ring test. *Acupuncture & Electro-therapeutics research*, *26*(3), 171-186. https://pubmed.ncbi.nlm.nih.gov/11761446/ .

766 Westcott, W. L. (2012, July/August). Resistance training is medicine: Effects of Strength Training on health. *Current Sports Medicine Reports*, *11*(4):p 209-216. https://doi.org/10.1249/JSR.0b013e31825dabb8 .

767 di Vico, R., Ardigò, L. P., Salernitano, G., Chamari, K., & Padulo, J. (2014). The acute effect of the tongue position in the mouth on knee isokinetic test performance: A highly surprising pilot study. *Muscles, Ligaments and Tendons Journal*, *3*(4), 318-323. https://pubmed.ncbi.nlm.nih.gov/24596696/ .

768 Teach Me Anatomy. The Vagus Nerve (CN 10). https://teachmeanatomy.info/head/cranial-nerves/vagus-nerve-cn-x/ .

769 Breit, S., Kupferberg, A., Rogler, G., & Hasler, G. (2018). Vagus nerve as modulator of the brain-gut axis in psychiatric and inflammatory disorders. *Frontiers in Psychiatry*, *9*, 44. https://doi.org/10.3389/fpsyt.2018.00044 .

770 Physiopedia. Sympathetic Nervous System. https://www.physio-pedia.com/Sympathetic_Nervous_System .

771 Breit, S., Kupferberg, A., Rogler, G., & Hasler, G. (2018).

772 Pavlov, V. A., Wang, H., Czura, C. J., Friedman, S. G., & Tracey, K. J. (2003). The cholinergic anti-inflammatory pathway: A missing link in neuroimmunomodulation. *Molecular Medicine (Cambridge, Mass.)*, *9*(5-8), 125-134.

773 Tiwari, R., Kumar, R., Malik, S., Raj, T., & Kumar, P. (2021). Analysis of heart rate variability and implication of different factors on heart rate variability. *Current Cardiology Reviews*, *17*(5), e160721189770. https://doi.org/10.2174/1573403X16999201231203854 .

774 Goren, E. (2023, December). Heart rate variability. *Komodo.* https://komodotec.com/what-is-hrv-heart-rate-variability/

775 Pavlov, V. A., Wang, H., Czura, C. J., Friedman, S. G., & Tracey, K. J. (2003).

776 Genetic Disease Investigators, LLC. (2016, January). Correcting the missing piece in chronic fatigue syndrome — Part 1. *Discovery Genetic Disease Investigators*. https://vagusnervesupport.com/wp-content/uploads/2017/11/Chronic-Disease-Digest-Text-Correcting-the-Missing-Piece-in-Chronic-Fatigue-Syndrome.pdf .

777 Cleveland Clinic. Valsalva maneuver. (2022, June 9). https://my.clevelandclinic.org/health/treatments/23209-valsalva-maneuver .

778 Jurvelin, H., Takala, T., Nissilä, J., Timonen, M., Rüger, M., Jokelainen, J., & Räsänen, P. (2014). Transcranial bright light treatment via the ear canals in seasonal affective disorder: A randomized, double-blind dose-response study. *BMC Psychiatry, 14*, 288. https://doi.org/10.1186/s12888-014-0288-6.

779 Breit, S., Kupferberg, A., Rogler, G., & Hasler, G. (2018). vagus nerve as modulator of the brain-gut axis in psychiatric and inflammatory disorders. *Frontiers in Psychiatry, 9*, 44. https://doi.org/10.3389/fpsyt.2018.00044

780 Khasar, S. G., Reichling, D. B., Green, P. G., Isenberg, W. M., & Levine, J. D. (2003). Fasting is a physiological stimulus of Vagus-mediated enhancement of nociception in the female rat. *Neuroscience, 119*(1), 215-221. https://doi.org/10.1016/s0306-4522(03)00136-2 .

781 Rominger, C., Weber, B., Aldrian, A., Berger, L., & Schwerdtfeger, A. R. (2021). Short-term fasting induced changes in HRV are associated with interoceptive accuracy: Evidence from two independent within-subjects studies. *Physiology & Behavior*, 241. https://doi.org/10.1016/j.physbeh.2021.113558 .

782 Billot, M., Daycard, M., Wood, C., & Tchalla, A. (2019). Reiki therapy for pain, anxiety and quality of life. *BMJ Supportive & Palliative Care, 9*(4), 434-438. https://doi.org/10.1136/bmjspcare-2019-001775 .

783 Demir Doğan, M. (2018). The effect of Reiki on pain: A meta-analysis. *Complementary Therapies in Clinical Practice, 31*, 384-387. https://doi.org/10.1016/j.ctcp.2018.02.020 .

784 Dyer, N. L., Baldwin, A. L., & Rand, W. L. (2019). A large-scale effectiveness trial of Reiki for physical and psychological health. *Journal of Alternative and Complementary Medicine (New York, N.Y.), 25*(12), 1156-1162. https://doi.org/10.1089/acm.2019.0022 .

785 McManus, D. E. (2017). Reiki is better than placebo and has broad potential as a complementary health therapy. *Journal of Evidence-Based Complementary & Alternative Medicine, 22*(4), 1051-1057. https://doi.org/10.1177/2156587217728644 .

786 DiBenedetto, J. (2022). Experiences with a distant Reiki intervention during the COVID-19 pandemic using the Science of Unitary Human Beings Framework. *ANS. Advances in Nursing Science, 45*(4), E145-E160. https://doi.org/10.1097/ANS.0000000000000441 .

787 Özcan Yüce, U., Arpacı, A., Kütmeç Yılmaz, C., Yurtsever, D., Üstün Gökçe, E., Burkev, F. G., Yıldırım, G., Gökşin, İ., Ünal Aslan, K. S., Bektaş Akpınar, N., Altınbaş Akkaş, Ö., & Yurtsever, S. (2024). The effect of distant Reiki sessions on holistic well-being. *Holistic Nursing Practice, 38*(1), 50-57. https://doi.org/10.1097/HNP.0000000000000557 .

788 Demir, M., Can, G., Kelam, A., & Aydıner, A. (2015). Effects of distant Reiki on pain, anxiety and fatigue in oncology patients in Turkey: A pilot study. *Asian Pacific Journal of Cancer Prevention: APJCP, 16*(12), 4859-4862. https://doi.org/10.7314/apjcp.2015.16.12.4859 .

789 Seto, A., Kusaka, C., Nakazato, S., Huang, W. R., Sato, T., Hisamitsu, T., & Takeshige, C. (1992). Detection of extraordinary large bio-magnetic field strength from human hand during external Qi emission. *Acupuncture & Electro-Therapeutics Research, 17*(2), 75-94. https://doi.org/10.3727/036012992816357819 .

790 Over the decade that I ran my holistic healing center, numerous men who were veterans or in the military came in at various times and told me that they had learned Reiki in the military. Some of them had impressive stories about the power of Reiki healing during their military career.

791 Argueta, D. A., Ventura, C. M., Kiven, S., Sagi, V., & Gupta, K. (2020). A balanced approach for cannabidiol use in chronic pain. *Frontiers in Pharmacology, 11*, 561. https://doi.org/10.3389/fphar.2020.00561 .

792 Meng, H., Johnston, B., Englesakis, M., Moulin, D. E., & Bhatia, A. (2017). Selective cannabinoids for chronic neuropathic pain: A systematic review and meta-analysis. *Anesthesia & Analgesia, 125*(5), 1638-1652. https://doi.org/10.1213/ANE.0000000000002110 .

793 Lynn, V. Dilution ratios for essential oils. https://www.vicki-lynn.com/dilution-ratio-oils.html .

794 Zhao, H., Ren, S., Yang, H., Tang, S., Guo, C., Liu, M., Tao, Q., Ming, T., & Xu, H. (2022). Peppermint essential oil: Its phytochemistry, biological activity, pharmacological effect and application. *Biomedicine & Pharmacotherapy — Biomedecine & Pharmacotherapie, 154*, 113559. https://doi.org/10.1016/j.biopha.2022.113559 .

795 Mei, N., Guo, L., Fu, P. P., Fuscoe, J. C., Luan, Y., & Chen, T. (2010). Metabolism, genotoxicity, and carcinogenicity of comfrey. *Journal of Toxicology and Environmental Health. Part B, Critical reviews*, *13*(7-8), 509-526. https://doi.org/10.1080/10937404.2010.509013 .

796 Błażowski, Ł., Majak, P., Kurzawa, R., Kuna, P., & Jerzyńska, J. (2021). A severity grading system of food-induced acute allergic reactions to avoid delay of epinephrine administration. *Annals of Allergy, Asthma & Immunology : Official Publication of the American College of Allergy, Asthma, & Immunology. 127.* 10.1016/j.anai.2021.04.015.

797 Gazit, Y., Jacob, G., & Grahame, R. (2016). Ehlers-Danlos Syndrome-Hypermobility Type: A much neglected multisystemic disorder. *Rambam Maimonides Medical Journal*, *7*(4), e0034. https://doi.org/10.5041/RMMJ.10261 .

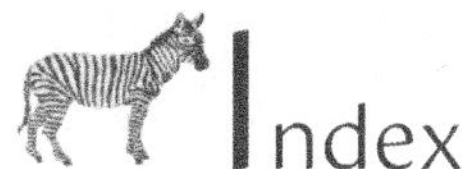

Index

About the Author

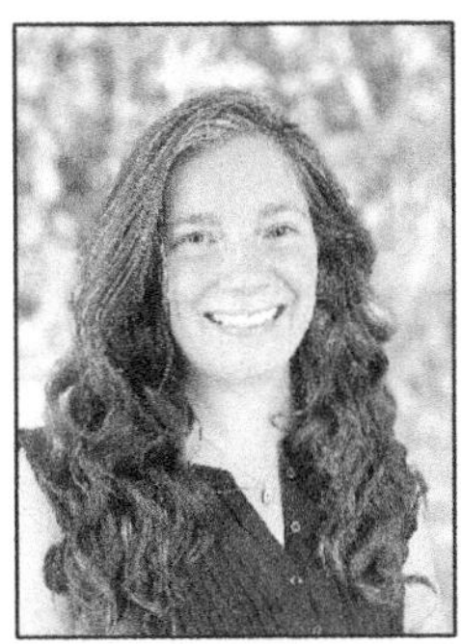

SHANNON ERIN GALE IS AN AUTHOR, homemaker, and homeschooling mom. She lives in Kentucky with her husband, son, and two dogs. She previously founded and directed the Vibrant Life holistic healing center, Gale Force Dance professional performance company, Frankfort School of Ballet, Helpful Editor professional services, and Circle Play and Learn Academy forest school. She has been published in numerous books, newspapers, and magazines. This is her first standalone book, but she has many more planned. Please visit her website: shannonegale.com.

Made in United States
Orlando, FL
26 September 2024

52005917R00241